DENTISTRY AND ORAL SCIENCES

CLINICAL REPORTS IN DENTISTRY

DENTISTRY AND ORAL SCIENCES

Additional books and e-book in this series can be found
on Nova's website under the Series tab.

DENTISTRY AND ORAL SCIENCES

CLINICAL REPORTS IN DENTISTRY

LISA R. AMIR
EDITOR

nova
Medicine & Health
New York

Library of Congress Cataloging-in-Publication Data

ISBN: 978-1-53617-328-4

Published by Nova Science Publishers, Inc. † New York

CONTENTS

PREFACE

The book presents extensive case reports covering various clinical dentistry disciplines. In Oral Medicine, cases of various oral lesions and their risk factors were reported, as well as the precautions of radiotherapy for oral condition. In Oral Surgery, various surgical techniques were discussed related to orbital cavity reconstruction, mandibular defect reconstruction, arthoplasty, management of tumors in maxillofacial region, management of Schneiderian membrane perforation and lateral sinus lifting procedures in severe bone loss case.

The use of CBCT on implant planning and identification of ameloblastoma tumor margin were reported. In Prosthodontics, treatment of removable partial denture and orbital defect reconstruction were discussed. In Conservative Dentistry, endodontics treatment and retreatment in rare cases were discussed, including management of fracture instruments and iatrogenic pulp exposure and replantation of avulsed teeth. In Pediatric Dentistry, various techniques related to intrusive luxation, treatment of lip sucking and approach for children in special need toward dental anxiety were addressed.

In Orthodontics, a case of management malocclusion of a difficult case was reported. In Forensic Dentistry, the importance of forensic odontology in burnt victim age estimation and post mortem reconstruction methods were reported. In Periodontology, cases of trauma from occlusion and the aesthetic of crown lengthening were reported. This large collection of case reports, discussing various treatments of clinical problems, identification of oral diseases that are frequently encountered in daily practice will surely give valuable information for general practitioners and dental specialists in order to achieve the highest standard in clinical dentistry.

Chapter 1 - *Introduction:* Oral infection caused by Herpes Simplex Virus (HSV) commonly occurs in childhood. However, recurrent infections are more common among adults with a prevalence of 70 – 80%. Stress is one of trigger factors that contributes to HSV reactivation. Stress is a condition that tends to disrupt the immune system, resulting in biological systemic alterations. This case report aimed to describe the importance of stress management in decreasing recurrence of HSV infection.

Case report: A 30-year-old female patient came to the oral medicine clinic at Universitas Indonesia with a chief complaint of a sore mouth, preceded by fever and malaise. Such symptoms caused difficulty in eating and swallowing over the last week. Similar symptoms occurred few times before. The patient was otherwise healthy, except recent fatigue and psychological stress postpartum. She felt very anxious about a possible oral malignant lesion. Clinical examination revealed poor oral hygiene, multiple ulcers surrounded by an erythematous area 0.5 – 6mm in size located throughout the oral cavity. Lympadenopathy of both submandibular regions was also noted. Result of IgG HSV-1 test was positive and she was diagnosed with recurrent intra-oral herpes (RIH). Therapy included 100mg doxycycline mouthwash, 200mg Acyclovir and 7 days of oral multivitamin. Patient was advised to take sufficient rest time, to eat more nutritious foods, increase fluid intake and manage possible underlying psychological disorders. The lesions were clinically resolved in the patients 4th visit to the clinic.

Conclusion: It is important to understand the association between psychological stress and recurrence of HSV infection. Adopting stress management with a cognitive psychotherapy approach may improve self-confidence in patients to have rational and positive thoughts and reduce future recurrence of HSV.

Chapter 2 - *Introduction*: Betel-quid chewing is habitually practiced in parts of Indonesia and comprises of various composition. It is a well-established risk factor of numerous oral mucosal lesions, including oral potentially malignant disorders (OPMDs) and oral squamous cell carcinoma. The present study aimed to discuss a case of suspected oral squamous cell carcinoma in an elderly patient with betel-quid chewing as a risk factor. *Case report*: A 76-year-old female presented to the dental hospital of Universitas Indonesia; she was referred from a private hospital with a working diagnosis of pseudomembranous candidiasis on the left buccal mucosa. She had chewed betel-quid, a mixture of betel-quid leaf, lime, areca nut, gambier, and tobacco, for more than 20 years. An intra-oral examination revealed mixed white nodular and plaque lesions on the left buccal and alveolar mucosa, an erythematous base, ulceration and induration in posterior part of the lesion adjacent to the retromolar pad, which led to the clinical suspicion of oral squamous cell carcinoma. Betel-quid chewing is believed to be a risk factor of oral squamous cell carcinoma. The betel-quid composition, long duration and moderately high frequency of chewing, the way betel-quid is kept in the mouth, increased patient's age, and poor oral hygiene increase the risk of oral squamous cell carcinoma. *Conclusion:* As dentists, we play a key role in the early detection of oral mucosal changes associated with betel-quid chewing, particularly OPMDs and oral squamous cell carcinoma, and to provide adequate education and treatment for the patients.

Chapter 3 - *Introduction*: Similarity exist between clinical and histopathological features of erosive oral lichen planus (EOLP) and discoid lupus erythematosus (DLE).

Case report: A 49-year-old woman presented to the Oral Medicine Clinic of Cipto Mangunkusumo General Hospital Jakarta with a 2-week-old pain on the right and left cheeks, which worsened when she ate spicy food and smoked. There were erosive areas with radiating white striae and dark pigmentations that spread from the commissure to the retromolar pads of the buccal mucosa. Based on intra-oral clinical features, the working diagnosis was EOLP with differential diagnoses were DLE and erythroleukoplakia. EOLP and DLE have similar clinical feature which is erythema or erosive areas with radiating keratotic striae. But the result of histopathological examination was consistent with lichen planus. Oral lesions were treated with topical dexamethasone.

Conclusion: EOLP and DLE have similar clinical and histopathological features that cause difficulties in diagnosis. Therefore, elaborating the result of both clinical and histopatological features is very important in the diagnosis of EOLP and DLE. In this case report the histopathological examination establish the diagnosis of EOLP.

Chapter 4 - *Introduction:* The present case report aimed to provide information on the oral manifestations and management of pemphigus vulgaris (PV) during pregnancy.

Case report: A 25-year-old woman diagnosed with PV was under dermatological treatment since 2011. In January 2018, she was referred to the oral medicine (OM) clinic of Dr. Cipto Mangunkusumo General Hospital due to oral ulcers. Her clinical examination revealed desquamation and crust on the lips, erosions, desquamation and sloughing of the gingiva, erosions on the palate and poor oral hygiene. She was treated with topical dexamethasone and chlorhexidine gluconate 0.2% mouth rinse as well as systemic methylprednisolone, azathioprine, $CaCO_3$ and ranitidine. The patient was pregnant after her fifth visit to the OM clinic and her PV was clinically worsening with eruption of new lesions on oral mucosa and skin. Although uncommon, oral manifestations of PV can occur during pregnancy which complicates its management and creates a therapeutic dilemma due to the need of higher dose of medication when the PV flares up, but on the other hand, the drugs used are known to have teratogenic effect.

Conclusion: Interdisciplinary comprehensive treatment is highly recommended to ensure maternal and fetal safety in such cases. Accordingly, the prescription of methylprednisolone was restricted, while azathioprine and $CaCO_3$ were discontinued. The patient's response to therapy was continuously monitored at each visit which showed continuous improvement and the fetus was growing well.

Chapter 5 - *Introduction:* To provide an overview of the predisposing factors for recurrent aphthous stomatitis (RAS) and geographic tongue (GT) in a young female patient.

Case report: A 21-year-old woman presented with a large, painful lesion on the left lip for seven days. The patient was used to experiencing canker sores 3 or 4 times a year. In addition, she complained of pain, sores, and heat on the tongue. Upon intra-oral examination, the authors found a single, irregularly shaped ulcer, with a white base and surrounded by erythema in the left labial mucosa and multiple erythematous lesions surrounded by white edges and migratory in the dorsal, ventral and lateral of her tongue. The authors diagnosed the patient as having a minor recurrent aphthous stomatitis (RAS) and symptomatic geographic tongue (GT) and prescribed chlorhexidine gluconate 0.2% and multi-vitamins. At the next visit a month later, the initial RAS lesions had disappeared but a few new ones had appeared; the GT lesions were still present. Suspecting that there could be psychological reason for prolonged duration of the oral lesions, the patient was then given Perceived Stress Scale (PSS) questionnaires. In search for other predisposing factors, the patient also was sent for CBC examination. PSS score showed mild stress in patient and CBC results of normal Hemoglobin (13.1g/dL), low count on MCV (71.8fL), and decrease count on MCH (23.4pg). From these results the authors concluded that stress, small average red blood cells and low average content of hemoglobin per red cells have contributed to the clinical picture. Without anemia, condition of low blood count as describe above called pre-anemic stage. The complete management for these cases should include communication, information and education and dietary recommendations, including taking multi-vitamins, and finding stressors to implement interventions to alleviate the stress.

Conclusion: Finding and eliminating stressors and pre-anemic stage as predisposing factors may influence the success of RAS and GT management.

Chapter 6 - *Introduction:* The oral cavity can be a site for pathological manifestations of many diseases and their treatments. One example is the head and neck cancer (HNC). Main treatment modalities for HNC are surgery, radiotherapy and chemotherapy. Head and neck cancer treatment by radiotherapy may induce pathological conditions in the oral cavity, both during treatment and after its conclusion. This case report described oral assessment before radiotherapy on a patient with HNC and briefly reviewed radiotherapy oral sequelae.

Case Report: A 56-year-old female was referred to the oral medicine clinic at Cipto Mangunkusumo National Hospital for evaluation and elimination of oral infection foci prior to radiotherapy for HNC. The patient underwent a thorough oral examination, where the authors noted poor oral hygiene with several necrotic dental roots, teeth requiring extractions, multiple dental caries, and ill-fitting denture with denture stomatitis. A treatment plan was generated, and the patient received proper dental management and was informed about the possibility of oral complications related to radiotherapy.

Conclusion: In patients with HNC, radiotherapy can induce various pathological conditions within the oral cavity, potentially decreasing the patient's quality of life and compromising treatment outcomes. However, those conditions can be mitigated or prevented by oral precautions, elimination of infection sources, and maintenance of good oral hygiene.

Chapter 7 - *Introduction:* This case report aimed to describe the oral lesions indicating hematinic deficiency.

Case report: The first case is a 20-year-old female patient with chief complaints of ulceration at the corner of her mouth. Laboratory examination revealed low haemogloblin, hematocrit, erythrocyte index, and RDW-CV levels. After clinical examination, she was diagnosed with angular cheilitis, related to iron deficiency anemia. She was prescribed 0.2% chlorhexidine gluconate mouthwash and multi-vitamins. The second case is 21-year-old male patient complaining of oral discomfort. Clinical examination revealed multiple ulcers in the oral mucosa. The working diagnosis was recurrent aphthous stomatitis and laboratory examination was conducted. Based on clinical and complete blood count, the patient was diagnosed recurrent aphthous stomatitis-related iron deficiency. He was prescribed 0.2% chlorhexidine gluconate mouthwash and multi-vitamins.

Conclusion: Recurrent aphthous stomatitis and angular cheilitis are common oral lesions that indicate signs of hematinic deficiency. The dentists must carry out subjective and objective examinations along with appropriate investigations to detect the presence of systemic factors of underlying diseases for adequate case management.

Chapter 8 - *Introduction:* PFAPA syndrome is characterized by periodic fever, aphthous stomatitis, pharyngitis and cervical adenitis. It usually happens to children younger than 5 years of age.

Case report: Herein, the authors present a case of 14-year-old Taiwanese male who had been suffering from periodic oral aphthous ulcerations and high fever almost every month since he was 1 year old. At the time of examination, yellowish crusts on upper and lower vermillions noted with pain, along with several ruptured vesicles over soft palate and pharyngeal area were seen. Multiple oral aphthous ulcers were noted throughout oral mucosa, including tongue border, buccal mucosa and labial mucosa. Under thorough history taking and medical records, the authors excluded other diseases, including cyclic neutropenia. A diagnosis of PFAPA syndrome with impetigo on upper and lower vermillion and herpangina was rendered. The patient was treated with supporting treatment on the first week until herpangina resolved, followed by oral prednisolone (5mg, 3 times per day for 5 days) and topical triamcinolone rinse (4mg in 20ml water, topical rinse, 4 times daily for 7 days) and the patient responded well. Thereafter the authors recommended ranitidine therapy (150mg, once per day for 3 months) as prophylaxis for the recurrent aphthous stomatitis. The patient was doing well without recurrence of aphthous ulcers. The patient is currently under close follow up and ranitidine therapy would be indicated if the symptoms recurred.

Conclusion: Through this case, the authors want to prove that typical PFAPA syndrome could be easily diagnosed through careful examination of patient's history and clinical features.

Chapter 9 - *Introduction:* The mandibular canal is a crucial anatomical indicator for implant planning in the posterior mandibular region. Implant positioning near the mandibular canal may result in damage to the inferior alveolar nerve, leading to paresthesia of the lower lip and chin.

Case report: A 38-year-old man with no relevant medical history presented to Pondok Indah Hospital for the replacement of his missing mandibular teeth, which had been removed 1 year prior to presentation. The patient wanted to have the missing dentition restored using a dental implant. The authors placed dental implants at the 1st, 2nd and 3rd right mandibular molars. The risk of damage to the trigeminal nerve branches is known as a complication of implant treatment in the posterior mandibular region. CBCT provides three-dimensional (3D) images with a moderate radiation dose, and numerous studies have reported its value in diagnosing spatial associations between anatomical structures.

Conclusion: The present report highlight the use of CBCT for assessing the distance between anatomical structures. CBCT is regarded as a credible and precise tool.

Chapter 10 - *Introduction*: The use of dental implants has gained popularity over the past few decades. However, sufficient vertical dimensions are a pre-requisite to warrant the success of these implants. Vertical bone defects including ridge resorption and sinus pneumatization frequently occur in the posterior maxillary region. Lateral sinus lift is one of the most extensively used augmentation procedures. The technique allows for the placement of an implant on the dorsal side of the maxilla where the quality of the alveolar bone is often poor due to the maxillary sinus. Herein the authors describe a case of vertical ridge augmentation using lateral sinus lift with simultaneous implant placement in the posterior maxillary region.

Case Report: A 52-year-old male with missing teeth (16 and 17) in the maxillary posterior region reported to the authors' clinic. The height of alveolar ridge in the area was measured at 2.1 mm. Two threaded implants (width, 4.1 mm; length, 10 mm) were placed immediately after performing the lateral sinus lift and were surrounded with bone graft material.

Conclusion: Lateral sinus lift appears to be a useful pre-prosthetic surgical procedure for vertical augmentation of atrophied alveolar ridges with low sinus floors.

Chapter 11 - *Introduction:* Temporomandibular joint ankylosis (TMJA) is characterized by a limited range of motion of the mandible and is mainly caused by untreated trauma, TMJ surgery, or other diseases such as rheumatoid arthritis. Treatment of choice for TMJA is surgery with the following techniques: (1) gap arthroplasty, (2) interpositional muscle graft arthroplasty, and (3) total TMJ replacement with an autogenous or alloplastic graft. The primary objective of TMJA treatment is to restore joint function and prevent reankylosis. *Case Report:* A 13-year-old female was referred to the authors' hospital with the chief complaint of having had difficulty in mouth opening over the past year. The patient had a history of a bicycle accident 2 years before presentation, during which she hit the sidewalk and suffered an open wound in the chin area without loss of consciousness. The wound was subsequently sutured at a hospital, and she was discharged without any medications. The authors performed bilateral interpositional temporal muscle graft arthroplasty. The patient showed uneventful postoperative healing with a 3-cm interincisal opening. *Conclusion:* Interpositional temporal muscle graft arthroplasty is suitable for the treatment of bilateral temporomandibular joint ankylosis provided that regular physiotherapy and close follow-up are continued.

Chapter 12 - *Introduction:* The authors reported a case of odontectomy of a Class C or grade 4 impacted upper left third molar (M3) that was surgically removed using alternative classification and technique.

Case Report: A 20-year-old woman presented with the chief complaint of pain in the upper left posterior jaw. Clinical examination showed a normal appearance without eruption of upper M3. Panoramic radiograph showed impacted 28 and 18 teeth at the apex region of 27 and 17. Odontectomy was performed in 15 minutes under general anesthesia. The incision was extended from the maxillary tuberosity to the mesial cervicobuccal region of teeth #28 and #16 and continued with a curved oblique buccal incision to the mucobuccal fold. The impacted upper M3 was clearly identified by the presence of bulging on the buccal maxillary bone. Finally, odontectomy and wound closure were performed.

Conclusion: An impacted upper M3 may be treated easily by understanding the surrounding anatomic structures. Oral surgery experts can also apply suitable surgical techniques to ease the odontectomy.

Chapter 13 - *Introduction:* Dental implants are widely used for replacing teeth loss. Sinus augmentation is one of the procedures used to obtain increased vertical height for dental implant placement when the proportional bone height is not achieved. The most common complication during this procedure is *Scheneiderian* membrane perforation, which can be managed using collagen membranes.

Case report: A case of *Schneiderian* membrane perforation that occurred during a sinus augmentation procedure and was subsequently managed using a collagen membrane. A 51-year-old female patient with missing teeth numbers 14, 15, 16, 17 and with an alveolar height less than 3 cm. The *Schneiderian* membrane perforation was managed using tissue additives and a collagen membrane followed by bone graft particulate and dental implant placement.

Conclusion: The treatment of *Schneiderian* membrane perforation can be effectively managed using collagen membrane.

Chapter 14 - *Introduction*: Oral squamous cell carcinoma (OSCC) of the mandible is characterized as tumors developing adjacent to the mandibular bone, including the mandibular alveolar ridge, lower buccal sulcus, sublingual sulcus and mandibular retromolar area. The first choice of therapy for most resectable stages is surgical treatment. However, mandibular reconstruction is a challenge associated with postoperative aesthetics and functional outcomes. Although aggressive treatment has improved local and regional tumor control, a number of patients still die of distant metastases.

Case Report: A 72-year-old male was diagnosed with OSCC of the inner mucosa of the lower lip, gingiva, cheek and mandible (cT4aN2bM0 stage IV in July 2017). Owing to an extensive lesion, induction chemotherapy was initially undertaken. Although the original mucosal lesion was nearly resolved after chemotherapy, a progressive bony lesion was observed. Accordingly, the patient underwent segmental mandibulectomy, bilateral neck dissection and reconstruction with free fibula flap and *deltopectoral* (DP) *flap*. The final pathology results showed moderately differentiated SCC pyT4aN2bM0 at stage IV. He underwent adjuvant treatment postoperatively. However, bilateral lung metastases occurred when palliative chemotherapy and supportive care were undergoing.

Conclusion: Early operative treatment should be an option for patients suffering from a progressive head and neck tumor, which may help achieve considerably better life expectancy and quality of life for a longer period.

Chapter 15 - *Introduction*: Fibrous dysplasia is a non-odontogenic bone disease wherein normal bone is replaced by fibrous tissue. The etiology is still unknown but seems to be linked to genetic factors. Patients with this condition typically manifest symptoms by their late teens or early twenties, the primary symptom being facial asymmetry. Herein, the authors described the management of 2 patients with fibrous dysplasia of the maxilla who underwent excision and surgical contouring, with 6 months of follow-up.

Case report: A 15-year-old male and a 22-year-old female presented to the Department of Oral and Maxillofacial Surgery at Tangerang Central Hospital. Both patients complained of asymptomatic swelling of the left maxilla. For the male, this swelling began 3 years prior to presentation, whereas for the female, there was a 10-year history of swelling. Each patient was bothered by facial asymmetry. On panoramic radiography, both patients exhibited a large radiopaque mass without a distinct border. Both histopathological examinations showed patterns suggestive of fibrous dysplasia and both patients were referred for excision and surgical recontouring.

Conclusion: Excision and surgical recontouring are effective in managing patients with fibrous dysplasia; however, extended follow-up is necessary.

Chapter 16 - *Introduction:* Ameloblastoma is a slow-growing, epithelial odontogenic benign tumor which is aggressive and locally invasive. It is commonly seen in the posterior lower jaw and is characterized by formation of dental embryonic residual. The etiology of ameloblastoma might be related to odontogenic cyst epithelial layer, dental lamina, enamel organ, stratified squamous epithelium of the oral cavity, or displaced epithelial residual. Many cases of ameloblastoma have been reported to have residual epithelial residues originally degenerated from dentigerous cysts.

Case report: Here the authors reported the surgical management of ameloblastoma mimicking a dentigerous cyst. A 14-year-old girl complained of experiencing swelling in the lower right jaw for one year. The lesion was hard and cystic with a well-defined border. She had no pain. Color and temperature of the lesion were equal to color and temperature of the surrounding tissue. There was no history of trauma and toothache and no pus or bloody discharge. Initial diagnosis was a dentigerous cyst and the patient underwent surgical enucleation of the mass followed by extraction of the involved teeth under general anesthetic. Histopathological examination of the removed specimen revealed a plexiform ameloblastoma pattern.

Conclusion: Ameloblastoma is a locally malignant tumor requiring enucleation and/or curettage and resection. Long-term follow-up is necessary to rule out recurrent tumor.

Chapter 17 - *Introduction:* Ameloblastomas are rare, benign, odontogenic tumors that mainly affect the mandible. They are slow-growing tumors with an affinity for bone, and they have a high recurrence rate if not adequately removed. Tumor removal needs attention with regard to the assessment of the correct free tumor margin. Computed tomography (CT), as the gold standard, allows good assessment and contrast enhancement is helpful. Advancements in imaging technology have resulted in the development of cone beam computed tomography (CBCT) as an alternative imaging approach. The authors present a patient with an ameloblastoma, who underwent both CT and CBCT. The authors compared the imaging characteristics and tumor margin between these imaging approaches in this patient.

Case Report: The patient was a 34-year-old woman with swelling in the right lower jaw. She underwent both CT and CBCT. The lesion was identified as an ameloblastoma. The authors found that both approaches provided good image quality with regard to anatomy; however, there was a slight difference in measurement results.

Conclusion: The authors' findings suggest that CBCT provides good image quality for surgical guidance with regard to measuring ameloblastomas and determining the free tumor margin and that CBCT results are as good as CT results in the assessment of ameloblastomas.

Chapter 18 - *Introduction*: Lipomas are common, benign, soft-tissue tumors containing mature adipose tissues that rarely develop in the head and neck region; however, these should be considered as one of the potential diagnoses of a neck mass. Most lipomas develop in subcutaneous tissues, but deeper tissues may also be involved. Between 15% and 20% of lipomas involve head and neck masses and between 1% and 5% involve benign oral cavity neoplasms. The authors reported the case of a patient with lipoma on the left sub-mandibular region of the face.

Case report: A 54-year-old man was admitted to Cipto Mangunkusumo hospital with an initial complaint of swelling on the left mandible with a painless, mobile, and smooth surface that had been present for 1 year prior to admission. Computed tomography revealed a radiolucent image of the left mandible. The diagnosis was a lipoma on the left mandible. Complete surgical excision should be performed on lipomas because of the potential for recurrence after inadequate surgery.

Conclusion: A submandibular incision can provide good visualization of the tumor and also lead to a better esthetic end result for the patient.

Chapter 19 - *Introduction:* Dentigerous cyst is the most common odontogenic cyst in the jaw after radicular cyst and more frequently occurs in males at the 20s – 30s years. This cyst is commonly associated with impacted or embedded teeth, such as the third mandibular molar. Dentigerous cyst is frequently discovered accidentally when radiographs are used to investigate a failed tooth eruption or missing tooth, and it can could grow to be an ameblastoma. This case report described the diagnosis and management of a right maxillary dentigerous cyst.

Case Report: A 14-year-old female visited the Oral and Maxillofacial Surgery Clinic of Cipto Mangunkusumo Hospital because she has had a swelling in her right maxilla from 3 months ago. Enucleation of the cyst along with odontectomy of the unerupted tooth were performed under general anesthesia. The diagnosis was a maxillary dentigerous cyst due to an impacted maxillary canine.

Conclusion: An adequate and appropriate treatment to prevent further maxillary damage and recurrence is necessary in the rare case of maxillary dentigerous cyst.

Chapter 20 - *Introduction*: Fibro-epithelial hyperplasia is a localized or generalized proliferative fibrous lesion of oral mucosa resulting from local irritation and response to injury. This pathological lesion can impair the gingival functions of mastication and their aesthetic appearance. This case study is a diagnostic and management report of a patient with 10-year-long slowly progressive gingival enlargement with several systemic complications. This patient has been managed by excisional surgery.

Case report: A 69-year-old female patient came to the oral and maxillofacial clinical department in Persahabatan Hospital with a chief complaint of gum enlargement starting 10 years ago, accompanied by systemic complications. Panoramic radiographic showed no bone destruction. The fibrous inflammatory gingival tissue was surgically excised under general anesthesia. Post-surgery, the enlarged gingival tissue was significantly reduced and no post-operative complications were noted.

Conclusion: Cognizant and careful treatments are needed in patients with large fibro-epithelial hyperplasia accompanied by systemic complications.

Chapter 21 - *Introduction*: Radicular cysts are the most common cystic lesions in the jaw, with a prevalence of approximately 52% to 68% cysts affecting the jaw. These cysts are associated with non-vital teeth. Nonsurgical treatment includes root canal therapy, where the lesion is localized, or surgical treatment such as enucleation of a large lesion. In this case report, the authors described the surgical approach of a right mandibular radicular cyst with relocation of the inferior alveolar nerve due to surgical enucleation.

Case Report: A 61-year-old female patient attended the division of oral and maxillofacial surgery at Jakarta Hospital with the chief complaint of pain, swelling and paresthesia of the right posterior jaw. Intra-oral clinical examination revealed swelling at the buccal mucosal region #44–46. Unilocular periapical radiolucency associated with teeth #44–46 was revealed on a panoramic radiograph. The patient was treated by surgical enucleation under general anesthesia.

Conclusion: Enucleation with relocation of the inferior alveolar nerve was performed to remove the radicular cyst. Depending on the size and extent of the lesion, surgical enucleation of a radicular cyst is necessary for optimal treatment and prevention of recurrence.

Chapter 22 - *Introduction*: Disfigurement associated with the loss of an eye causes significant physical and emotional complications. Prosthetic rehabilitation of such patients leads to improvement in their appearance as well as psychological status. Growth of adolescent patients and disease recurrence are important considerations when managing such cases. The present report described the ocular and orbital prostheses fabricated for an adolescent over the course of several years.

Case Report: A 13-year-old female was referred to the Department of Prosthodontics, Faculty of Dentistry, Universitas Indonesia in 2015 for ocular prosthesis fabrication for the rehabilitation of orbital meningioma. Her medical history revealed tumor recurrence requiring several surgeries. Enucleation of the left eye had been performed in 2009, followed by a second surgery in 2010. Tumor debulking and radiation therapy had been performed in 2014 due to recurrence. In early 2015, the defect area did not provide sufficient space for inserting an ideal ocular prosthesis, but for psychological reasons, the first ocular prosthesis was fabricated at this time. In mid-2015, a second ocular prosthesis was fabricated. In 2017, the patient visited the department with a loose-fitting ocular prosthesis. By this time, the defect area was large enough to accommodate an orbital prosthesis. Lastly, an adhesive-retained silicone orbital prosthesis utilizing the anatomical undercut was fabricated.

Conclusion: Selection of a maxillofacial prosthesis should follow the patient's condition to achieve optimal results. Several factors should be taken into consideration, such as the patient's tissue condition, defect size, disease behavior, age and economic status. Over several years, different types of prostheses may be indicated.

Chapter 23 - *Introduction:* Orbital trauma often occur in patients with multiple facial traumas. On the other side, injury of the soft tissue in the facial region must consider ocular trauma as one of the most significant factors contributing to visual impairment. Accurate diagnosis of eye injury requires expertise in ophthalmology, which makes it possible to identify mild ocular injury in maxillofacial trauma patients. Computed Tomography is the main modality used for orbital trauma because of its sensitivity to detect fracture and soft tissue injury accurately.

Case Report: The authors reported a case of ocular trauma with eyeball rupture and medial orbital wall fracture. This case was treated by eyeball enucleation and orbital wall reconstruction. Material used for orbital wall reconstruction was titanium mesh because it was superior to autogenous bone graft and porous polyethylene sheets (PPE). Surgery was performed carefully by opportune manipulating of bone, reconstruction material, and soft tissue.

Conclusion: Proper healing at the surgical approach site was observed, patient had no complaint and no post-surgery complication was noted. Eyeball prosthesis will be cast to reach an optimum aesthetic result.

Chapter 24 - *Introduction*: A highly resorbed mandibular ridge poses an inevitable challenge for prosthodontists. Denture base is required to be extended adequately. A good and retentive set of dentures is a desirable outcome besides good aesthetic and functional values.

Case report: A female aged 72 years visited Our Hospital and reported about losing her old dentures. She required a new set of dentures. Her examination revealed highly resorbed mandibular ridge or an order V pattern of alveolar ridge resorption, as described by *Atwood*. Closed mouth technique was used to develop border molding, where the patient's muscle and muscular activity provided maximum support to the denture-bearing area. This technique aimed to obtain an accurate impression of undisturbed and uncompressed tissues. Impression using a soft liner has also shown a wider denture support area. A new set of dentures was confirmed showing good retention and stability despite the resorbed ridge, by functional and speaking examination.

Discussion: Various methods have been used to achieve retention, stability, and support. The closed mouth technique was chosen owing to the stability of the material when stored.

Conclusion: The proposed method is an excellent option to overcome highly resorbed mandibular ridge in a fully edentulous patient.

Chapter 25 - *Introduction*: The pulp stones are calcified mass in the pulp chamber and often present in teeth that have experienced trauma or injury. The pulp stones can cover part or all of the pulp chamber so that it can close access to the root canal.

Case report: A 27-year-old man came to the Conservative Dentistry Clinic, Faculty of Dentistry, Universitas Indonesia with a chief complain of severe pain in the upper left and right back teeth since last week. The patient experienced intermittent pain even though he has been taking pain killer medication. The radiographic examination showed the presence of stone-like formation in the pulp chamber that covers some areas of root canals in bilateral maxillary first molar. The precise combination of magnification and minimal invasive instrument will remove the multiple pulp stones entirely till the root canal treatment in this patient has done very well in single visit on each tooth. During 1-year follow-up, there was no more pain and cone beam computed tomography (CBCT) evaluation demonstrated good tissue healing.

Conclusion: The successful treatment in a difficult endodontic case can be obtained through proper magnification and minimally invasive instruments.

Chapter 26 - *Introduction:* Retreatment of root canals due to a previously failed endodontic treatment on chronic apical periodontitis e.c. pulp necrosis was reported. The aim of this case report was to present the technique that used for retreatment of a failure endodontic therapy of maxillary incisive.

Case report: Patient male, 32-year-old came with the broken post on his maxillary anterior incisor. The failure was due to inadequate restoration made the reinfection of bacteria in the root canal apex. Retreatment procedures for the case of a failure endodontics was performed. Success criteria on retreatment was accomplished one-month post retreatment combined with a appropriate restoration.

Conclusion: The success on retreatment depends on technique used to remove old post, restoration and obturation materials, leaving much of the residual tooth structure intact. If done properly, this increases prognosis of the case.

Chapter 27 - *Introduction*: Successful endodontic treatment depends on knowledge of root canal morphology, interpretation of radiograph, biomechanical preparation and obturation of root canal system. The possibility of root/canal variation should be considered, although the maxillary first premolar is commonly a bi-rooted tooth with an uncomplicated endodontic anatomy. This case report described the non-surgical endodontic retreatment on a maxillary first premolar with type V Vertucci canal configuration. ProTaper next instruments were used to remove the old gutta percha and to clean and shape all root canals, followed by the complete obturation with *cold lateral condensation* technique with *gutta percha* and accessory cone of root canal system.

Case report: A 21-year-old female patient came to specialist clinic of conservative dentistry Universitas Indonesia with the chief complaint of dull pain in upper right middle region of jaw. The patient had her previous endodontic treatment approximately two years ago. The patient also complained on the unpleasant feeling when eating. Intra-oral examination revealed a large cavity on her 14 tooth. Intra-oral periapical radiograph confirmed that the tooth had a previous root canal treatment, with incomplete root canal filling and chronic apical abscess. The tooth was diagnosed with a chronic apical abscess caused by inadequate endodontic treatment. Treatment planning was root canal retreatment and dowel crown restoration. The condition was a consequence of the failure of the first treatment, where the palatal canal was undetected and untreated.

Conclusion: This case highlight the need to understand, interpret the maxillary first premolar with a Vertucci type V canal configuration to achieve successful results.

Chapter 28 - *Introduction*: This was a case report on the usage of calcium hydroxide $Ca(OH)_2$ as an intracanal medicament for the treatment of chronic apical lesions caused by pulp necrosis. Chronic apical lesions generally are asymptomatic, sensitive to percussion, and often has established sinus tract. The purpose was to report the calcium hydroxide intracanal medicament for the treatment of chronic apical lesions.

Case report: Patient is female, 24-year-old, diagnosed with a chronic apical lesions e.causa pulp necrosis on tooth #16. Root canal treatment was performed using intracanal medicament calcium hydroxide/$Ca(OH)_2$. Six months after root canal treatment, there were no signs of infection clinically and decreased radiolucency on the mesial apex was observed. Post-core crown were applied as the final restoration.

Conclusion: Calcium hydroxide as intracanal medicament can induce regeneration process on chronic apical lesions cases.

Chapter 29 - *Introduction*: The *goal* of endodontic treatment is the prevention or cure of apical periodontitis. Biomechanically, this means cleaning, shaping and disinfection that enable three dimensional obturation of root canal systems. Evaluation of one or more periapical radiographs is mandatory. Here, the authors discuss the endodontic treatment of a Vertucci type II (2-1) J-shaped root canal identified radiographically.

Case report: A 29-year-old woman visited the Specialist Clinic of Conservative Dentistry University of Indonesia. The patient was referred there to continue dental treatment of the mandibular first molar. The mandibular first molar had undergone root canal treatment 9 months previously; however, the procedure had not been completed. One month previously, she started experiencing discomfort in the area while eating. A complete history was taken, and clinical and radiographic examinations were performed. She was diagnosed with a chronic apical abscess caused by inadequate endodontic treatment, and she underwent non-vital root canal treatment with post-endodontic onlay ceramage restoration.

Conclusion: Endodontic management in this case was successful because of adequate diagnosis, preparation, obturation and restoration. The treatment restored tooth morphology and function. Further evaluation are needed at 1, 3, 6 and months postoperatively.

Chapter 30 - *Introduction*: Permanent maxillary canines can present with an unusual length. This case report described a clinical case of endodontic treatment of a 32 mm upper cuspid, with the emphasis on the adjustments to the preparation and obturation steps of the root canal procedure.

Case report: A 66-year-old male patient presented to Conservative Dentistry Clinic, Faculty of Dentistry, Universitas Indonesia with pain sensation in his upper left canine upon biting on tooth #23. This tooth was previously restored with amalgam and has a secondary caries. During the root canal treatment, the tooth was found to have an unusual length of 32 mm. Adjustments of the instruments used, root canal preparation technique and fabrication of custom-made gutta-percha were needed to suit the working length of the tooth and obtain good root canal preparation and obturation results.

Conclusion: Successful endodontic treatment of an unusually long tooth can be achieved if adjustments are made to provide proper disinfection, preparation, obturation of the root canal as well as preservation of the remaining tooth structure.

Chapter 31 - *Introduction*: External resorption of tooth may occur following dental trauma and pulp necrosis and result in loss of apical constriction. This will complicate the endodontic treatment since there is a risk of endodontic obturation material to extrude beyond the apex to the periodontal tissue. Mineral Trioxide Aggregate (MTA) has been known for its bioactivity, biocompatibility, antibacterial potential and ability to induce tissue regeneration and repair. This case report aimed to present the non-surgical treatment of apical external resorption using MTA.

Case report: A 23-year-old male came to Conservative Clinic Faculty of Dentistry Universitas Indonesia with a chief complaint of his discolored front tooth. The diagnosis of tooth #11 was chronic apical periodontitis e causa pulp necrosis with open apex due to external resorption. The treatment plan was non-vital root canal treatment, apical plug using MTA, internal bleaching using 30% hydrogen peroxide for the tooth discoloration followed with post-endodontic restoration using resin composite.

Conclusion: MTA is still one of the materials of choice that can be used for apical plug. At 3-months follow up, the tooth was asymptomatic and functional. No re-darkening of tooth color occurred after internal bleaching. There were no signs of gingival inflammation. Radiographic examination showed lesion regression, increased alveolar bone density and successful healing at tooth #11. In this case, MTA has successfully repaired apical external resorption and induced hard tissue formation in the apical area.

Chapter 32 - *Introduction*: Knowledge on the anatomy of the root canals and an accurate interpretation of radiograph results are required before endodontic treatment. The mesial roots of the mandibular first molars commonly have two canals. These canals, however are merged in the apical root. This variation is called the Vertucci's type II configuration, and it has an incidence rate of 41.87%. Such variation was identified via clinical and radiographic examinations obtained using various angles. This study aimed to identify and manage the root canal treatment of the mandibular first molar with Vertucci's type II configuration.

Case report: A 25-year-old female patient complained of pain in the left mandibular molar. In tooth 36, filling and a metal post were observed, and radiographic results showed that the tooth has been initially treated. Moreover, a radiolucency was observed in the distal root. Based on history taking and clinical examination, chronic apical abscess caused by non-hermetic endodontic treatment was observed in tooth 36. Endodontic retreatment was provided and the removal of the gutta-percha and metal post, root canal treatment, adequate obturation and restoration with fiber post and porcelain fused to the metal crown were initiated.

Conclusion: Complex knowledge about the anatomy and morphology of the tooth is required for chemo-mechanical preparation to remove necrotic tissues and bacteria in the root canal and to produce adequate obturation. Thus, adequate post-treatment restoration can prevent root canal failure and maintain teeth for as long as possible in the jaw.

Chapter 33 - *Introduction*: The aim of this paper was to present the management of the fractured instrument on curvature of the Vertucci's type V canal in a maxillary lateral incisor by means of bypass techniques.

Case report: A-50-year-old male was referred with a history of lingering pain mainly at night in the upper left front teeth. The examination revealed secondary caries beneath the composite restoration, sensitive to vitality test, insensitive to percussion, and the tooth was confirmed radiographically to have a single root canal with curvature in the apical third. The patient was diagnosed with Irreversible pulpitis e causa secondary caries. The treatment plan was a vital root canal treatment combined with fiber post and direct composite restoration. During instrumentation, there was a fractured instrument due to a narrowed canal, and the dental radiograph confirmed the root canal has divided into 2 canals in the curvature. The fractured instrument was successfully bypassed with K-File, and the obturation was done using the GuttaCore obturation system.

Conclusion: The bypass technique is a favorable alternative to remove the fracture instruments in the apical third and the GuttaCore obturation system can be used to reach both canals branches in Vertucci's type V canal.

Chapter 34 - *Introduction:* This case report described the management of iatrogenic pulp exposure with Biodentine as direct pulp capping material.

Case report: A 19-year-old female patient complained about discomfort associated with thermal stimulation on the permanent mandibular left first molar. Pulp sensitivity was confirmed by thermal pulp vitality tests. The radiograph revealed a deep caries lesion close to the pulp and a lack of periapical radiolucency and periodontal ligament widening. Based on the examinations, the treatment plan was to cover the left dentine with pulp capping material indirectly, but iatrogenic pulp exposures occurred. Clinical procedures were taken consisted of caries removal, bleeding control, the Biodentine application as a direct pulp capping material, and resin composite application as the overlying restoration. Biodentine was the choice of treatment because of its high biocompatibility and bioactivity that can encourage protective hard formation and healing on the site of injury.

Conclusion: Clinical success for six months follow-up was confirmed by sensitivity over vitality test and lack of radiographic pathological findings.

Chapter 35 - *Introduction*: The first permanent molar has a very high rate of caries in children with mixed dentition mostly due to deep pits and fissure of the occlusal surface, morphological features and developmental enamel defects. In case of deep caries lesions, the pulp can become infected leading to irreversible pulpitis. The managements of irreversible pulpitis include pulpectomy, root canal treatment, and tooth restoration. Adhesive restoration with an indirect resin composite onlay, offers many advantages for endodontically treated teeth. The case report aimed to present an indirect composite resin restoration onlay for a broken-down molar tooth of a pediatric patient.

Case Report: This paper described the clinical management of irreversible pulpitis in a first permanent molar of a 9-year-old girl from pulpectomy to placement of a composite resin onlay as a definitive restoration. On follow-up, the resin composite restoration remained in place with no fracture or subjective complaints.

Conclusion: Functional and aesthetic restoration of an endodontically-treated first permanent molar tooth of a pediatric patient can be achieved with the use of an indirect composite resin onlay and will directly impact the success of the root canal treatment and the longevity of the restoration.

Chapter 36 - *Introduction*: The authors reported a case of delayed replantation of two avulsed maxillary central incisors.

Case Report: A 12-year-old boy attended the dental clinic because of avulsed teeth due to a bike accident. The accident occurred while the child was cycling on paved roads. His parents brought the avulsed teeth to the clinic 2 h later in dry condition as they kept the teeth in a plastic bag after they cleaned the teeth using detergent. Intra-oral examination showed the blood was continuously discharged from the tooth socket and the maxillary permanent central incisors were avulsed. Radiograph revealed no alveolar bone wall fracture or other hard tissue injuries. The avulsed teeth showed large canals with closed apex and endodontic treatment was extra-orally performed just before they were replanted into the sockets.

Conclusion: Six-month observation after the replantation showed no pathological symptoms such as no mobility, negative palpation test and different sound in percussion test on the avulsed teeth.

Chapter 37 - *Introduction:* Dental avulsion is defined as a complete removal of tooth from the alveolar socket resulting in the complete disruption of blood supply to the pulp. Dental replantation is indicated for avulsed teeth with viable and aseptic periodontal ligament cells. Replantation is associated with the insertion and temporary fixation of avulsed teeth and aims to prevent tooth loss, so the function and aesthetic value of the tooth can be maintained as well as the height of alveolar ridges.

Case report: A 9-year-old male patient with the chief complaint of the first maxillary incisor having been released due to a fall. The avulsed tooth was carefully replanted in its original position after an extra oral root canal treatment, and a semi rigid splinting was consequently performed using the Ivy eyelet wiring ligation technique.

Conclusion: The risk of root resorption in replantation case is relatively high and relays on the clinical conditions of the periodontal ligament, apical foramen closure, duration of extra oral time and the age of patient.

Chapter 38 - *Introduction*: Pulp inflammation can extend to the periodontium causing damage to the periodontal tissue. The relationship between pulp and periodontium occurs due to their interconnected vascularization and their close proximity to each other. Diagnosing endo-perio lesions can be challenging because pulp tissue and periodontium previously have been studied separately, and one primary disease had characteristics similar to the other.

Case report: This case reported two cases of endo-perio lesions that were performed in a conventional root canal treatment via sequential endodontic and periodontal treatments. Follow-up radiographs demonstrated the complete healing of the hard and soft tissue lesions.

Conclusion: Endodontic treatment performed with proper cleaning and shaping and specific medication, followed by periodontal treatment could be successful in treating endo-perio lesions.

Chapter 39 - *Introduction:* Application of fixed prosthetics can cause periodontal problems. Improper sizing and placement of fixed prosthetics can endanger the periodontal system in several ways, including causing gingival inflammation problems or trauma from occlusion that inhibits attachment and causes bony defects. The authors reported the treatment of occlusional trauma caused by improper prosthetic crown sizing.

Case report: A 75-year-old man presented with complaints of pain when chewing and eating. He underwent anamnesis, dental, periodontal examinations and radiography. Treatment planning was made from initial therapy through the rehabilitation phase. After 3 months he was re-evaluated. The patient's main complaint of pain disappeared after coronoplasty, but this treatment did not reduce the pocket depth. A flap operation that used a combination of DFDBA and pericardium membrane successfully reduced pocket depth, loss of attachment and intrabony defects after 3 months of follow-up.

Conclusion: Improper fixed prosthetic sizing can cause trauma from occlusion, pain, increased pocket depth and loss of attachment. In this case, coronoplasty successfully eliminated pain. Flap surgery is an effective means of reducing pocket depth and mitigating loss of attachment. Periodontal professionals should consider the prosthetic implant's size, placement and the occlusal loading of periodontal ligament as a result of prosthetic placement so as to prevent traumatic occlusion.

Chapter 40 - *Introduction:* It is believed that the smile represents personality and appearance. The common cause of excessive gingival display is altered passive eruption (APE), which was resulted from incomplete natural migration of the gingiva during tooth eruption.

Case report: A 30-year-old female was referred from Orthodontist in private practice. At the first visit, the patient chief complaint was her tooth arrangement, and asked any treatment to help her in order to minimize her gummy emergence when she was smiling. From the clinical examination, there was an excessive gum appearance of about 5 millimetres (mm) in her upper jaw. This case showed the unequal proportion of the teeth, including the square shape of central incisive, the proportion of lateral incisive and canine. The ratio of intra-tooth relationship for the central incisive was 8 mm:8 mm (height :width). In addition, the gingival zenith level was also not ideal. The management of this case was divided into the preparation phase, surgery phase and follow-up phase. In the preparation phase, the authors examined the biological width, anatomical consideration and esthetic consideration. In the surgery phase, the authors prepared for crown lengthening procedure with gingivectomy and bone reduction by 2 - 3 mm. From the result, the patient was very satisfied with her new tooth shape and smile.

Conclusion: Crown lengthening procedure is one of the alternative treatments for altered passive eruption cases. Bone reduction estimation was calculated by the evaluation of biological width, anatomical and esthetic consideration.

Chapter 41 - *Introduction*: An intrusive luxation is a severe type of dental trauma that may destruct the periodontal ligament, pulp, and alveolar bone. However, the position of the intruded primary teeth may be close to the developing permanent successors; thus, any traumatic injuries may result in multiple complications, and an appropriate treatment should be established, including waiting for spontaneous re-eruption, surgical repositioning, and extraction. This study aimed to present a successful conservative management of intrusive luxation in tooth 61 in a 23-month-old girl.

Case report: A 23-month-old girl and her parents were referred to the Pediatric Dentistry Clinic of Universitas Indonesia. The patient presented with a history of falling while playing, and she was then diagnosed with intrusive luxation in the left maxillary primary incisor. Spontaneous re-eruption was observed 4 weeks after injury. Periodic evaluation was conducted until 6 months after injury, and no complications were observed on the affected tooth.

Discussion: The successful treatment of intrusive luxation in the primary teeth was influenced by the child's age, severity and direction of intrusion, and/or involvement of permanent tooth bud. Conservative management, including waiting for spontaneous re-eruption, is a treatment option for intrusive luxation if the permanent tooth bud is not damaged.

Chapter 42 - *Introduction:* Pulp capping in carious teeth has been considered unpredictable and therefore contraindicated. Mineral trioxide aggregate (MTA) known as new material can resist bacterial leakage and may provide protection for the pulp, allowing repair and continued pulp vitality in teeth when used in combination with a sealed restoration.

Case report: A 15-year-old boy patient reported to the Pedodontic Clinic at the Dental hospital Faculty of Dentistry Universitas Indonesia with an extensive destruction of coronal tooth on maxillary left second premolar.

Methods: Teeth were treated with MTA Angelus®. MTA material that has been manipulated according to the manufacturer's instructions was placed in the exposed area until closed. Upon completion, GIC material to cover the top surface of MTA was applied.

Results: MTA produced a white layer similar to hydroxyapatite in the upper layer and provide chemical bonds between the cavity wall and MTA layer. It was attached to the MTA surface and continues to grow. They also produce mineralized matrix on the MTA.

Conclusion: Case selection is necessary in determining the type of treatment that fits the caries conditions and the rest of the dental tissue. Exposure to the pulp due to caries involvement can be done with MTA material closure.

Chapter 43 - *Introduction:* Class II division 1 malocclusion is the most frequent problem in the orthodontic practice. It is characterized with a retrognathic mandible, and repositioning the mandible forward is needed to enhance its growth and improve dentoskeletal relationships. Functional twin block appliance is a widely used functional appliance for the management of Class II malocclusion.

Case report: a 10-year-11-month old girl patient attended Dental Hospital of Faculty of Dentistry, Universitas Indonesia with a chief complaint of her upper anterior teeth were more protrude than lower anterior teeth. On clinical examination, her facial profile is convex, symmetry. She had proclined maxillary anterior teeth with a 10mm overjet and a 5mm overbite. The lateral cephalometric radiography indicated a skeletal class II pattern with hyper-divergent growth which was due to mandibular retroposition and maxillary protrusion. The initial treatment objective was reduce overjet by skeletal improvement, thus promoting mandibular growth by correction class II relationship, attain normal overjet and overbite by using functional twin block appliance and then consider fixed orthodontic treatment after functional appliance treatment. The use of twin block functional appliances have skeletal effects such as increase mandibular growth (increase height of mandibular ramus and length of mandible), the SNB value was improved to 2°. The ANB value was reduce 2°, decrease overjet 4.5mm and overbite 1mm.

Conclusion: This case has demonstrated the successful management of the first phase of treatment of a patient with Angle Class II Division 1 malocclusion using the Twin Block appliances in 6 months. The Second phase of treatment will be continued with fixed appliances.

Chapter 44 - *Introduction*: Intrusive luxation is commonly seen in primary dentition as young children have wide medullar spaces in their alveolar bone. The management of intruded primary incisors recommended by the American Academy of Pediatric Dentistry is to wait for spontaneous re-eruption or extract the tooth, depending on the degree and the direction of intrusion as well as the presence of alveolar bone fracture. Comprehensive examination is essential for determining the most appropriate approach. Here the authors report their experience with a case of intrusive luxation in the left maxillary lateral incisor of a 6-year-old patient.

Case Report: Intrusive luxation of left maxillary lateral primary incisor (tooth #62) was diagnosed, the tooth was in contact with the underlying permanent tooth and the treatment of extraction of the intruded tooth was performed. Recall examination was regularly conducted to monitor the eruption of the permanent successor. Direct trauma caused by simulation of deciduous teeth can impact the permanent successor. By extracting tooth #62, direct trauma to permanent successor tooth #22 was minimized so the development can be continued normally. Recall examination post extraction on week 1 and 4 revealed no unusual symptoms such as abscess, fever, fistula or soft tissue swelling.

Conclusion: Intrusive injuries need a careful examination owing to their close anatomical association with the developing permanent successors. In the case of intrusive luxation of tooth #62, due to the root impacting the underlying permanent tooth, extraction was selected as the ideal treatment approach.

Chapter 45 - *Introduction*: The goals of orthodontic treatment are correcting the malocclusion especially bilateral constriction of upper and lower arch, achieving good occlusion and also improve the esthetic. *Case report*: This case report described the treatment of class I malocclusion with bilateral arch constriction. The 33-year-old female patient presented with class I malocclusion, mesofacial, retrognathic chin, convex profile, and bilateral constriction of both arch. She was treated by pre-adjusted appliances and no teeth was extracted. The upper arch had 2 phases treatment, segmental method and continuous method to correct the constriction. After 18 months of treatment, the malocclusion was corrected with successful aesthetic improvement, class I canine and molar relationship in the left and right side, and also ideal overjet and overbite. *Conclusion*: Treatment for bilateral arch constriction could be corrected by pre-adjusted appliances. An accurate examination will result in a proper diagnosis and an effective and efficient treatment plan. However, expansion for bilateral arch constriction should consider the limits of expansion because excessive expansion leads to instability.

Chapter 46 - *Introduction*: A case of age estimation on burnt victim using tooth development and attrition analyses was reported. *Case Report*: A burnt body was brought to Forensic Department of National Cipto Mangunkusumo Hospital (RSCM), Jakarta, for identification. The authorities instructed minimal invasive identification procedure to avoid more damage to the body. Teeth were the only evidence available in the victim that could be used for age estimation. Victim's age was estimated from the third molar eruption status and attrition severity.

Discussion: All teeth had reached the occlusal plane except the left lower third molar, which had not fully erupted. Attrition was found on almost all teeth especially on all first molars, but not on any third molar. By comparing these findings to American Dental Association (ADA) eruption diagram and the findings of Firdaus (2014) and Tuteja (2012) studies and by analyzing the severity of the attrition, it could be concluded that the estimated age range of victim was 20 to 30 years with a clenching or bruxism habit.

Conclusion: This case illustrated the importance of tooth development and attrition analyses in burnt victim age estimation.

Chapter 47 - *Introduction:* Forensic odontology is primarily concerned with dental findings or evidence analysis which can help investigators determine victim identification including gender, race, and age in a justice context. According to studies, the accuracy is high enough (up to 43-89%) because of the dental resilience from the decomposition process and its ability to survive an extreme conditions such as high temperature in burn cases.

Case report: The postmortem procedure in this child fire victim case was done as requested by the police department by only examining the overall external body as well as the extra-oral and intra-oral conditions, taking routine photographs, and estimating victim's age by using the dental eruption chart. As there was no radiograph caused by the limited postmortem procedure, clinical examination with dental chart method was used and the estimation result was then matched to the victim's document.

Conclusion: Forensic odontology could give better information with more detailed antemortem data and postmortem procedure.

SECTION 1: ORAL MEDICINE

In: Clinical Reports in Dentistry
Editor: Lisa R. Amir
ISBN: 978-1-53617-328-4

Chapter 1

STRESS MANAGEMENT FOR DECREASING RECURRENCE OF HERPES SIMPLEX VIRUS INFECTION

***Rolis A. Wuriyanti*[1], *Marco Meleti*[2] *and Yuniardini S. Wimardhani*[3,*]**

[1]Oral Medicine Residency Program, Faculty of Dentistry,
Universitas Indonesia, Jakarta, Indonesia
[2]Department of Medicine and Surgery,
Center of Laser Surgery and Oral Pathology,
Dental School, University of Parma, Parma, Italy
[3]Department of Oral Medicine, Faculty of Dentistry,
Universitas Indonesia, Jakarta, Indonesia

ABSTRACT

Introduction: Oral infection caused by Herpes Simplex Virus (HSV) commonly occurs in childhood. However, recurrent infections are more common among adults with a prevalence of 70 – 80%. Stress is one of trigger factors that contributes to HSV reactivation. Stress is a condition that tends to disrupt the immune system, resulting in biological systemic alterations. This case report aimed to describe the importance of stress management in decreasing recurrence of HSV infection.

Case report: A 30-year-old female patient came to the oral medicine clinic at Universitas Indonesia with a chief complaint of a sore mouth, preceded by fever and malaise. Such symptoms caused difficulty in eating and swallowing over the last week. Similar symptoms occurred few times before. The patient was otherwise healthy, except recent fatigue and psychological stress postpartum. She felt very anxious about a possible oral malignant lesion. Clinical examination revealed poor oral hygiene, multiple ulcers surrounded by an erythematous area 0.5 – 6mm in size located throughout the oral cavity.

* Corresponding Author's Email: yuniardini@ui.ac.id.

Lympadenopathy of both submandibular regions was also noted. Result of IgG HSV-1 test was positive and she was diagnosed with recurrent intra-oral herpes (RIH). Therapy included 100mg doxycycline mouthwash, 200mg Acyclovir and 7 days of oral multivitamin. Patient was advised to take sufficient rest time, to eat more nutritious foods, increase fluid intake and manage possible underlying psychological disorders. The lesions were clinically resolved in the patients 4th visit to the clinic.

Conclusion: It is important to understand the association between psychological stress and recurrence of HSV infection. Adopting stress management with a cognitive psychotherapy approach may improve self-confidence in patients to have rational and positive thoughts and reduce future recurrence of HSV.

Keywords: Herpes Simplex Virus, reactivation, recurrent intra-oral herpes, stress management

1. Introduction

The Herpes Simplex Virus (HSV) is responsible for most viral infections in the oral and perioral regions. HSV consists of two different serotypes: HSV-1, which is associated with oral and labial lesions, and HSV-2, which is associated with genital lesions. Both serotypes can infect both sites due to sexual transmission [1]. In the United States, HSV-1 is found in up to 53% of the adult population, and 60 – 80% of cases are detected through the research of HSV-1 antibodies [2]. The immune-response to viruses are thought to last life following infection [3]. In Europe, half of the population is seropositive for HSV-1 infection. In developing countries, almost all people are infected with this virus [4].

HSV-1 is a pathogen able to cause either primary, latent, recurrent, or persistent infection during the host's lifetime [2]. This virus is transmitted by direct contact with infected secretions and the majority of primary infections usually occur sub clinically [5]. After primary infection, the virus moves along sensory axons, replicates, and becomes latent in the trigeminal ganglion in the head and neck region. During this phase, there is a decrease in the regulation of the replication process, and the virus is not infectious. Consequently, it is undetected as an antigen such that it escapes the immune surveillance [5]. The quiescent virus in the trigeminal host ganglion can be stimulated and reactivated by several factors, such as external stimuli, emotional stress, menstruation, sun exposure, and immunosuppressive conditions [5, 6]. Emotional or psychological stress can suppress some components of the immune response with the increase in cortisol secreted by the adrenal cortex, resulting in homeostatic and biological disturbances [7]. Recurrent herpes infection on lips is also termed herpes labialis and has clinical features of coalescent blisters on the vermillion border. Intra-oral herpes consists of small-sized ulcers that usually involve keratinized mucosa, predominantly in the palatal area [8].

Social problems and environmental demands to improve self-existence and the personal inability to fulfill these needs can cause emotional stress. Some common causes of stress include occupational problems, exams, domestic problems, illness, and sleep deprivation. In addition, stress conditions can be inherited resulting in worsening of psychological status [9]. Here we reported the case of a patient with frequent episodes of HSV infection recurrence which were possibly related to inability to cope with fatigue and postpartum psychological stress.

2. Case Report

A 30-year-old female patient came to the Dental Hospital at the Faculty of Dentistry, Universitas Indonesia with chief complaints of mouth soreness and ulcers throughout the oral cavity. Symptoms were also accompanied by malaise and fever, inducing some difficulties in eating and swallowing in the last week. The patient is a housewife with two boys aged 4 years and 6 months. Antibiotics, steroids and multivitamins were already administered by her previous physician. Consuming warm water did not ameliorate the clinical condition. Anamnesis revealed a history of similar symptoms occurring almost monthly, predominantly affecting lips and buccal mucosa. It was not possible to obtain full anamnestic data during the first appointment, because of the emotional stress and anxiety of the patient.

Extra-oral examination revealed that left and right submandibular lymph nodes were tender. Intra-oral examination revealed poor oral hygiene with sub and supragingival calculus and debris, as well as multiple ulcers with irregular borders 0.5 – 5mm in size, white erythematous borders and base in keratinized and non-keratinized mucosa (Figure 1A-C). The working diagnosis of intra-oral herpes infection with differential diagnosis of herpetiform type of recurrent aphtous stomatitis was made. After the first visit, the patient was given 100mg doxycycline mouthwash and was tested for anti HSV-1 and 2 antibodies (IgG and IgM) and complete blood count. Based on the results of the serological test, anti HSV-1 IgG were positive, therefore 200mg Acyclovir 5 times a day for a week were prescribed. The patient returned for one-week follow up without complaint or new lesions. She felt more calm and was able to communicate better, thus allowing us to obtain comprehensive information about her condition and medical history.

However, oral discomfort and multiple sores appeared after coming back from a trip last month. Her pain levels increased, which lead to fear and anxiety.

The patient claimed that she had difficulties in controlling her mood when she was presented with an uncomfortable situation. Intra-oral examination revealed that most of the lesions improved, but ulcers at the floor of the mouth and soft palate did not (Figure 2A-D). Doxycycline mouthwash and multivitamin were continued, while acyclovir was discontinued. Encouragement and motivation was given to cope with her situation, and she was advised to get sufficient rest to accelerate the healing process.

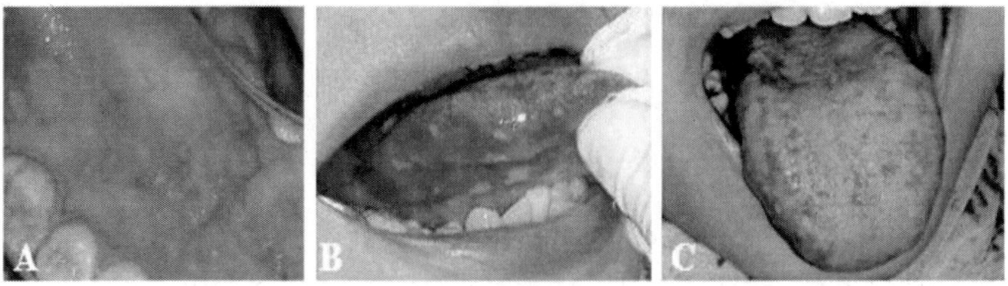

Figure 1. Intra-oral condition during the 1st visit. Multiple ulcers on the labial mucosa (A); multiple ulcers on the hard and soft palate (B); multiple ulcers on ventral and lateral part of the tongue (C).

On her 3rd visit, new painful ulcers under tongue were observed. The patient reported them first appeared 3 days prior. She reported significant fatigue and psychological stress associated with her housework and the recent birth of a child.

We administered the Depression Anxiety Stress Scale Questionnaire which confirmed the presence of mild anxiety.

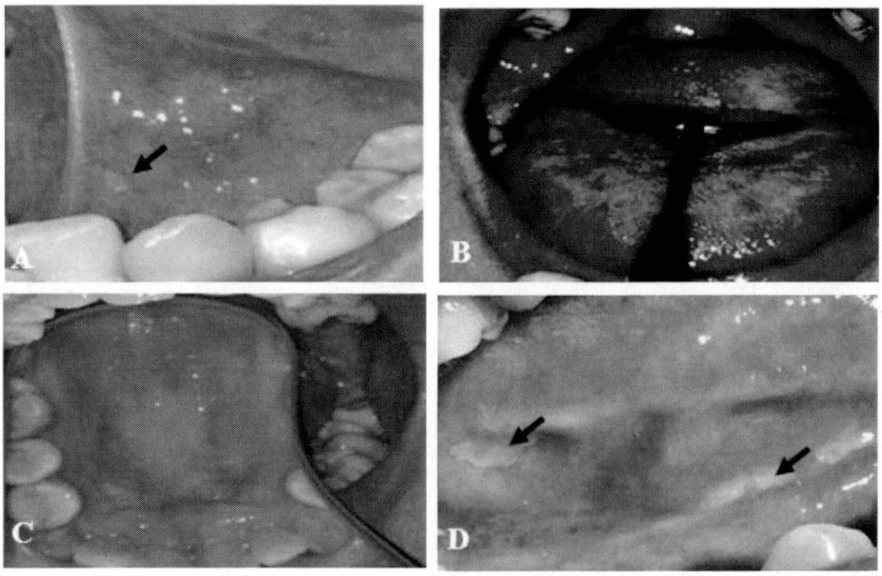

Figure 2. Intra-oral condition during the 2nd visit. Single ulcer on the floor of the mouth (A); multiple ulcers on the soft palate (B); multiple erythema on the hard palate (C); multiple ulcers on the ventral and lateral aspects of the tongue (D).

Intra-oral examination revealed multiple ulcers with a white base, erythematous borders 0.5 – 1mm in size on the tongue and gingiva (Figure 3A-C). Acyclovir was re-administered as well as doxycycline mouthwash and multivitamin.

On the 4th visit, improvement was observed, however there were still some healing ulcers. (Figure 4A-D).

At the last visit, objective improvement of the oral ulcers was observed. No new oral ulcers appeared (Figure 5A-C) and the pain was decreasing. The patient was referred for elimination of focal infection to improve her oral hygiene.

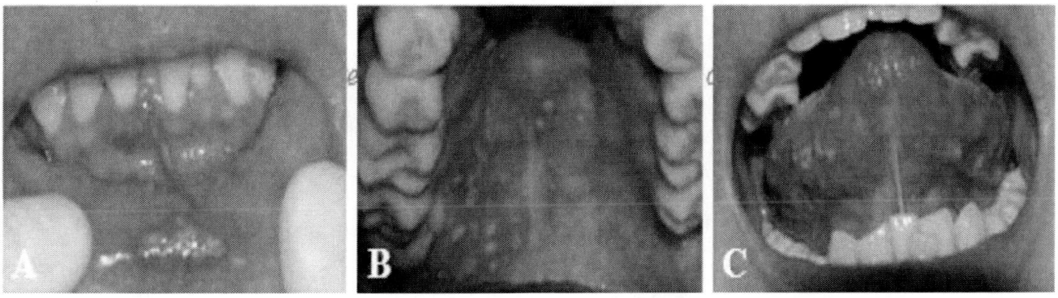

Figure 3. Intra-oral condition of the 3rd visit. Multiple ulcers on hard palate (A); multiple ulcers on ventral and lateral aspects of the tongue (B); multiple ulcers on the tongue (C).

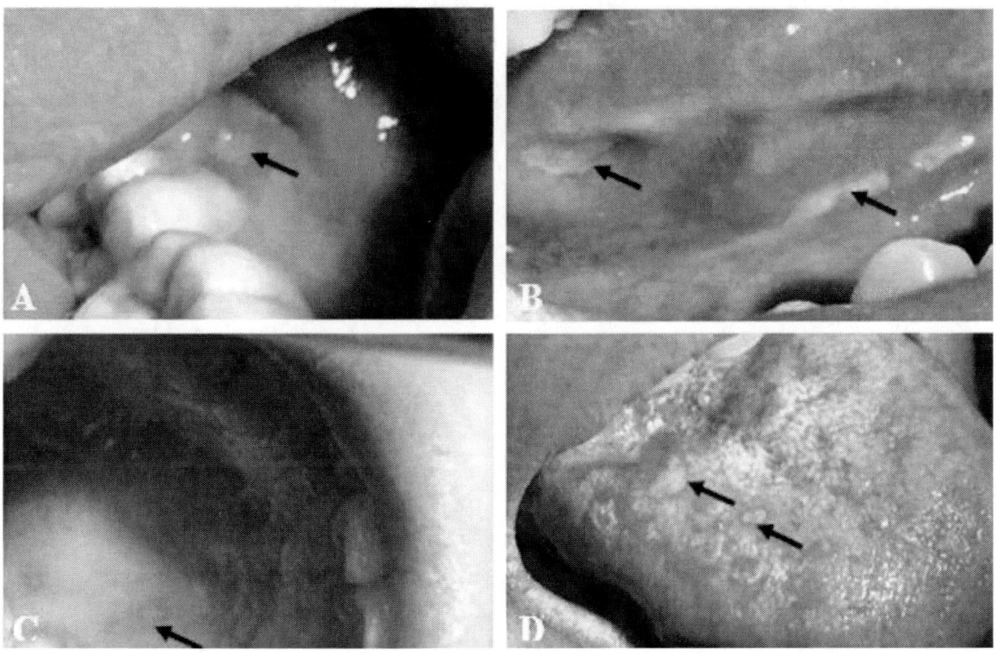

Figure 4. Intra-oral condition the 4th visit. Single ulcer on the gingival 38 region (A); multiple ulcer on ventral and lateral of the tongue (B); multiple ulcer on the hard palate (C); multiple ulcer on dorsal of the tongue (D).

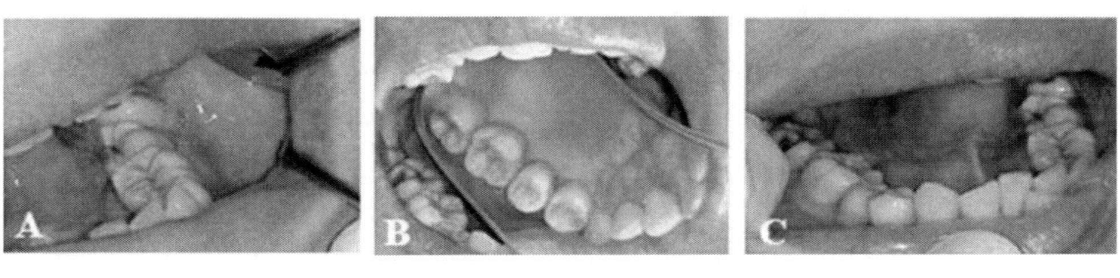

Figure 5. Intra-oral condition the 5th visit. The lesion was healed (A); (B); and (C).

All medications were discontinued and she was suggested to keep up her stress management to maintain mood balance and psychological condition to prevent recurrence of HSV infection. This case management was declared successful. It was proven that until this case report was published, the patient has not come for any complains.

3. Discussion

Viral infection is generally well recognizable on the basis of the clinical manifestations. Most viruses that have a long-term evolutionary relationship with hosts are usually less pathogenic. Due to their dependence on the host for replication, the evolution of the virus is slow. Viruses are divided into three groups based on their replication-adaptive strategy: latent, "hit-and-run", and "slow-and-low". The Human Herpes Viruses (HHVs) are considered to have latent replication strategy [5]. The HHVs are a group of viruses that contain double-stranded DNA genome that is covered by protein, termed "the envelope". It has an ability to manipulate the host's immune system by creating molecular mimicry similar to interleukin, chemokine, or chemokine receptors that interfere with the host's cytokine response, or by reducing antigen recognition by Major Histocompatibility Complex (MHC) of infected cells. In addition, HHV is divided into several subfamily groups: *alpha*, *beta*, and *gamma*. HSV belongs to the *alpha* subfamily, which not only primarily targets neurons for long-term residency but also replicates in epithelial cells for transmission through skin and mucosa. *Beta* and *gamma* subfamilies prefer leukocytes as targets [5].

The HSV is a member of HHV family, consisting of two types: HSV-1 and HSV-2. HSV-1 is particularly associated wither current intra-oral herpes (RIH) and recurrent herpes labialis, whereas HSV-2 is associated with genital lesions. The intensity of the host immune response plays an important role to mitigate or aggravate clinical symptoms. Infection can either persist for the lifetime of neurons or "walk along" the axon into the oral mucosa. Oral ulcers are the most common signs of active HSV infection, and sometimes the skin around the nails of the hands and toes can be affected *(Herpetic Whitlow)* [5]. HSV can live with latent RNA form for the duration of the host's life in the sensory nerve ganglion, predominantly in the trigeminal ganglia [6, 7]. Latency is a reversible condition of decreasing viral genome transcription, such that it can be undetected by routine immune surveillance. Interferon produced by CD8+ plays a major role to maintain latency stage. When interferon secretion stops due to decreased CD8+ counts, negative feedback regulation will gradually trigger viral replication [5]. However, previous work has demonstrated that HSV apparently has a periodic replication lytic phases that can regularly produce new viral progeny [6, 8, 10]. The HSV reactivation may be affected by the path of c-Jun N-terminal kinase (JNK) protein, a member of MAP family kinase. This protein is activated before the viruses begin to leave neurons. If the JNK path is inhibited, HSV cannot be reactivated, leading some to conclude that the activation of JNK protein plays a key role in HSV reactivation [6]. Besides that, the progression of the reactivation can also be influenced by external factors that may interfere with immune T-cell function, such as an immunosuppressive condition (HIV/AIDS, organ transplant recipient), fatigue, psychological stress, and aging [7, 9, 10].

Fatigue is often associated with circadian or photoperiodic changes due to sleep deprivation that leads to affective disturbances, psychosomatic disorders, and other pathological conditions, including the alteration of immune and endocrine properties [5]. Meanwhile, psychological stress tends to stimulate the hypothalamus–pituitary–adrenal axis and sympathetic nerves system, which normally maintains homeostasis, through the release of cortisol and catecholamines [7, 10, 11]. Both hormones support the shifting of cytokines from Th1 CD4+ to Th2 CD4+ production. As a result, the number of CD8+ decreases while antibodies production increases. This condition reduces the latency phase of HSV. Moreover, the increase in epinephrine can suppress macrophage function to destroy HSV-infected cells [12]. The prodromal symptoms of HSV infection include pain, tingling, and itching prior to the appearance of initial lesions. These lesions are erythematous papules which evolve into fluid-filled blisters [4]. Oral lesions initially appear accompanied by an unusual sensation of lack of tactile perception or sensory feelings progressing to tingling, burning, or throbbing in affected area. After 24 – 48 hours, vesicles which are easily disrupted arise and develop to form ulcers. Sites of predilection of oral ulcers are generally in the keratinized mucosa (vermillion border, lip, hard palate, attached gingival and alveolar crest) but in some cases can also appear in non-keratinized mucosa (labial, buccal mucosa and tongue) [13]. The same thing happens in this case, so the herpetiform type of recurrent aphthous stomatitis is used as a differential diagnosis. But this can be eliminated based on the prodromal symptoms and was supported by the results of serological examinations, that the herpes virus was activated.

The stress condition is a negative factor that can disturb the host's performance [14]. It is often associated to either HSV-1 or HSV-2 reactivation from the latency state. As reported recently, the entity of psychological stress related not only depending on how great external pressure is experienced, but also by genetic factors such as mood disorders. Inherited psychological disturbances may make a host more vulnerable to HSV reactivation even with small stressor influences. In the case presented here, the patient was a self-described perfectionist who quickly became anxious if a situation was out of her control, such as the recent child birth. Thus, stress management became essential for her to decrease the recurrence her HSV infection [7].

Initial approach to manage stress includes techniques to reduce internal or external pressure. There are two ways to cope with stress: passive and active. The passive way is when the patient decides to suffer or reject the reality, compared to the active way, in which a patient decides to face reality, clarify the problem, and ask for help. To overcome the problem, the patient needs to employ strategies to trouble shoot and handle emotions. Trouble shooting focuses on attempting to change a stressful situation through problem solving, while handling emotion is based on self-acceptance without changing the situation [15].

Antiviral prophylaxis was apparently not necessary in the case reported here, because the patient was immunocompetent. We felt that reassuring herself-confidence was needed to improve her chances of managing any situation, which would attenuate predisposing factors of virus reactivation. Finally, an explanation about the negative effects of prolonged fatigue and psychological stress was also given to her.

Conclusion

This case report has shown that a psychological approach such as cognitive psychotherapy can reduce stress and increase self-confidence, which can lead patient to positive thoughts to cope with the stress of daily living. Such a strategy can likely reduce the recurrence rate of HSV infection. However, some more evidence based on the same case reports or researches were still needed.

References

[1] Siegel, M. A. (2002). "Diagnosis and management of recurrent herpes simplex infections". *J. Am. DenT. Assoc.,* 133:1245 - 1249.

[2] Egan, K. P., Wu, S., Wigdahl, B., Jennings, S. R. (2013). "Immunological control of herpes simplex virus infections". *J. Neurovirol.,* 19:328 - 345.

[3] Gilbert, S. C. Oral shedding of herpes simplex virus type 1 in immunocompetent persons (2006). *J. Oral Pathol. Med.,* 35:548 - 553.

[4] Wald, A., Corey, L. (2007). *Human herpesviruses: Biology, Therapy, and Immunoprophylaxis.* In: Arvin, A., Campadelli-Fiume, G., Mocarski, E. et al. Persistence in the population: epidemiology, transmission Immunocompetent host. Cambridge: Cambridge University Press. 1 - 21.

[5] Grinde, B. (2013). "Herpesviruses: latency and reactivation - viral strategies and host response". *J. Oral Microbiol.,* 1:1 - 9.

[6] Cliffe, A. R., Arbuckle, J. H., Vogel, J. L., Geden, M. J., Rothbart, S. B., Cusack, C. L., Strahl, B. D., Kristie, T. M., Deshmukh, M. (2015). "Neuronal stress pathway mediating a histone methyl/ phospho switch is required for herpes simplex virus reactivation". *Cell Host Microbe,*18:649 - 58.

[7] Chida, Y., Maom, X. (2009). "Does psychosocial stress predict symptomatic herpes simplex virus recurrence? A meta-analytic investigation on prospective studies". *Brain Behav. Immun.,* 23:917 - 925.

[8] Bhateja, S., Arora, G., Mastud, S. K. (2017). "Recurrent Intra-oral Herpes (RIH) infection–A case report". *Biomed. J. Sci. Tech. Res.,* 1:3 - 5.

[9] Perng, G.-C., Jones, C. (2010). "Towards an understanding of the herpes simplex virus type 1 latency-reactivation cycle". *Interdiscipl. Perspect. Infect. Dis.,*1 - 18.

[10] Glaser, R., Kiecolt-glaser, J. K. (2005). “Stress-induced immune dysfunction: implications for health". *Immunol.,* 5:243 - 51.

[11] Elenkov, I. J., Chrousos, G. P. (1999). "Stress hormones, Th1/Th2 patterns, pro/anti-inflammatory cytokines and susceptibility to disease". *Trends Endocrinol. Metab.,* 10: 359 - 68.

[12] Logan, H. L., Lutgendorf, S., Hartwig, A., Lilly, J., Berberich, S. L. (1998). "Immune, stress, and mood markers related to recurrent oral herpes outbreaks". *Oral Surg., Oral Med., Oral Pathol. Oral Radiol.,* 86:48 - 54.

[13] Lugito, M. D. H. L., Pradono, S. A. (2014). "Valacyclovir in the management of recurrent intra-oral herpes infection". *J. Dent. Indones.,* 21(1):21 - 6.

[14] Kurebayashi, L. F. S., Miyuki Do Prado, J. M., Paes da Silva, M. J. (2012). "Correlations between stress and anxiety levels in nursing students". *J. Nursing Edu. Pract.,* 2:128 - 134.

[15] Baqutayan, S. M. S. (2015). “Stress and coping mechanisms: A historical overview". *Mediter. J. Soc. Sci.,* 6:479 - 488.

In: Clinical Reports in Dentistry
Editor: Lisa R. Amir
ISBN: 978-1-53617-328-4

Chapter 2

SUSPECT ORAL SQUAMOUS CELL CARCINOMA IN AN ELDERLY PATIENT WITH BETEL-QUID CHEWING HISTORY: A CASE REPORT

Felicia Paramita[1], Gus P. Subita[2,*] and Harum Sasanti[2]
[1]Oral Medicine Residency Program, Faculty of Dentistry,
Universitas Indonesia, Jakarta, Indonesia
[2]Department of Oral Medicine, Faculty of Dentistry,
Universitas Indonesia, Jakarta, Indonesia

ABSTRACT

Introduction: Betel-quid chewing is habitually practiced in parts of Indonesia and comprises of various composition. It is a well-established risk factor of numerous oral mucosal lesions, including oral potentially malignant disorders (OPMDs) and oral squamous cell carcinoma. The present study aimed to discuss a case of suspected oral squamous cell carcinoma in an elderly patient with betel-quid chewing as a risk factor. *Case report*: A 76-year-old female presented to the dental hospital of Universitas Indonesia; she was referred from a private hospital with a working diagnosis of pseudomembranous candidiasis on the left buccal mucosa. She had chewed betel-quid, a mixture of betel-quid leaf, lime, areca nut, gambier, and tobacco, for more than 20 years. An intra-oral examination revealed mixed white nodular and plaque lesions on the left buccal and alveolar mucosa, an erythematous base, ulceration and induration in posterior part of the lesion adjacent to the retromolar pad, which led to the clinical suspicion of oral squamous cell carcinoma. Betel-quid chewing is believed to be a risk factor of oral squamous cell carcinoma. The betel-quid composition, long duration and moderately high frequency of chewing, the way betel-quid is kept in the mouth, increased patient's age, and poor oral hygiene increase the risk of oral squamous cell carcinoma. *Conclusion:* As dentists, we play a key role in the early detection of oral mucosal changes associated with

* Corresponding Author's Email: guspermana11@gmail.com.

betel-quid chewing, particularly OPMDs and oral squamous cell carcinoma, and to provide adequate education and treatment for the patients.

Keywords: betel-quid chewing, oral squamous cell carcinoma, elderly patients

1. INTRODUCTION

Betel-quid chewing is a common practice in parts of Indonesia. Betel-quid is usually kept or chewed in the mouth. The betel-quid composition greatly varies according to where the betel-quid is used. Common betel-quid composition includes Piper betle leaf, lime, and areca nut. Betel-quid chewing can cause numerous oral mucosal lesions. Mucosal desquamation and yellowish or reddish-brown crusts that result from the incorporation of the betel-quid are observed in chewers (betel chewer's mucosa). Areca nut–associated lesions display a grayish-white discoloration with a diffuse border and cannot be rubbed off. Quid-induced lesions are characterized by discoloration, wrinkles, thickening of the oral mucosa, and ulceration. Betel-quid lichenoid lesions are white, wavy, non-elevated parallel lines with a central erythematous area at the site of quid placement. Oral submucous fibrosis is characterized by fibrosis of the oral mucosa, which causes limited jaw opening (trismus) [1]. In addition to all these oral mucosal lesions, betel-quid chewing is a risk factor of oral potentially malignant disorders (OPMDs) including leukoplakia and oral squamous cell carcinoma [2, 3].

Oral squamous cell carcinoma may be preceded by OPMDs with an increased risk of malignancy development [4]. Of all OPMDs, leukoplakia has received significant attention. According to the World Health Organization in 1978, leukoplakia is defined as a white plaque that cannot be characterized as other lesions clinically or pathologically [5]. Clinically, leukoplakia is divided into homogenous and non-homogenous types. Homogenous leukoplakia is characterized by a white plaque, flat or wavy surface, and fissures or fine cracks.

Non-homogenous leukoplakia has a varied clinical appearance and may appear as nodules, verrucous, or speckled. It is generally accepted that non-homogenous leukoplakia presents a higher risk of malignant transformation than its homogenous counterpart [6]. In the present study, we report a case of suspected oral squamous cell carcinoma with betel-quid chewing as the primary risk factor.

2. CASE REPORT

A 76-year-old female patient presented to the dental hospital of the Universitas Indonesia. She was referred from a private hospital with a working diagnosis of pseudomembrane candidiasis of the left buccal mucosa. The patient had experienced pain in the left cheek for three years. The patient was administered antibiotics upon admission. Two months prior to this visit, the patient had been administered antifungal oral suspension, topical corticosteroid, and diclofenac, but there was no improvement.

The patient had chewed betel-quid for more than 20 years. The betel-quid composition included Piper betle leaf, lime, areca nut, gambier, and tobacco; this mixture was chewed three to four times a day. The betel-quid was usually kept in her left cheek. The patient had stopped chewing betel-quid for three months after being warned by her dentist.

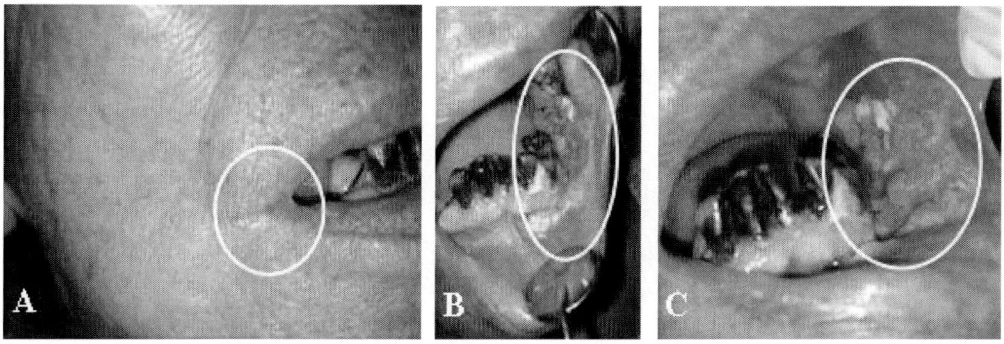

Figure 1. Fissured lesion at the right lip commissure (A); Intra-oral examination revealed a mixed white nodular and plaque lesions on the left buccal and alveolar mucosa, an erythematous base (B); ulceration and induration in posterior part of the lesion adjacent to the retromolar pad (C).

The extra-oral examination identified a fissured lesion at the right lip commissure (Figure 1A). The intra-oral examination showed that the patient had poor oral hygiene as observed by the deposits of plaque and calculus, tooth mobility, and several missing teeth. Mixed white nodular and plaque lesions on the left buccal and alveolar mucosa, an erythematous base, ulceration and induration in posterior part of the lesion adjacent to the retromolar pad (Figure 1B, C). The patient had obtained complete blood count results from the previous hospital. Hemoglobin, hematocrit, and erythrocyte levels were all lower than previously measured (11.5 g/dL, 34.2%, and 3.58×10^6 μL, respectively). The erythrocyte sedimentation rate had increased to 29 mm/hour. The other blood counts remained in normal range.

The clinical examination led to suspicion of oral squamous cell carcinoma and the patient was referred to an oncologist for further evaluation. Two weeks later, the patient visited an oncologist who suggested that she undergo biopsy for histopathological examination. The oncologist also explained the treatment modalities and the risks. The patient's family decided to refuse the biopsy retrieval procedure and the treatment. The oncologist prescribed paracetamol and tramadol for pain control.

3. Discussion

The clinical signs of the lesion were suggestive of oral squamous cell carcinoma and the suspicion was further confirmed by betel-quid chewing history which is a known risk factor. The betel-quid composition used greatly vary according to the place where the betel-quid habit presents. The specific composition are divided into three basic categories: (a) betel-quid nuts with no tobacco products, (b) betel-quid with tobacco products without betel nuts and (c) betel-quid nuts with tobacco and tobacco products [1]. The contents of nitrosamines in tobacco and arecoline in betel-quid nuts may be carcinogenic [2, 7]. Nitrosamines found in tobacco are genotoxic and may affect the DNA repair pathway [8]. Arecoline is an alkaloid that is cytotoxic, genotoxic, and mutagenic. Arecoline triggers alterations in genes that are believed to play an important role in malignant transformation. The decreased regulation of p21 and p27 through reactive oxygen species pathways causes a G1/S cell cycle transition that can result in faulty DNA replication. Arecoline also suppresses the tumor suppressor genes BRCA1 and BRCA2 [9].

In addition to betel-quid composition, the duration and frequency of betel-quid chewing also affects the risk of oral squamous cell carcinoma. Chewing 10 times per day increases the relative risk by 7.5 times compared with chewing once a day, which only increases the risk by 2.5 times [10]. Chewing betel-quid for over 30 years is associated with a six-fold increased risk of malignancy [10]. Moreover, there is an increased risk of malignancy even when the betel-quid is not chewed but are merely placed in the oral cavity and come in contact with the oral mucosa [1].

The patient is presently 76 years old and according to literature, age is also a risk factor of squamous cell carcinoma because of the accumulation of mutations over time. DNA repairing abilities decrease with increasing age, as does the immune system; consequently, the immune surveillance of cancer cells is reduced. In addition, age also affects the treatment options and prognosis [11, 12]. The patient also had poor oral hygiene and never brushed her teeth. According to some studies, oral hygiene, which is characterized by the habit of brushing, affects the risk of oral squamous cell carcinoma. Thus, daily tooth brushing may be a protective factor against oral squamous cell carcinoma, with an odds ratio of 0.42 [13-15]. In this case, the betel-quid composition combined with tobacco, the long duration and high frequency of betel-quid use, the way betel-quid was in direct contact with the oral mucosa, the patient's age, and poor oral hygiene together increased the risk of oral squamous cell carcinoma. However, a histopathological examination is required to confirm the diagnosis.

Thus, preventing the lesion from undergoing malignant transformation is the most important action in this situation. This action begins with providing information and education to patients regarding the risk factors associated with betel-quid chewing. The patients must receive this information for improving self-awareness of the condition of their oral cavities. Early detection and diagnosis before reaching stage II can improve survival in patients with oral squamous cell carcinoma [12, 16]. Individuals with suspected oral malignancy are referred for histopathological evaluation.

CONCLUSION

We as dentists have the important role of evaluating the condition and detecting the changes that occur in the oral cavity of patients with betel-quid chewing habits. In addition, patients should be educated about the effect of their habits and possible oral lesions, including the potential for oral squamous cell carcinoma.

REFERENCES

[1] Zain RB, Ikeda N, Gupta PC, Warnakulasuriya S, van Wyk CW, Shrestha P, et al. (1996). Oral mucosal lesions associated with betel quid, areca nut and tobacco chewing habits: consensus from a workshop held in Kuala Lumpur, Malaysia, November 25-27, 1996. *J. Oral Pathol. Med.*

[2] Sharan RN, Mehrotra R, Choudhury Y, Asotra K. (2012). Association of Betel nut with carcinogenesis: Revisit with a clinical perspective. *PLoS One,* 7(8).

[3] Syafriadi M. (2008). Pathogenesis of oral cancer. *J. Dent. Indones.* 15(2):104-110.

[4] Goodson ML, Sloan P, Robinson CM, Cocks K, Thomson PJ. (2015). Oral precursor lesions and malignant transformation - who, where, what, and when? *Br. J. Oral Maxillofac. Surg.* 53(9):831-835.

[5] van der Waal I. (2018). Historical perspective and nomenclature of potentially malignant or potentially premalignant oral epithelial lesions with emphasis on leukoplakia - some suggestions for modifications. *Oral Surg. Oral Med. Oral Pathol. Oral Radiol.* 125(6):577-581.

[6] Speight PM, Khurram SA, Kujan O. (2018). Oral potentially malignant disorders: risk of progression to malignancy. *Oral Surg. Oral Med. Oral Pathol. Oral Radiol.* 125(6):612-627.

[7] Narayan T, Shilpashree S. (2016). Meta-analysis on clinicopathologic risk factors of leukoplakias undergoing malignant transformation. *J. Oral Maxillofac. Pathol.* 20(3):354-361.

[8] Chandirasekar R, Kumar BL, Sasikala K, Jayakumar R, Suresh K, Venkatesan R, et al. (2014). Assessment of genotoxic and molecular mechanisms of cancer risk in smoking and smokeless tobacco users. *Mutat. Res.* 767:21-27.

[9] Arakeri G, Patil SG, Aljabab AS, Lin KC, Merkx MAW, Gao S, et al. (2017). Oral submucous fibrosis: An update on pathophysiology of malignant transformation. *J. Oral Pathol. Med.* 46(6):413-417.

[10] Guha N, Warnakulasuriya S, Vlaanderen J, Straif K. (2014). Betel quid chewing and the risk of oral and oropharyngeal cancers: A meta-analysis with implications for cancer control. *Int. J. Cancer.* 135(6):1433-1443.

[11] Gugić J, Strojan P. (2013). Squamous cell carcinoma of the head and neck in the elderly. *Rep. Pr. Oncol. Radiother.* 18(1): 16-25.

[12] Yamada SI, Kurita H, Tomioka T, Ohta R, Yoshimura N, Nishimaki F, et al. (2017). Healthy life expectancy of oral squamous cell carcinoma patients aged 75 years and older. *Oral. Oncol.* 64:22-26.

[13] Oji C, Chukwuneke F. (2012). Poor oral hygiene may be the sole cause of oral cancer. *J. Maxillofac. Oral Surg.* 11(4): 379-383.

[14] Balaram P, Sridhar H, Rajkumar T, Vaccarella S, Herrero R, Nandakumar A, et al. (2002). Oral cancer in southern India: The influence of smoking, drinking, paan-chewing and oral hygiene. *Int. J. Cancer.* 98(3):440-445.

[15] Moreno-López LA, Esparza-Gómez GC, González-Navarro A, Cerero-Lapiedra R, González-Hernández MJ, Domínguez-Rojas V. (2000). Risk of oral cancer associated with tobacco smoking, alcohol consumption and oral hygiene: a case-control study in Madrid, Spain. *Oral Oncol.* 36(2):170-174.

[16] Rakhmania H, Sufiawati I. (2017). Impact of delay on diagnosis and treatment of oral squamous cell carcinoma: Three cases report. *J. Int. Dent. Med. Res.*, 10(3):1017-102 2.

In: Clinical Reports in Dentistry
Editor: Lisa R. Amir

ISBN: 978-1-53617-328-4

Chapter 3

DIFFICULTIES IN DIAGNOSIS OF ORAL LICHEN PLANUS AND DISCOID LUPUS ERYTHEMATOSUS: A CASE REPORT

***Wiwik Mayanti*[1], *Gus P. Subita*[2,*], *Endah A. Wulandari*[3] and *Diah R. Handjari*[4]**

[1]Oral Medicine Residency Program, Faculty of Dentistry, Universitas Indonesia, Jakarta, Indonesia

[2]Department of Oral Medicine, Faculty of Dentistry, Universitas Indonesia, Jakarta, Indonesia

[3]Division of Oral Medicine, Department of Dentistry, Faculty of Medicine, Universitas Indonesia/Dr. Cipto Mangunkusumo General Hospital, Jakarta, Indonesia

[4]Department of Anatomical Pathology, Faculty of Medicine, Universitas Indonesia/ Dr. Cipto Mangunkusumo General Hospital, Jakarta, Indonesia

ABSTRACT

Introduction: Similarity exist between clinical and histopathological features of erosive oral lichen planus (EOLP) and discoid lupus erythematosus (DLE).

Case report: A 49-year-old woman presented to the Oral Medicine Clinic of Cipto Mangunkusumo General Hospital Jakarta with a 2-week-old pain on the right and left cheeks, which worsened when she ate spicy food and smoked. There were erosive areas with radiating white striae and dark pigmentations that spread from the commissure to the retromolar pads of the buccal mucosa. Based on intra-oral clinical features, the working diagnosis was EOLP with differential diagnoses were DLE and erythroleukoplakia. EOLP and DLE have similar clinical feature which is erythema or erosive areas with radiating keratotic striae. But the result of histopathological examination was consistent with lichen planus. Oral lesions were treated with topical dexamethasone.

* Corresponding Author's Email: guspermana11@gmail.com.

Conclusion: EOLP and DLE have similar clinical and histopathological features that cause difficulties in diagnosis. Therefore, elaborating the result of both clinical and histopatological features is very important in the diagnosis of EOLP and DLE. In this case report the histopathological examination establish the diagnosis of EOLP.

Keywords: erosive oral lichen planus, discoid lupus erythematosus, clinical feature, histopathological feature

1. INTRODUCTION

Oral lichen planus (OLP) is a chronic inflammatory autoimmune disease that may affect mucosal and cutaneous tissues [1]. The prevalence of OLP is approximately 1%-2% in the general population, mainly affects middle-aged people and is more common among women than among men, with a female-to-male ratio of 2:1 [1, 2].

Classically, the presentation OLP is divided into six types clinically: reticular (fine white striae cross each other in the lesion), atrophic (areas of erythematous lesion surrounded by reticular components), papular type, bullous type, plaque type, erosive or ulcerative type (characterized by erosive or ulcerative areas surrounded by reticular components) [3].

Lupus erythematous (LE) is an inflammatory autoimmune disease and is considered a disease of collagen vascular or connective tissue [4]. LE is divided into two categories: chronic discoid type (DLE), which is localized in the skin or mucosa, and systemic type (SLE), which may involve any organ of the body [5]. Discoid lupus erythematosus (DLE) is commonly found in women, with a female-to-male ratio of 4:1 and usually affects women aged 21-40 years [5]. Oral lesions in LE, such as acute ulceration or chronic mucosal plaques, may present in 9%-45% of patients [6]. Clinically, DLE appears as erythematous, ulcerated, or atrophic central area surrounded by fine, white radiating striae [7].

Clinically, erosive oral lichen planus (EOLP) has similar features with the oral manifestation of DLE [8]. EOLP and DLE present as a combination of erythematous and ulcerated areas surrounded by radiating keratotic striae [9]. To confirm the diagnosis of EOLP and DLE, both clinical and histopathological features should be evaluated [10]. Histopathological features are used as important criteria in establishing the diagnosis of DLE and OLP. However, in some cases, the histopathological examination result shows inadequate characteristic features, thereby making it challenging to differentiate between DLE and EOLP [8]. The objective of the present case report is to describe the similarity in clinical and histopathological features of EOLP and DLE in making the definitive diagnosis.

2. Case Report

The patient is a 49-year-old woman who visited the Oral Medicine Clinic of Dr. Cipto Mangunkusumo General Hospital, Jakarta. She experienced pain and discomfort at both side of buccal mucosa since a month ago which got worse in the past 2 weeks whenever she ate spicy food and smoked cigarette.

Her previous dentist gave her 0.1% triamcinolone acetonide ointment, anti-allergy and anti-inflammatory drug which soothed the pain temporarily, but the pain immediately recurred after she stopped the drugs. In addition, she complained that her lower lip felt rough, and thickened, with dark pigmentations. Her medical and family histories were unremarkable. She had been smoking 3-5 cigarettes per day for approximately 25 years, and never consumes alcohol.

Clinical examination revealed white patches with dark pigmentations on the lower lip (Figure 1A) and on the buccal gingiva (Figure 1B). The right buccal mucosa showed an erosive area with the white patches and dark pigmentations (Figure 1C). Meanwhile, the left buccal mucosa showed erosive areas with diffused white patches and dark pigmentations (Figure 1D). In addition, the dark pigmentation was found throughout the hard palate (Figure 1E). The working diagnosis was suspected EOLP, and differential diagnoses were DLE and erythroleukoplakia. For definitive diagnosis, the patient was referred for biopsy and serology tests such as anti-dsDNA antibody, hepatitis C virus (HCV) antibody test, and antinuclear antibody (ANA) test. The case management at the first gave the suggestion to quit smoking, benzydamine hydrochloride oral rinse three times a day and apply Vaseline album ointment topically applied three times a day on the lower lip.

Complete blood count test revealed increased mean corpuscular volume at 93.9 fl (reference value: 82.0-92.0 fl), mean corpuscular hemoglobin at 33.1 pg/cell (reference value: 27.0-31.0 pg/cell), and decreased erythrocyte values at 4.4×10^6 µl (reference value: $4.5\text{-}5.5 \times 10^6$ µl). The serology test showed positive results for ANA test with titer >1/1000, HCV antibody was non-reactive, and anti-dsDNA antibody was negative. The histopathological examination result revealed stratified squamous epithelium which partially eroded, elongation of rete pegs, intact basement membrane, and no signs of malignancy.

The patient was referred to the Allergy and Immunology Clinic of Internal Medicine Department to confirm the diagnosis. The case management at the second visit was dexamethasone oral rinse two times a day (6 mg in the morning and 3 mg in the evening) and mixture of Vaseline album (20 gr) and dexamethasone (6 mg) ointment topically applied four times a day on the lower lip.

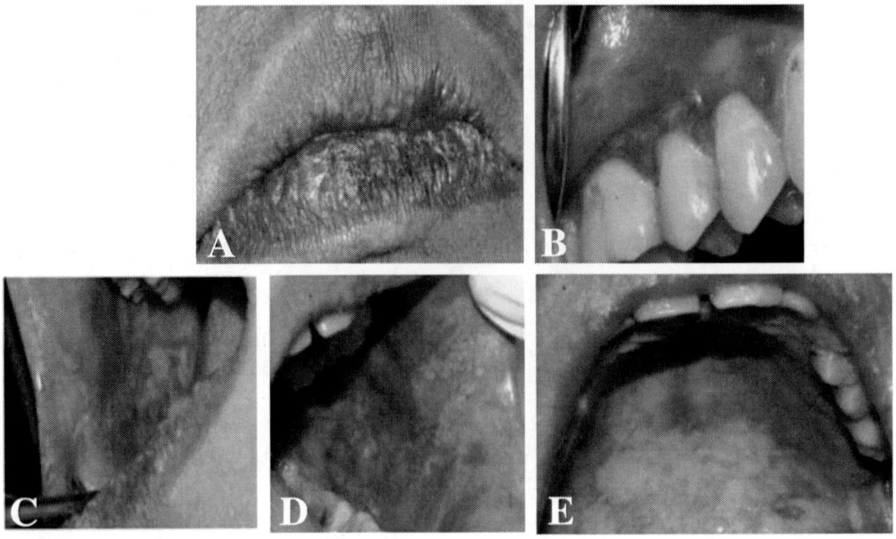

Figure 1. White patch with dark pigmentation was observed on the lower lip (A); buccal gingiva (B); and hard palate (E). Erosive area and white patch with dark pigmentation on the right and left buccal mucosa (C and D).

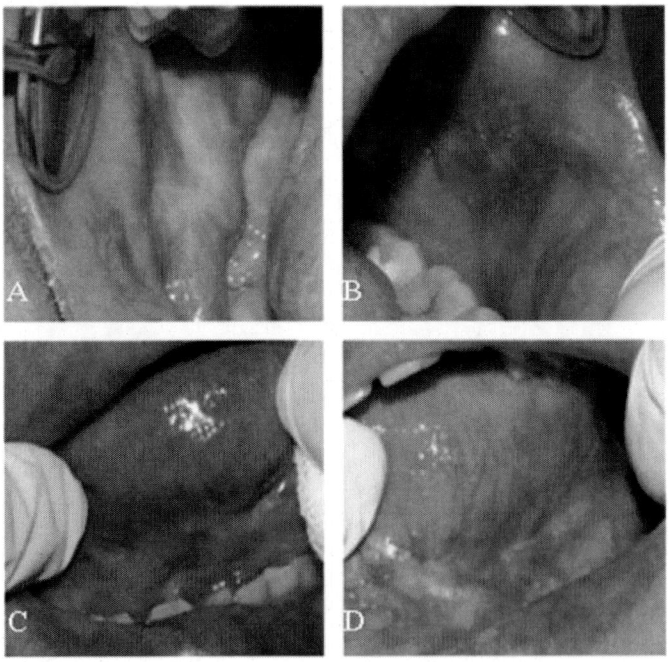

Figure 2. White striae and dark pigmentation on the right buccal mucosa (A); white patch and dark pigmentation on the left buccal mucosa (B); white patch and dark pigmentation on the ventral tongue (C and D).

The Allergy and Immunology Clinic diagnosed the lesions as lichen planus and the patient was administered systemic methyl prednisolone (8 mg) twice a day for 2 weeks.

Clinical examination showed improvement of lesions. The lower lip showed dark pigmentation, and the right buccal mucosa showed white striae and dark pigmentation (Figure 2A). On the left buccal mucosa, white patches and diffuse dark pigmentations were found (Figure 2B). There were striae on the palate, and the dark pigmentation was reduced. White patches and dark pigmentation were found on the ventral tongue around right and left mandibular canine to premolar regions (Figure 2C,D). To confirm the diagnosis of suspected EOLP, histopatological examination result from previous biopsied tissue was reevaluated at the Department of Anatomical Pathology. The treatment with dexamethasone oral rinse was continued twice a day with topical application of a mixture of Vaseline album and dexamethasone ointment on the lower lip. Furthermore, topical application of a mixture of aloe vera, sodium hyaluronate, glycyrhettinic acid, poly vinylpyrrolidone gel (8 ml), and dexamethasone (6 mg) ointment for the intraoral lesion four times a day was added.

Reevaluation of histopathological examination result which came out at the fourth visit showed stratified squamous epithelium which partially eroded, partially interconnected elongation of the rete ridge, and intact basement membrane with infiltrated lymphocytes.

(Figure 3A). The infiltrated lymphocytes presented on the surface of the lamina propria (Figure 3B). Degeneration in basal cell layer was found (Figure 4). The result of reevaluation of histopathological examination was consistent with EOLP.

3. Discussion

OLP and DLE are chronic inflammatory and immunological mucocutaneous disorders [2, 11]. OLP is common in women in the perimenopausal period aged >40 years, and it may affect the buccal mucosa, tongue, gingiva, palate, and lower lip [4, 12, 13]. Some factors associated with OLP are stress; drugs such as antimalarial, diuretics, gold salts, antiretroviral, beta blockers, and penicillamine; dental materials such as dental amalgam, composite and resin-based materials, and metals; chronic liver disease; HCV; genetics; and tobacco chewing [9]. In this patient, the only risk factor identified was smoking as she had smoking history for 25 years. In Indian communities, cigarette smoking is suggested to be an etiological factor of OLP [14]. Furthermore, any form of tobacco use is associated with OLP exacerbation [15]. Although DLE usually occurs in individuals aged 30-50 years, it affects women more often than it affects men and shows a peak prevalence in the late 30s [16]. DLE is commonly seen in the buccal mucosa, gingiva, labial mucosa, and vermilion border [5]. In the presented case, the lesion was found in a 49-year-old woman who was in perimenopausal period, and the lesions were present on the lower lip, buccal mucosa, palate, and ventral tongue, which are the common locations for both OLP or DLE lesions.

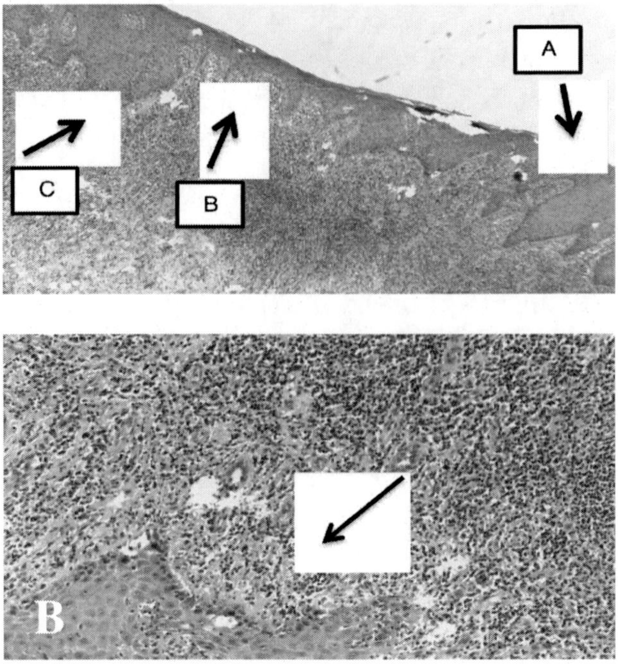

Figure 3. Stratified squamous epithelium which partially eroded (A). Atrophic rete pegs (B). Elongation of rete ridge (C); Infiltration of lymphocytes on the surface of lamina propria (D) (100× magnification).

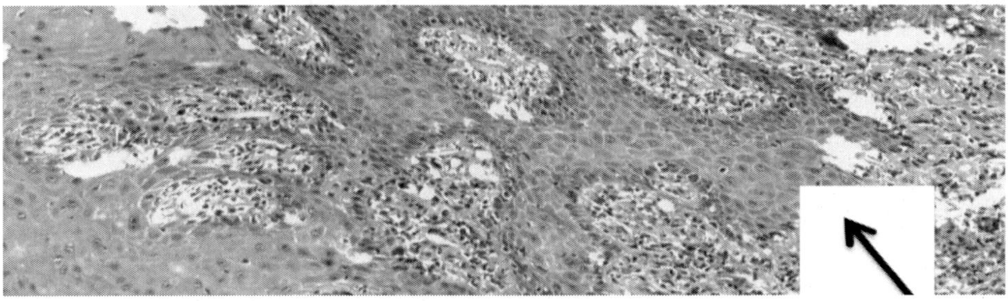

Figure 4. Degeneration in basal cell layer (40x magnification).

EOLP can affect the patient's quality of life because it is symptomatic and has a risk of developing into squamous cell carcinoma [1]. EOLP symptoms range from intermittent mild pain to severe pain, discomfort of the oral mucosa, sensitivity of the oral mucosa to spicy foods and hot or oral hygiene products, and pain that interferes with mastication [4, 10, 16]. Frequent symptoms of DLE are burning sensation during intake of hot and spicy foods and tenderness from tooth brushing [17]. In our case, the patient complained of worst pain when consuming spicy foods and smoking. These symptoms can occur in both EOLP and DLE lesions.

EOLP and DLE have a similar clinical feature [8]. Clinically, EOLP can manifest as atrophic and erythematous areas frequently surrounded by fine radiating striae [10]. On the contrary, DLE is clinically characterized by the presence of a central atrophic red area with small white dots surrounded by a border zone of radiating white striae and peripheral telangiectasia [5]. The characteristic of OLP is bilateral symmetrical lesions or multiple lesions [10]. In contrast, DLE is frequently asymmetrically distributed [16]. This asymmetry in lesion distribution in DLE is important to differentiate it from OLP, because OLP is commonly symmetrical [16]. OLP and DLE occasionally can occur as an overlap syndrome, it is defined as the presence of OLP and DLE in the same lesion, whereas the presence of OLP features in one lesion and DLE features in other one should be considered as a coexistence [17]. The clinical resemblance allows EOLP and DLE to become a primary differential diagnosis [16]. In this case, the erosive area and fine, white radiating striae lesions are symmetrical and bilateral, leading to the diagnosis of OLP.

Both EOLP and DLE, an increased ANA titer can be found [18]. ANA is a group of autoantibodies, including anti-dsDNAantibodies, anti-Sm antibodies, anti-RNP antibodies, anti-Ro/SSA antibodies, and anti-La/SSB antibodies [19]. Each autoantibody has specific properties of its determinant antigen, originating from a damaged cell nucleus [18]. Several studies showed a significantly higher serum ANA positive rate in EOLP than in other types of OLP [18]. EOLP lesion causes more destruction to the oral mucosa, which may consequently release more nuclear antigens into the local tissues and blood circulation [18]. In the presented case, the ANA titer increased to 1/1000. Furthermore, the increasing production of antibodies to nuclear antigens is one of the characteristic features of LE [18]. Previous studies had suggested that patients with DLE show a lower titer in ANA test than those with SLE, who usually has a remarkably increased ANA titer [11]. In our patient, HCV antibody test was non-reactive. HCV infection is often associated with OLP; in some countries such as Italy and Japan, routine screening for hepatitis C and other liver disorders is recommended in patients with OLP [19]. There is a hypothesis that HCV is suspected to trigger an autoimmune process in OLP [19].

EOLP and DLE share some histopathological examination features, including hyperkeratosis in the epithelium, degeneration in basal cell layers, and the infiltration of lymphocytesin the lamina propria [20]. In this case report, the histhopathological examination results was consistent with EOLP because hyperkeratosis in the epithelium with presence of elongation of rete ridge, atrophy of rete ridge and damage to the basement membrane. In the basement membrane, there was a localized damage due to the infiltration of lymphocytes. In addition, the infiltration of lymphocytes was found on the surface of the lamina propria.

Although corticosteroid therapy gives positive result in both erosive oral lichen planus and discoid lupus erythematosus cases, but the risk of malignant transformation in OLP make it very important to establish the diagnosis. Some literature had suggested that the risk of developing squamous cell carcinoma in patients with OLP is approximately 10 times higher than that in the unaffected general population. Although malignant transformation is rare in DLE [21], clinicians should closely observe such suspicious lesions and confirmed the diagnosis histopathologically at the earliest [9].

Conclusion

EOLP and DLE are oral manifestations of chronic inflammatory autoimmune diseases which are commonly found in women. The clinical features of EOLP and DLE are similar and characterized by radiating keratotic striae and atrophic or erosive area; therefore, histopathological examination is highly required to establish the diagnosis. Evaluation of clinical and histopathological features is strongly important in making the diagnosis of EOLP.

References

[1] Keloth M. I., Chatra L. (2016). Oral erosive lichen planus - A case report and review on the management. *IOSR J. Dent. Med. Sci.,* 5:82-86.

[2] van der Waal I. (2015). Oral Lichen Planus: diagnosis and management. *J. dent. Indones.,* 22:89-92.

[3] Krupaa R. J., Sankari S. L., Masthan K., et al. (2015). Oral lichen planus: An overview. *J. Pharm. BioallSci.*, 7:158-161.

[4] Scott S. S., Rossi D. E. (2012). Glick M. Lupus Erythematosus: Consideration For Dentistry. *J. Am. Dent. Assoc.,* 129:330-339.

[5] Ranginwala A. M., Chalishazar M. M., Panja P., et al. (2012). Oral discoid lupus erythematosus: a study of twenty-one cases. *J. Oral Maxillofac. Pathol. J.,* 16:368-373.

[6] Lourenc S. V., Sotto N., Vilela A. C., et al. (2008). Lupus erythematosus: clinical and histopathological study of oral manifestations and immuno-histochemical profile of epithelial maturation. *J. Cutan Pathol. J.,* 33: 657-662.

[7] Rai H., Dayakar A., Supriya H., et al. (2017). Discoid lupus erythematosus with epithelial dysplasia: a case report. *Int. J. Res. Med. Sci.,* 5:2833-2835.

[8] Schiodt M., Pindborg J. J., (1976). Histologic differential diagnostic problems for oral discoid lupus erythematosus. *Int. J. Oral Surg.*, 5:250-252.

[9] Balraj L., Nagaraj T., Nigam H., et al. (2017). Erosive lichen planus: A case report. *J. Med. Radiol. Pathol. Surg.,* 4:11-14.

[10] Chitturi R. T., Devy A. S., Nirmal R. M., et al. (2014). Oral Lichen Planus: A Review of Etiopathogenesis, Clinical, Histological and Treatment Aspects. *J. Interdiscipl. Med. Dent. Sci.,* 2, 1-5.

[11] Bajaj D. R., Devrajani B. R., Matlani B. L. (2014). Discoid Lupus Erythematosus: A Profile. *J. Coll. Physicians Surg. Pakistan*, 20, 361-364.

[12] Usatine R. P., Tinitigan M. (2011). Diagnosis and Treatment of Lichen Planus. *Am. Fam. Physician*, 84, 53-60.

[13] Nico M. M., Fernandes J. D., Lourenço S. V. (2015). Lichen Planus Affecting the Lips. *Clin. Exp. Dermatology Res.,* 6, 1-4.

[14] Gupta S., Jawanda M. K. (2015). Oral Lichen Planus an Update on Etiology Pathogenesis Clinical Presentation Diagnosis and Management. *Indian J. Dermatol.,* 60, 222-229.

[15] Garcia de Sousa F. A. C., Rosa L. E. B. (2008). Oral lichen planus: clinical and histopathological considerations. *Rev. Bras. Otorrinolaringol.,* 74, 284-292.

[16] Amitabha S., Karthikeyan R., Pradhuman V. (2011). Lupus Erythematosus Localized to Oral Cavity - A Case Report. *BFUDJ,* 2, 1-4.

[17] Demirci G. T., Altuna I. K., Sarikaya S, et al. (2011). Lupus erythematosus and lichen planus overlap syndrome: a case report, *Case Rep. Dermatol.,* 3, 107-108.

[18] Lin H., Wang Y., Chia J., et al. (2011). Modulation of Serum Antinuclear Antibody Levels by Levamisole Treatment in Patients with Oral Lichen Planus. *J. Formos. Med. Assoc.,* 110, 316-321.

[19] de Sousa F. A. C. G., Rosa L. E. B. (2008). Oral lichen Planus: clinical and histopathological consideration. *Rev. Bras. Otorrinolaringol.*, 74.

[20] Tuomo K. K., Charles E. T. (1989). A histopathologic study of oral mucosal lupus erythematosus. *Oral Surg. Oral Med. Patho.,* 67, 547-554.

[21] Ganesh D., Sreenivasan P., Ohman J. (2018). Potentially Malignant Oral Disorders and Cancer Transformation. *Anticancer Res.,* 38, 3223-3229.

In: Clinical Reports in Dentistry
Editor: Lisa R. Amir

ISBN: 978-1-53617-328-4

Chapter 4

A Therapeutic Dilemma of Oral Pemphigus Vulgaris in Pregnancy: A Case Report

Andi A. Putri[1], Gus P. Subita[2,*] and Endah A. Wulandari[3]

[1]Oral Medicine Residency Program, Faculty of Dentistry,
Universitas Indonesia, Jakarta, Indonesia

[2]Department of Oral Medicine, Faculty of Dentistry,
Universitas Indonesia, Jakarta, Indonesia

[3]Division of Oral Medicine, Department of Dentistry,
Dr. Cipto Mangunkusumo General Hospital/Faculty of Medicine,
Universitas Indonesia, Jakarta, Indonesia

Abstract

Introduction: The present case report aimed to provide information on the oral manifestations and management of pemphigus vulgaris (PV) during pregnancy.

Case report: A 25-year-old woman diagnosed with PV was under dermatological treatment since 2011. In January 2018, she was referred to the oral medicine (OM) clinic of Dr. Cipto Mangunkusumo General Hospital due to oral ulcers. Her clinical examination revealed desquamation and crust on the lips, erosions, desquamation and sloughing of the gingiva, erosions on the palate and poor oral hygiene. She was treated with topical dexamethasone and chlorhexidine gluconate 0.2% mouth rinse as well as systemic methylprednisolone, azathioprine, $CaCO_3$ and ranitidine. The patient was pregnant after her fifth visit to the OM clinic and her PV was clinically worsening with eruption of new lesions on oral mucosa and skin. Although uncommon, oral manifestations of PV can occur during pregnancy which complicates its management and creates a therapeutic dilemma due to the need of higher dose of medication when the PV flares up, but on the other hand, the drugs used are known to have teratogenic effect.

Conclusion: Interdisciplinary comprehensive treatment is highly recommended to ensure maternal and fetal safety in such cases. Accordingly, the prescription of

* Corresponding Author's Email: guspermana11@gmail.com.

methylprednisolone was restricted, while azathioprine and $CaCO_3$ were discontinued. The patient's response to therapy was continuously monitored at each visit which showed continuous improvement and the fetus was growing well.

Keywords: pemphigus vulgaris, pregnancy, oral manifestation, therapeutic dilemma

1. Introduction

Pemphigus is a chronic inflammatory autoimmune bullous disease, with the highest incidence reported in the fifth and sixth decades of life and the male-to-female ratio of 1:2. On the basis of its type, pemphigus can be classified as pemphigus vulgaris (PV), pemphigus vegetans, pemphigus foliaceus, pemphigus erythematosus, paraneoplastic pemphigus, and drug-related pemphigus [1].

PV is the most common form of pemphigus (constitutes >80% of total cases) and is considered fatal before the introduction of corticosteroids [1, 2]. PV is an autoimmune disease, with autoantibodies directed against desmoglein, a cell-to-cell adhesion molecule, resulting in blistering and/or ulceration of the affected surfaces with a mortality rate of 5 – 10% [3, 4]. In most of the cases, manifestations are observed in the oral mucosa [1]. Oral mucosa involvement may result in extensive mucosal erosion, which leads to low food intake [5].

The occurrence of PV is considered rare in pregnancy [6]. In one retrospective study by Ouahes, et al. Eight out of nine patients suffering from PV, only one patient was pregnant but only during full remission [7]. None of the eight patients who experienced pregnancies even after discontinuation of the drug (corticosteroids, azathioprine, or cyclophosphamide) [7]. Although uncommon, PV may appear or worsen during pregnancy, with the risk of fetal morbidity and mortality [5]. Several studies have suggested that PV can cause complications during pregnancy as well as serious harm to both the mother and fetus [3, 8]. The effect of PV on fetus during pregnancy varies ranging from stillbirth, intrauterine growth retardation to preterm birth, although it is also possible to deliver a completely healthy neonate [6]. Transplacental transmission of Ig-G PV antibodies from infants to fetus can present a risk of developing clinical manifestations of PV in neonates [7].

Inadequate treatment and control of PV can endanger the lives of patients because of the risk of severe infections therefore the severity of PV must be controlled to ensure patient and fetal health [9]. The onset of PV during pregnancy creates a therapeutic dilemma that needs to be addressed immediately [10]. Systemic corticosteroids treatment is considered as the first-line of therapy in pemphigus, including azathioprine, mycophenolate mofetil, methotrexate, rituximab, intravenous immunoglobulin, and topical corticosteroid, albeit their use in pregnancy remain controversial [8].

The etiology of preterm premature rupture of membranes which led to preterm delivery in the reported case may be related to the vigorous steroid therapy administered to the patient during pregnancy [7].

In this report, we presented a complicated case of pregnancy that occurred in a long-term-treated PV patient, which offered two challenges at once for clinicians. First, the medication used is believed to increase the risk to the health and safety of the patient and the fetus. Second, the drug is needed in higher dose to control the PV. In this report, we discussed the oral manifestations and clinical management of PV during pregnancy, which required interdisciplinary comprehensive treatment.

2. Case Report

In January 2018, a 25-year-old woman was referred from the Dermatology clinic of Dr. Cipto Mangunkusumo General Hospital (RSCM) to the oral medicine (OM) clinic due to oral ulcers since the past 1 month. The patient complained of gum bleeding during toothbrushing and mouth soreness on eating spicy food. The patient brushed her teeth thrice a day and gargled with honey dissolved in warm water to relieve the pain, which resulted in burning sensation instead.

The patient was diagnosed with PV in 2011 and had received past treatment in the OM clinic of RSCM for the oral manifestations of PV in 2013. Her skin and oral lesions were resolved between the end of 2013 and the middle of 2017. However, the condition reappeared in the middle of 2017, including blisters on the face and head and the subsequent appearance of oral ulcers in late 2017.

The patient claimed to be under stress due to lack of rest. She had been under systemic methylprednisolone therapy since 2011. Until date, the patient has been under routine medication of 8mg methylprednisolone (once a day), 50mg azathioprine (twice a day), 500mg $CaCO_3$ (twice a day), and a topical ointment for the head and skin lesions. Her extra-oral examination revealed dryness in the upper and lower lips, with desquamation and a reddish-brown crust on the right lower lip, as shown in Figure 1. Her intra-oral examination revealed poor oral hygiene; erythema at the overall gingival margin; erosive and sloughing on the left maxillary gingiva around premolar to molar teeth; desquamation on the left mandibular gingiva around premolar to molar teeth; erosion on the right maxillary gingiva around molar teeth; yellowish coat on one third of the posterior dorsal tongue; fissure on one third of the anterior tongue; and hairy tongue (Figure 1). Based on her clinical examination, the patient was diagnosed with oral manifestation of PV.

The patient was treated with dexamethasone swish and spit twice daily and a mixture of Vaseline album and dexamethasone to be topically applied on the lips four times daily.

In addition, the patient was referred to a periodontist for her tooth scaling.

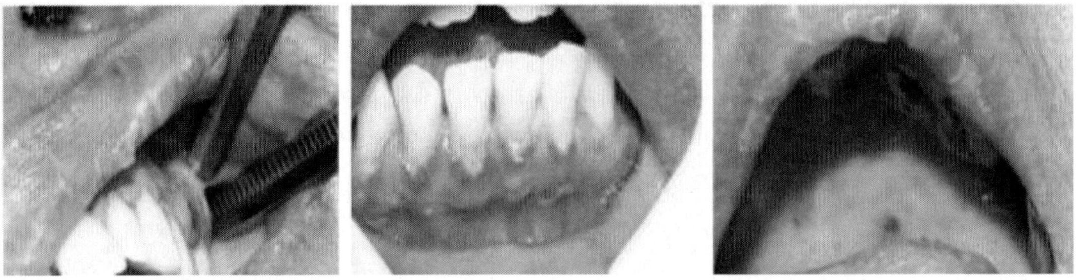

Figure 1. Clinical examination at the first visit. Desquamation and erosion on various sites of oral mucosa and gingiva with poor oral hygiene.

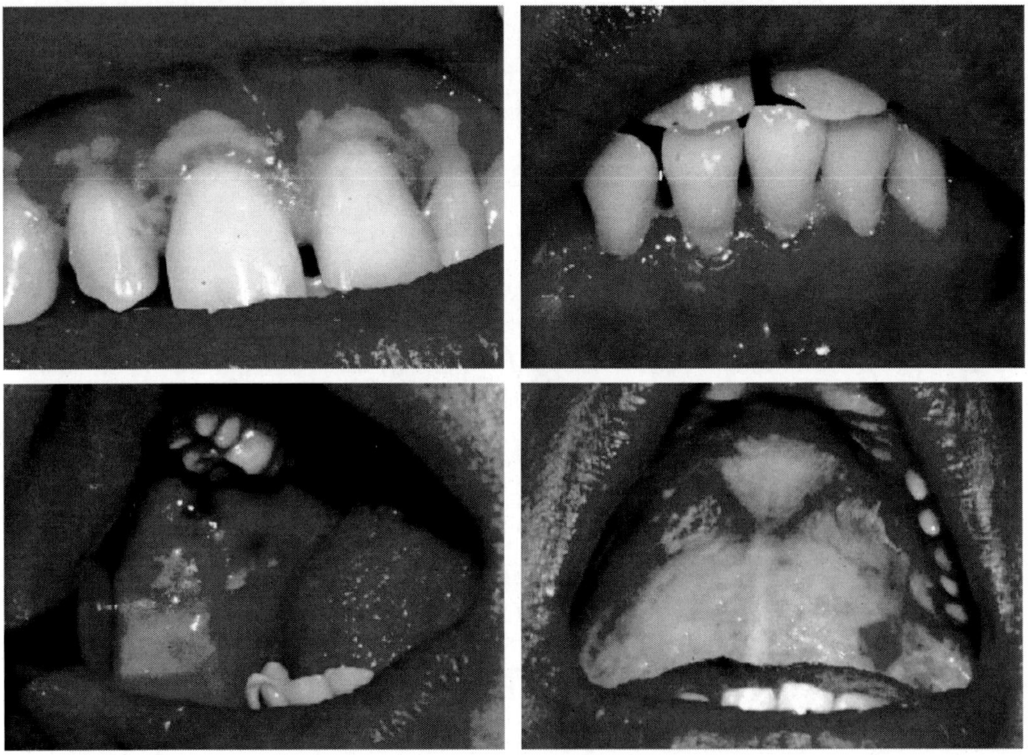

Figure 2. Clinical examination at the fourth visit. Note that improvement can be seen in the oral lesions.

The patient was routinely followed up at 2-week intervals without any significant improvement. An improvement in the oral mucosal condition was noted on the fourth visit. Clinical examination revealed improvement in all oral lesions without the occurrence of any new lesions (Figure 2).

Accordingly, the dose of dexamethasone for swish and spit and the mixture of topical ointment for lip lesion were tapered down. Similarly, the dose of systemic methylprednisolone was tapered down from 8 to 4mg daily. However, her oral mucosal condition worsened on her fifth visit, 2 months after her first visit (Figure 3).

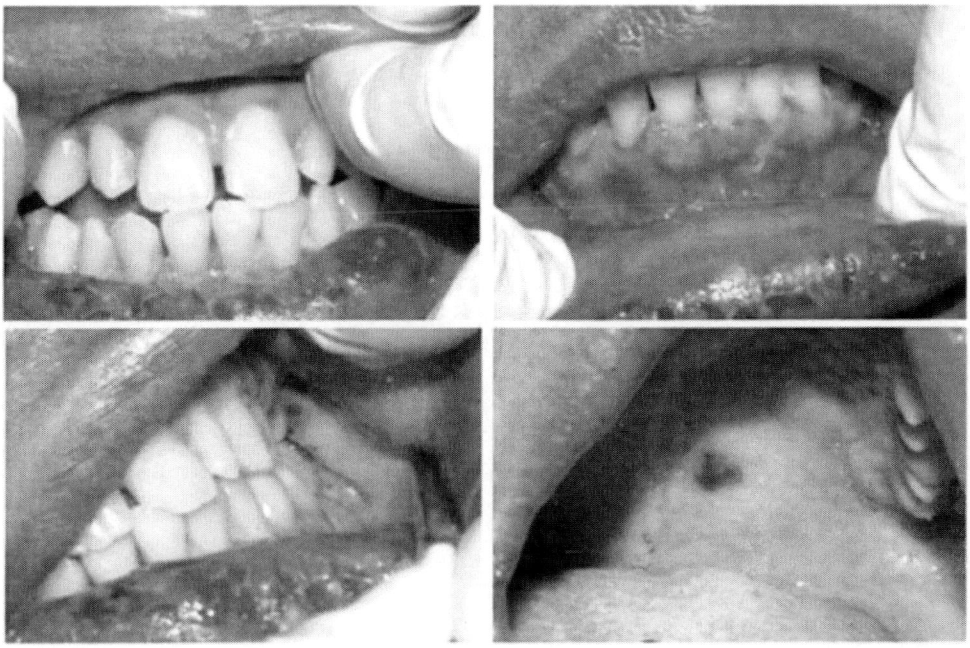

Figure 3. Clinical examination at the fifth visit. The oral conditions can be seen to have worsened.

New blisters arose on the ear, abdomen, thighs, and scalp. On this visit, the patient informed of being 6 weeks pregnant. The drug used for treating her oral lesion was not changed, but the dose of dexamethasone for swish and spit and that of the mixture of topical ointment for lip lesion was tapered up. The lip lesion was managed with the application of 0.9% NaCl lip dressing prior to the topical application of Vaseline album ointment.

The systemic methylprednisolone dose was tapered down, and the use of azathioprine and $CaCO_3$ was discontinued by the dermatologist. The patient, at this time point, had lost her appetite, often felt nauseous, and experienced anxiety related to the pregnancy. In regard to the anxiety issues, we referred the patient for psychiatric counseling, but the patient refused it.

On her sixth visit (at 8 weeks of pregnancy), the patient was hospitalized because of her worsening conditions. The patient complained of mouth soreness, swollen lips, and the occurrence of new blisters on the fingers, hands, feet, armpits, scalp, and eyelids.

The patient had difficulty in eating and could only consume liquids and porridge, which worried her with regard to the development of the fetus, ultimately leading to an idea of aborting her pregnancy. On this visit, yellow crust was observed on the upper and lower lips, with a bleeding fissure on the lower lip. Her intra-oral examination was difficult to perform because of pain on opening the mouth (Figure 4).

Moreover, oral malodor was evident because of poor oral hygiene, and the patient experienced mouth soreness on eating and drinking. The therapy from her last visit was continued.

On her seventh visit at 3 weeks after the last visit, the patient's overall condition had improved, with no new lesion found on her mouth or skin. She could also eat comfortably, without feeling soreness and nausea. The systemic treatment was tapered up to a high dose of systemic methylprednisolone (32mg in the morning and 24mg in the afternoon).

Despite the clinical improvements both in the extra-oral and intra-oral conditions, desquamations of the upper and lower gingiva and the left and right buccal mucosa persisted (Figure 5).

Three-dimensional ultrasonography revealed an 11-week-old fetus growing normally, albeit of a larger than average size.

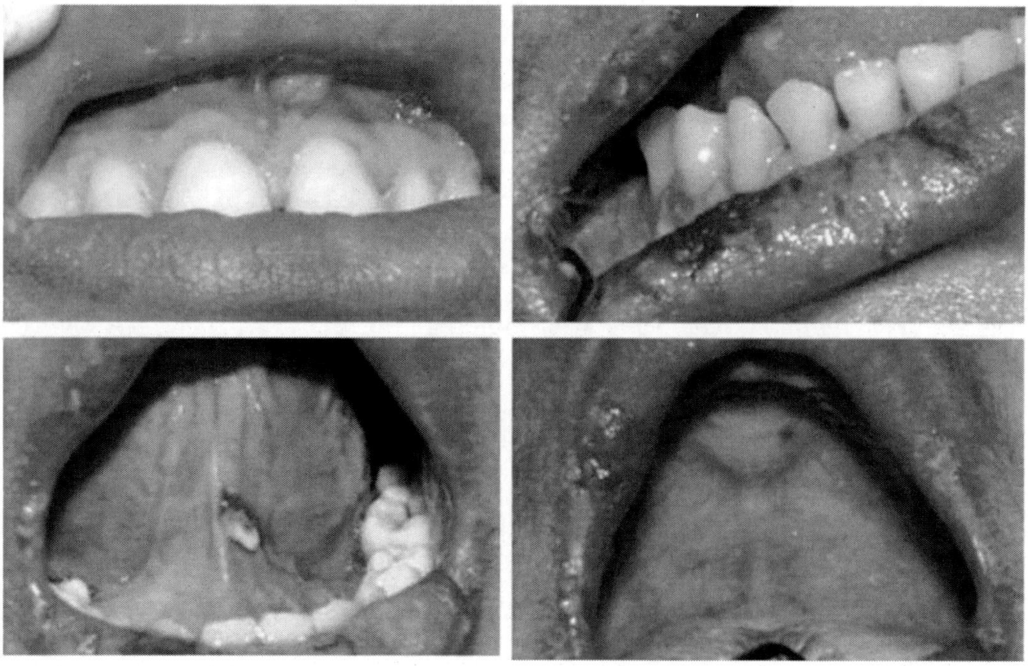

Figure 4. Clinical examination at the sixth visit. Oral and systemic conditions could be seen to have worsened.

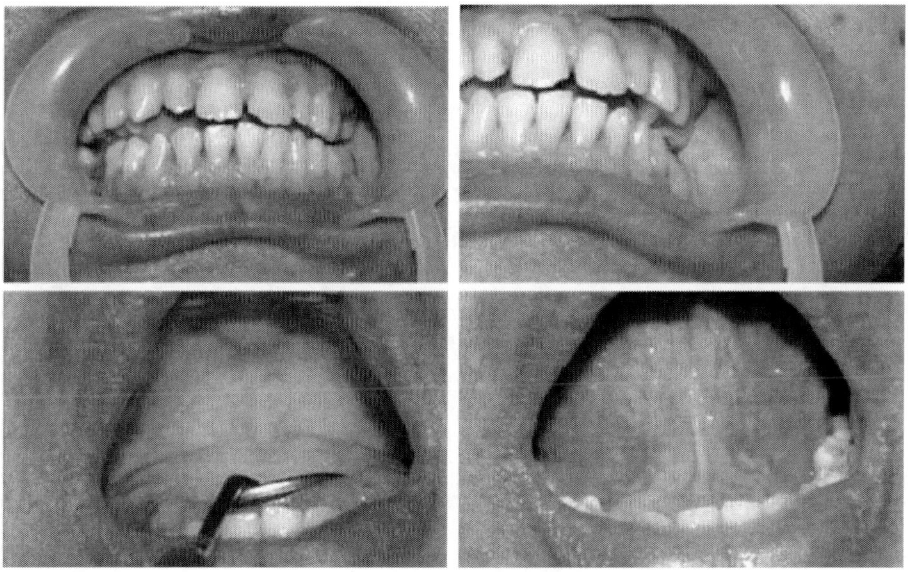

Figure 5. Clinical examination at the seventh visit. Improvement could be seen in all lesions.

The patient's fetal condition was continuously monitored, and interdisciplinary collaborations were continued. The doses of dexamethasone for swish and spit, the mixture of topical ointment for lip lesion, and systemic methylprednisolone were tapered down. On her last visit, the patient was only treated with dexamethasone swish and spit with a minimal dose, whereas her lips were moisturized with a topical application of Vaseline album. The overall clinical condition of the patient showed continuous improvement at every follow-up visit.

3. Discussion

PV is a chronic, intraepithelial, and potentially fatal autoimmune blistering disease that is characterized by the loss of attachment between keratinocytes (acantholysis), which induces blister formation in the suprabasal layer of the mucosal epithelium [11, 12]. This process was mediated by circulating reactive-desmoglein autoantibodies that directly attack the desmoglein/molecular surface of the layer of keratinocyte cells [13]. PV has two phenotypes, the mucosa dominant and the mucocutaneous dominant, with the possibility of shifting from one form to another. The oral mucosa is the first site of involvement in most of PV cases [14].

In general, intra-oral lesions in PV may involve the entire mucosal area of the oral cavity, although the most affected area is the buccal mucosa, followed by the involvement of the palatal, lingual, and labial mucosa [2, 15]. The gingiva is the least affected region, and desquamative gingivitis is the most common manifestation of PV when it involves the gingival area [15]. Several past literatures have mentioned that PV cases during pregnancy are rare and probably related to the risk of infertility in the active phase of PV [7, 9, 16]. The present case patient became pregnant during the course of the active phase of the disease, which further complicated the case. It has been reported that this disease may appear or worsen during pregnancy [5, 9]. In the present case, the oral and systemic conditions showed improvement initially, worsened at 6 weeks of pregnancy, and improved again at 11 weeks of pregnancy. Changes in this disease activity are more common in the first and second trimesters of pregnancy. The condition is usually stabilized in the third trimester, allegedly in association with endogenous corticosteroid production by the placenta in the late stages of pregnancy [17, 18].

Literatures on the oral manifestation of PV in pregnancy are rare. However, some studies have reported intra-oral findings, such as gingival lesions, particularly erosion and desquamative gingivitis in such cases [16, 18]. Our experience in the present case is in accordance with the clinical findings of past reports in that the lesions of gingival erosion and desquamation of the gingival margins could be found at each visit. Lopez-Jonet et al. reported that the occurrence of lesions of the gingiva is the first symptom of PV in pregnancy [16]. In this case, other than gingiva, intra-oral lesions also presented in various oral mucosal areas, such as buccal mucosa, palate, and tongue which clinically showed better improvement compared to gingiva lesions, which had occurred prior to the pregnancy. Hence, none of the oral lesions could be used as the marker of pregnancy in PV.

The treatment of PV without or with pregnancy is similar [17]. The use of high doses of systemic corticosteroid or other systemic immunosuppressive agents may be effective [18] but may become a dilemma because most of the medical interventions can cause adverse reactions to the conceived fetus or child [19]. In this case, the patient was followed up 6 times within 13 weeks. We educated the patient on improving her oral hygiene status as well as about the use of topical corticosteroids. The use of topical corticosteroids in active oral PV is considered as the first-line therapy [18]. However, the present patient's condition continued to deteriorate and less responsive to the topical medications; therefore, we consulted dermatologists and obstetric gynecologists for the consideration of increasing the dose of systemic corticosteroids. This intervention required close interdisciplinary collaboration among the dermatologists, obstetric gynecologists, and OM specialists.

Systemic corticosteroids in moderate doses are considered safe in pregnant women with autoimmune diseases [19]. However, each drug belongs to a different category as per the Food and Drug Administration guidelines. For instance, prednisone and prednisolone are in class B (do not present any risk to the fetus and pregnant woman), whereas dexamethasone and betamethasone are in grade C (have adverse effects on the fetus/teratogenic, although well-controlled studies in humans are limited). On the basis of the report of some researchers, prednisone is selected during pregnancy because its penetration through the placenta is limited by the enzyme, whereas dexamethasone almost entirely passes through the placenta, so that the effect on the fetus becomes greater. The grade C drugs may be given systemically only if the benefit is greater than the risk to the fetus [19]. In this case, the systemic corticosteroid used was methylprednisolone, whereas dexamethasone was used only topically.

Immunosuppressants, such as azathioprine, are steroid-sparing agents that extend the remission period and reduce the complications of steroids [14]. However, some studies have suggested that the use of immunosuppressant agents always lead to fetal death and that their use is not recommended during pregnancy [10, 14]. Therefore, the use of azathioprine was immediately discontinued as soon as the patient reported pregnancy. However, in cases where its use is necessary, it is advisable to maintain a low dose to prevent fetal defects [6]. Furthermore, cyclosporine is believed to be less effective in the treatment of pemphigus, but it is the safest corticosteroid-sparing agent in pregnancy [17].

In pregnant women, it is advisable to start treatment with systemic corticosteroids after the 12th week of pregnancy in order to avoid the risk of teratogenesis and the inhibition of intra-uterine growth [16]. In this case, both the topical and systemic corticosteroids were being used even before pregnancy occurred. Therefore, the condition of the mother and fetus continues to be monitored regularly until now. In the most recent follow-up, the patient's condition showed improvement and the fetus was growing well. Although systemic steroid therapy is required during pregnancy, after becoming symptom free, only a low dose of prednisolone (5mg/day) is needed to maintain good oral health and function [10]. If the disease worsens during the first trimester, medical termination of pregnancy may be considered, and if it happens during the second and third trimester, it is recommended to use aggressive topical therapy and application of corticosteroids is a safe treatment [17, 20]. Furthermore, the condition of desquamative gingivitis it is necessary to improve oral hygiene and avoid irritation of the lesion [21].

Another important thing to consider in the management of PV with pregnancy is the side effects of long-term steroid use, such as diabetes mellitus, myopathy, depression, and delayed wound healing [7]. Patients should be closely monitored considering that all drugs used in PV treatment greatly affect the safety of the mother and fetus.

CONCLUSION

Although uncommon, oral manifestations of PV can present during pregnancy, which makes the management more complicated and creates a therapeutic dilemma as the treatment drugs have known teratogenic effect. Therefore, it is recommended that interdisciplinary treatment strategy be employed to ensure maternal and fetal safety in such cases.

REFERENCES

[1] Arpita, R., Monica, A., Venkatesh, N., Atul, S., Varun, M. (2015). Oral pemphigus vulgaris: case report. *Ethiop. J. Heal. Sci.,* 25:367 - 372.

[2] Navarro, Claudia M., Sposto, M. R., Onofre, M. A., Scully, C. (1999). Gingival lesions diagnosed as pemphigus vulgaris in an adolescent. *J. Periodontol.,* 70:808 - 812.

[3] Elmuradi, S., Ojeda, D., Stoopler, E. T. (2018). Oral pemphigus vulgaris in pregnancy. *JOGC,* 37:951.

[4] Ibrahim, S. B. K., B. M. Yashodhara, Umakanth, S. (2012). Pemphigus vulgaris in a pregnant woman and her neonate. *BMJ Case Rep.,* 28:1 - 5.

[5] Torgerson, R. R., Marnach, M. L., Bruce, A. J., III R. S. R. (2006). Oral and vulvar changes in pregnancy. *Clin. Dermatol.,* 24:122 - 132.

[6] Nageswaramma, S., Swarnakumari, G., Lakshmisarojini, V., Sailaja, D., Glory, G. R. (2015). Pemphigus vulgaris in pregnancy: a rare case report. *IJCMAAS,* 7:191 - 193.

[7] Fainaru, O., Mashiach, R., Kupferminc, M., Shenhav, M., Pauzner, D., Lessing, J. B. (2000). Pemphigus vulgaris in pregnancy: a case report and review of literature. *Hum. Reprod.,* 15:1195 - 1197.

[8] Tavakolpour, S., Sadat, H., Saeid, M. (2017). Management of pemphigus disease in pregnancy. *Am. J. Reprod. Immunol.,* 77:5 - 9.

[9] Salzberg, K. W., Gero, M. J., Ragsdale, B. D. (2014). Pemphigus vulgaris in pregnancy. *Cutis,* 94:206 - 209.

[10] Muhammad, J. K., Lewis, M. A. O., Crean, S. J. (2002). Oral pemphigus vulgaris occurring during pregnancy. *J. Oral Pathol. Med.,* 31:121 - 124.

[11] Voegeli, A. C., Muniz, F., J. R. Mascaro, J. M., Garcia, M. C. F., Arimany, J. L., Amagais, M., Camps, A. (2002). Neonatal pemphigus vulgaris with extensive mucocutaneous lesions from a mother with oral pemphigus vulgaris. *Br. J. Dermatol.,* 147:801 - 805.

[12] Cholera, M., Chainani-Wu, N. (2016). Management of pemphigus vulgaris. *Adv. Ther.,* 33(6):910 - 958.

[13] Gregoriou, S., Efthymiou, O., Stefanaki, C., Rigopoulos, D. (2015). Management of pemphigus vulgaris: challenges and solutions. *Adv. Ther.,* 8:521 - 527.

[14] Gharote, H. P., Nair, P. P., Kasetty, S., Thomas, S., Kulkarni, A. (2012). Pemphigus vulgaris – a report of three cases. *BMJ Case Rep.,* 8:6 - 11.

[15] Ohta, M., Osawa, S., Endo, H., Kuyama, K., Yamamoto, H., Ito, T. (2011). Pemphigus vulgaris confined to the gingiva: a case report. *Int. J. Dent.,* 2011:4 - 7.

[16] López-Jornet, P., Bermejo-Fenoll, A. (2005). Gingival lesions as a first symptom of pemphigus vulgaris in pregnancy. *Br. Dent. J.,* 198:1 - 2.

[17] Lin, L., Zeng, X., Chen, Q. (2015). Pemphigus and pregnancy. *Saudi Med. J.*, 36:1033 - 1038.

[18] Ramos-e-silva, M., Martins, N. R., Kroumpouzos, G. (2006). Oral and vulvovaginal changes in pregnancy. *Clin. Dermatol.*, 24:122 - 132.

[19] Brzezińska-wcisło, L., Zbiciak-nylec, M., Wcisło-dziadecka, D., Salwowska, N. (2017). Pregnancy: a therapeutic dilemma. *Adv. Dermatol. Allergol.*, 34:433 - 438.

[20] Bhagat, N., Raj, R., Arora, R. (2017). Pemphigus vulgaris in pregnancy with transient neonatal pemphigus-can psychological stress be culprit?. *Int. J. Reprod. Contracept. Obs. Gynecol.*, 6:4703 - 4707.

[21] Wahyuni, I. S., Dewi, T. S., Herawati, E., Zakiawati, D. (2016). Profil lesi oral pada penderita penyakit autoimun penyakit autoimun. *Maj Kedokt Gigi Indones.*, 2(3):1 - 3.

In: Clinical Reports in Dentistry
Editor: Lisa R. Amir

ISBN: 978-1-53617-328-4

Chapter 5

PREDISPOSING FACTORS IN RECURRENT APHTHOUS STOMATITIS AND GEOGRAPHIC TONGUE: A CASE REPORT

Dwi K. Sari[1], Gus P. Subita[2,*] and Ambar K. Astuti[2]
[1]Oral Medicine Residency Program, Faculty of Dentistry, Universitas Indonesia, Jakarta, Indonesia
[2]Department of Oral Medicine, Faculty of Dentistry, Universitas Indonesia, Jakarta, Indonesia

ABSTRACT

Introduction: To provide an overview of the predisposing factors for recurrent aphthous stomatitis (RAS) and geographic tongue (GT) in a young female patient.

Case report: A 21-year-old woman presented with a large, painful lesion on the left lip for seven days. The patient was used to experiencing canker sores 3 or 4 times a year. In addition, she complained of pain, sores, and heat on the tongue. Upon intra-oral examination, we found a single, irregularly shaped ulcer, with a white base and surrounded by erythema in the left labial mucosa and multiple erythematous lesions surrounded by white edges and migratory in the dorsal, ventral and lateral of her tongue. We diagnosed the patient as having a minor recurrent aphthous stomatitis (RAS) and symptomatic geographic tongue (GT) and prescribed chlorhexidine gluconate 0.2% and multi-vitamins. At the next visit a month later, the initial RAS lesions had disappeared but a few new ones had appeared; the GT lesions were still present. Suspecting that there could be psychological reason for prolonged duration of the oral lesions, the patient was then given Perceived Stress Scale (PSS) questionnaires. In search for other predisposing factors, the patient also was sent for CBC examination. PSS score showed mild stress in patient and CBC results of normal Hemoglobin (13.1g/dL), low count on MCV (71.8fL), and decrease count on MCH (23.4pg). From these results we concluded that stress, small average red blood cells and low average content of hemoglobin per red cells have

* Corresponding Author's Email: guspermana11@gmail.com.

contributed to the clinical picture. Without anemia, condition of low blood count as describe above called pre-anemic stage. The complete management for these cases should include communication, information and education and dietary recommendations, including taking multi-vitamins, and finding stressors to implement interventions to alleviate the stress.

Conclusion: Finding and eliminating stressors and pre-anemic stage as predisposing factors may influence the success of RAS and GT management.

Keywords: Recurrent Aphthous Stomatitis (RAS), Geographic Tongue (GT), Stress, perceived tress scale, pre-anemic stage

1. INTRODUCTION

Lesions in the oral cavity may be the manifestations of systemic conditions or psychological disorders. Stress is the most common predisposing factor. Recurrent aphthous stomatitis (RAS) presents characteristic of spontaneous ulcers in the oral mucosa that occur at least twice a year, do not occur in other parts of the body and are not associated with a specific systemic disease [1, 2]. The cause of RAS is still unknown but is thought to be related to the host and environmental factors [3-8]. RAS severity can be assessed using the Ulcer Severity Score (USS) developed by Tappuni et al. [1]. Other lesions in the oral cavity (affecting 4.8% of the world's population) include geographic tongue (GT) or benign migratory glossitis. Symptomatic GT occurs with discomfort, heat and soreness in the affected areas.

GT is a chronic inflammatory condition characterized by an area of atrophy and erythema surrounded by a yellowish white line with a migratory location (usually involving the dorsum region of the tongue). Studies have described the systemic conditions, including psoriasis, diabetes, allergies, the presence of nutritional disorders, and even psychological disorders (such as stress) as the causative factors of GT [9-13].

Stress is defined as a form of tension that manifests emotionally, mentally, psychically, and physically when an individual cannot fulfill his needs and wants [3, 12, 13]. In patients with RAS, stress predisposes to the emergence of lesions [14, 15], while in GT stress will aggravate the clinical condition (number of lesions) and complaints [11, 13]. The Perceived Stress Scale (PSS) has been used in studies on psychological illness, stressful situations, and stress management with three interpretation values ranged from mild (0 - 13), moderate (14 - 26) and severe (27 - 40) stress [15-19]. In addition to stress, nutritional deficits leading to hemoglobin, iron, B_{12} and folic acid deficiencies are predisposing factors for RAS [20]. Stress, nutritional deficiency of zinc and HLA-B15 factor levels also play a role in the development of GT [21].

Measurements of the pre-anemic stage can be done with a complete blood test, including hemoglobin values, mean cell volume (MCV), mean cell hemoglobin (MCH) and mean cell hemoglobin concentration (MCHC). The normal examination value ranges vary depending on place of the examination done. In the present case, the normal range of examination values goes from 11.5 to 16.5g/dL for Hemoglobin, from 80 – 100fL for MCV, from 26.0 – 34.0pg for MCH, and from 31.0 – 37.0g/dL for MCHC. Pre-anemic stage is a condition when there was no anemic stage with decrease value in cells blood count [22].

The purpose of this case report was to show a typical case of RAS and GT on the oral cavity with stress as a predisposing factor by showing results of PSS questionnaires and pre-anemic stage, based on measurement values from complete peripheral blood tests.

2. Case Report

A 21-year-old woman came to the Universitas Indonesia Dental Hospital with the chief complaint of a large, painful ulcer on the left lip of seven days of evolution. She referred to a history of canker sores 3 to 4 times a year, not preceded by a fever and healed in less than 2 weeks. Other family members had similar experienced of canker sores. The patient is a fresh graduate and is currently just beginning to work. The canker sores usually appeared close to exam taking times. The patient also complained of pain, sores and heat on the tongue. She consumed more than 8 glasses of water a day; however, her diet was less regular, and she rarely ate fruits or vegetables. She did not have a history of systemic disease (other than gastritis) or of drug allergies.

We found no abnormalities in the extra-oral examination. The intra-oral examination revealed good oral hygiene, and a single, irregular ulcer with a white base and surrounded by erythema with a 7-mm diameter in the left labial mucosa (Figure 1A). In the dorsum, lateral and ventral areas of the tongue, we found multiple erythematous lesions surrounded by white edges and slightly prominent (Figure 1B, C). We diagnosed the patient as having minor RAS and symptomatic GT. The patient was given a dental health education (DHE) and the minor RAS was treated by applying a sterile gauze wetted with chlorhexidine gluconate 0.2% 10ml for 3 - 4 minutes 4 times a day. In addition, the patient was given the education on GT and she was later instructed to avoid hot and spicy foods.

Furthermore, we prescribed multivitamin therapy containing Vitamins E, C, B_1, B_2, B_5, B_6, B_{12}, niacin, zinc, and folic acid once daily. At the follow-up visit a month later, the initial minor RAS lesions had disappeared, but a few new lesions had appeared (Figure 2A-E). We found a single, irregular, ulcerated lesion surrounded by a 5mm-sized erythematous halo on the left mandibular premolar area. We noted a single ulcer in the right buccal mucosa with irregular clearly-defined borders, and a white base surrounded by a 2-mm halo erythema. In the ventral tongue we also found a single ulcerated lesion with irregular edges, a borderless clear yellowish white base surrounded by a halo erythema and a 1-mm diameter (Figure 2C).

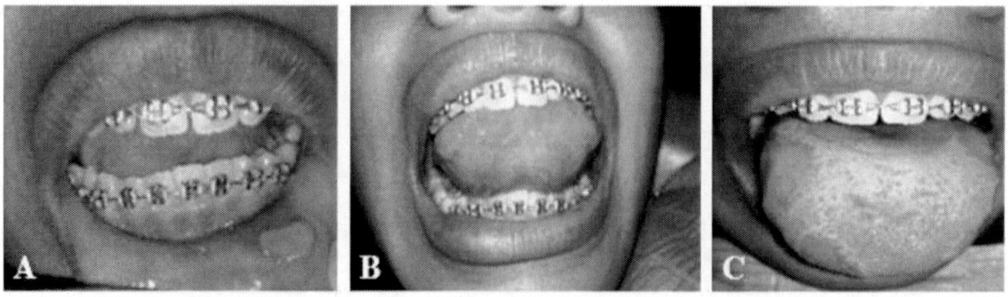

Figure 1. Minor recurrent aphthous stomatitis on the first visit (A); Geographic tongue at first visit (B, C).

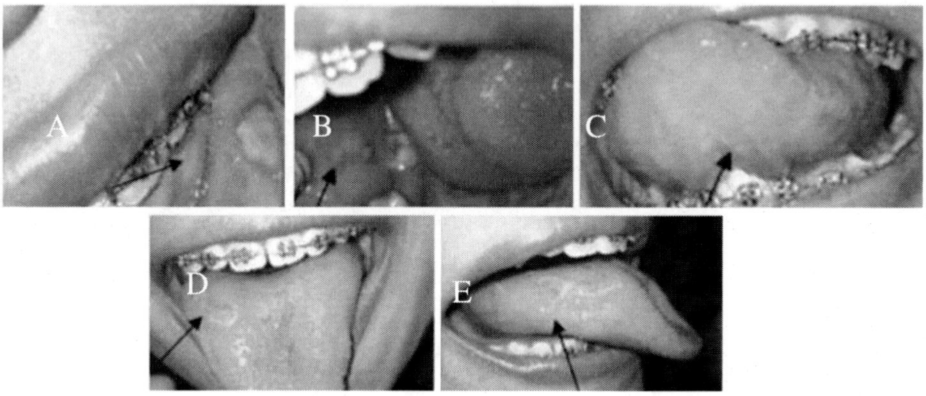

Figure 2. Minor recurrent aphthous stomatitis on second visit (A-C); Geographic tongue on second visit (D, E).

In the dorsal and ventral areas of the tongue, we still observed the presence of papillary atrophy surrounded by multiple hyperkeratosis areas; however, the number of areas were fewer in number than at the first visit (Figure 2D, E).

As the number of ulcerations increased, we used an Ulcer Severity Score (USS) and the patient obtained a score of 26. The calculations were done by counting (1) the number of ulcers that had appeared in the patient during the 3 preceding months; (2) the ulcer mean diameter in millimeters; (3) the duration of the lesion per half-weeks; (4) the ulcer-free period (calculated by the value of ten minus the mean ulcer-free period within a week); (5) whether the lesion was located on the keratin or non-keratin mucosa; and (6) the degree of pain felt by the patient. At this point, we suspected psychological involvement and pre-anemic stage condition to be present; therefore, we ordered a complete peripheral blood test and scores after a Perceived Stress Scale (PSS) questionnaire. The PSS score showed mild stress and the CBC showed normal hemoglobin at 13.1g/dL, reduce count on MCV at 71.8fL, and low amount of MCH at 23.4pg. We modified the treatment by prescribing triamcinolone acetonide (0.1%) 4 times daily in the ulcer areas, but we continued the multi-vitamin. We advised the patient on stress management and educated her about the foods that need to be consumed to improve nutrition associated with our findings of the complete peripheral blood tests. After that, the patient could not show up for a follow-up visit; however, a telephonic anamnesis revealed the disappearance of the canker sores and the lack of complaints of heat and sore on the tongue.

3. DISCUSSION

At the first visit our diagnosis of minor RAS was established based on the history of recurrent ulcers 3 to 4 times a year without preceding febrile symptoms and the lack of ulceration lesions involving other parts of the body. The minor RAS type was supported by our finding of 3-10-mm ulceration lesions, ranging from 1 to 5 lesions, a healing time of 7 to 14 days and a predilection to appear in the non-keratinous mucosa (labial and buccal mucosa). From our anamnesis we also found the existence of a family history (father) of canker sores. Genetic factors have been shown to contribute to RAS [1, 2, 23, 24]. The multiple erythemas surrounded by white edges and slightly prominent in the dorsum, lateral, and ventral tongue and the patient's complaints about her tongue feeling hot, sore and uncomfortable supported our diagnosis of geographic tongue.The pathogenesis of RAS can be divided into three mechanisms that include the dysregulation of the primary immune system (that can be precipitated by stress), the dysfunction of the mucosal barrier, and an increase in the exposure to antigen. Primary immune system dysregulation changes the distribution, proliferation and activity of lymphocytes, monocytes, natural killer cells, phagocytosis, production of cytokines, and lymphocyte CD8 and CD4 ratios. Trauma, pre-anemic stage, smoking habits, and menstrual cycle disruptions are factors that can affect mucosal barrier function [4, 6, 22-24]. In the body, stress will activate the sympathetic system resulting in dilation of the blood vessels and recruitment of leukocytes (hypersensitivity reaction). Psychological stress acts as a predisposing factor for RAS and is not an etiological factor [25]. The pathogenesis of GT is unclear, but it is thought to be related to epithelial displacement. Epithelial displacement consists of a desquamation phase and a balanced turnover of the oral mucosal basal layer. In GT, there is an imbalance between the two processes, with an overactive desquamation phase, giving the image of an ulcer with a decrease in keratin maturation. Failure of the control mechanisms of epithelial cell desquamation, the regeneration process and the epithelial keratinization contributes to the occurrence of GT [8].

The severity of RAS could be assessed using the Ulcer Severity Score (USS). To assess the anxiety level of our patient, we used the PSS questionnaire adapted to the Indonesian language; it contains ten questions, where only those numbered as 4, 5, 7, and

8 are related to stress. In the present case, the therapy at the first visit was done with 10ml of chlorhexidine gluconate (0.2%) for 3 - 4 minutes for 4 times a day on the ulcer areas, and we included education instructing the patient to avoid hot and spicy foods and prescription of a daily multi-vitamin supplement. Chlorhexidine gluconate is an antiseptic, antifungal and also has an analgesic effects. Antibacterials should be given to RAS patients because bacteria can contribute to the pathogenesis of RAS. Based on this theory, bacteria contribute antigens that can trigger the body's defense system and cross-react with keratinocyte cells in the oral mucosa [25]. In addition, we prescribed a multi-vitamin supplement containing vitamin E 30 iU, vitamin C 750mg, folic acid 400mcg, vitamin B_1 15mg, vitamin B_2 15mg, vitamin B_3 100mg, vitamin B_6 20mg, vitamin B_{12} 12mcg, pantothenic acid 20mg, and zinc 22.5mg. Improved nutrition is expected to help cure RAS and relieve GT symptoms.

On the follow-up visit a month after the first encounter, we observed an improvement in GT lesions, but not in RAS lesions. The old RAS lesions had disappeared, but three new ones were apparent. We believe the improvement seen was due to the patient following our recommendations to avoid spicy, hot foods, and to the presence of high content of Zinc on the multivitamin supplement. Zinc intake has been associated with GT lesion improvements [16]. At this follow-up visit, the patient was then given USS, PSS questionnaire and was sent for CBC examination. We obtained a USS score of 26, indicating the need to replace the RAS management by using triamcinolone acetonide (0.1%) 4 times daily in the ulcer regions. Based on research conducted by Tappuni et al. (2013), the USS score decreases significantly with therapy using topical steroids.We obtained a PSS total score of 11 indicating mild stress criteria. From the results of CBC, our patient had normal hemoglobin levels at 13.1g/dL, MCV at 71.8fL, and MCH at 23.4pg. The normal level of the hemoglobin may be due to the consumption of a multi-vitamin supplement; however, the MCV and MCH results were below normal [26]. Small average red blood cells and low average content of hemoglobin per red cells have contributed to the clinical picture. Without anemia, condition of low blood count as describe above called pre-anemic stage [22]. Patients with pre-anemic stage can display oral mucosa atrophy as a result of a lack adequate oxygen transport amounts in the oral mucosa [22]. This could explain why the patient's RAS condition had not improved by the time of the second visit. We intervened and educated the patient to change her diet, continuing giving multi-vitamins and also interventions to alleviate the stress. Stress management is encourage in this patient because stress can cause various abnormalities in the oral cavity [27].

The final follow-up of our patient was done by a telephone interview; however, the patient confirmed her canker sores had healed and she was not experiencing heat, pain, or sores on her tongue. In cases of RAS and GT a practitioner should look for the main cause or for predisposing factors to take appropriate action to reduce the severity of RAS and GT. Stress and pre-anemic stage play major roles in the pathogenesis of both lesion types.

CONCLUSION

Stress and pre-anemic stage contributed to the development of some oral cavity lesions. Dentists rarely assess the degree of stress in their patients and do not consider the factor in the management of the lesions. Laboratory tests are usually considered unnecessary in cases of RAS or GT. However, the treatment provided without eliminating etiological or predisposing factors does not guarantee the cure of the oral cavity lesions. Through this case report we hope to spread awareness among practitioners on the importance of considering stress and pre-anemic stage for the management of oral cavity lesions.

REFERENCES

[1] Tappuni, A. R.; Kovacevic, T.; Shirlaw, P. J.; Challacombe, S. J. (2013). Clinical assessment of disease severity in recurrent aphthous stomatitis. *J. Oral Pathol. Med.*, 42; 635 - 641.

[2] Arun, K. M.; Ananthakrishnan, V.; Goturu, J. (2014). Etiology and pathophsiology of recurrent aphtous stomatitis: A review. *IJCRR*, 06; 18 - 22.

[3] Kunikullaya, U. K.; Kumar, M. A.; Ananthakrishnan, V.; Jaisri, G. (2017). Stress as a cause of recurrent aphthous stomatitis and its correlation with salivary stress markers. *Chin. J. Physiol.*, 60; 226 - 230.

[4] Huling, L. B.; Baccaglini, L.; Choquette, L.; Feinn, R. S.; Lalla, R. V. (2012). Effect of stressful life events on the onset and duration of recurrent aphthous stomatitis. *J. Oral Pathol. Med.*, 41; 149 - 152.

[5] Khan, N. F.; Ghafoor, F.; Khan, A. A. 2006). Pathogenesis of recurrent aphthous stomatitis: A review of literature. *Proceeding SZPGMI*, 20; 113 - 118.

[6] Sun, A.; Chen, H.; Cheng, S.; Wang, Y.; Chang, J. Y. (2015). Significant association of deficiencies of hemoglobin, iron, vitamin B12, and folic acid and high homocysteine level with recurrent aphthous stomatitis. *J. Oral Pathol. Med.*, 44; 300 - 305.

[7] Chen, H.; Sui, Q.; Chen, Y.; Ge, L.; Lin, M. (2015). Impact of haematologic deficiencies on recurrent aphthous ulceration: A meta-analysis. *Br. Dent. J.*, 218; 8 - 13.

[8] Chaubal, T.; Bapat, R. (2017). Geographic tongue. *Am. J. Med.,* 130, e533 - e534.

[9] Picciani, B.; Santos, V. D. C.; Teixeira-souza, T.; Izahias, L. M.; Curty, Á.; Avelleira, J. C.; Azulay, D.; Pinto, J.; Carneiro, S.; Dias, E. (2017). Investigation of the clinical features of geographic tongue: Unveiling its relationship with oral psoriasis. *Int. J. Dermatology*, 56; 421 - 427.

[10] Gonzaga, H. F. S.; Chaves, M. D.; Gonzaga, L. H. S.; Picciani, B. L. S.; Jorge, M. A.; Dias, E. P. (2015). Environmental factors in benign migratory glossitis and psoriasis: retrospective study of the association of emotional stress and alcohol and tobacco consumption with benign migratory glossitis and cutaneous psoriasis. *J. Eur. Acad. Dermatology Venereol.*, 29; 533 - 536.

[11] Alikhani, M.; Khalighinejad, N.; Ghalaiani, P.; Khaleghi, A. (2014). Immunologic and psychologic parameters associated with geographic tongue. *Oral Surgery, Oral Med. Oral Pathol. Oral Radiol.*, 1 - 4.

[12] Ebrahimi, H.; Pourshahidi, S.; Tadbir, A. A.; Shyan, S. B. (2010). The relationship between geographic tongue and stress. *Iran Red. Crescent Med. J.*, 12; 313 - 315.

[13] Deshpande, T. S. (2015). Stress related oral diseases: A review abstract. *Clinical Dentistry,* 8 - 12.

[14] Pakfetrat, A.; Delavarian, Z.; Rasekhi, J.; Seyyedi, A.; Salah, S. (2014). Psychological assessment of patients with oral aphthous ulcers. *J. Islam Dent. Assoc. Iran*, 26; 271 - 277.

[15] Andreou, E.; Alexopoulos, E. C.; Lionis, C.; Varvogli, L. (2011). Perceived stress scale: reliability and validity study in Greece. *Int. J. Environ. Res. Public Health*, 8, 3287 - 3298.

[16] Reis, R. S.; Fereira Hino, A. A.; Rodriguez Anez, C. R. (2010). Perceived stress scale: reliability and validity study in Brazil. *J. Health Psychol.*, 15; 107.

[17] Saraswati, K. D. H. (2017). Perilakukerja, perceived stress dan social support pada mahasiswa internship. *Jurnal Muara Ilmu Sosial, Humaniora dan Seni*, 1; 216 - 222.

[18] Gilliani, S. W.; Syed, S. A.; Sari, Y. O.; Sariff Azmi (2011). Perceived stress scale psychometric validation for Malaysian diabetic patients. *British journal of pharmaceutical research,* 1(4); 156 - 163.

[19] Wardani, D. A. K.; Huriyati, Emy; Mustikaningtyas; Hastuti, J. (2015). Obesitas, body image dan perasaan stress pada mahasiswa di Daerah Istimewa Yogyakarta. *Jurnal Gizi Klinik Indonesia*, 11; 161 - 169.

[20] Chavan, M.; Jain, H.; Diwan, N.; Khedkar, S.; Shete, A.; Durkar, S. (2012). Recurrent Aphthous Stomatitis: A Review. *J. Oral Pathol. Med.,* 41; 577 - 583.

[21] Mehta, V. (2017). Benign migratory glossitis: report of a rare case with review of literature. *J. Dent. Heal. Oral Disord. Ther.*, 6; 4 - 6.

[22] Shin-Yu Lu. (2016). Perception of iron deficiency from oral mucosa alterations that show a high prevalence of candida infection. *JFMA*, 115; 619 - 627.

[23] Challacombe, S. J.; Alsahaf, S.; Tappuni, A. R. (2015). Recurrent aphthous stomatitis: towards evidence-based treatment? *Curr. Oral Heal. Rep.*, 2, 158 - 167.

[24] Bankvall, M.; Sjoberg, F.; Gale, G.; Wold, A.; Jontell, M.; Ostmar, S. (2014). The oral microbiota of patients with recurrent aphthous stomatitis. *J. Oral Microbiol.,* 6, 25739.

[25] Jain, K.; Mehendiratta, M.; Kardam, P.; Yadav, J. (2016). Crosstalk between mind and oral cavity: an insight into pathogenesis, classification, presentation and management of oral psychosomatic disorders. *Int. Neuropsyciatric Dis. J.*, 5; 1 - 12.

[26] Hoffbrands, V. A. (2016). *Hoffbrand's Essential Haematology*. 7th Ed. New Jersey: Wiley-Blackwell. Chapter 2; 19 - 22.

[27] Irmagita, A.; Subita, G. P. (2003). Beberapatipe lichen planus oral yang dipicu oleh ramipril dan stress emosional (laporankasus). *Jurnal Kedokteran Gigi Universitas Indonesia*, 10; 805 - 810.

In: Clinical Reports in Dentistry
Editor: Lisa R. Amir
ISBN: 978-1-53617-328-4

Chapter 6

ORAL PRECAUTIONS IN PATIENT WITH HEAD AND NECK CANCER UNDERGOING RADIOTHERAPY: A CASE REPORT

Masita Mandasari[1] and Anandina I. Soegyanto[2,*]
[1]Oral Medicine Residency Program, Faculty of Dentistry,
Universitas Indonesia, Jakarta, Indonesia
[2]Department of Oral Medicine, Faculty of Dentistry,
Universitas Indonesia, Jakarta, Indonesia

ABSTRACT

Introduction: The oral cavity can be a site for pathological manifestations of many diseases and their treatments. One example is the head and neck cancer (HNC). Main treatment modalities for HNC are surgery, radiotherapy and chemotherapy. Head and neck cancer treatment by radiotherapy may induce pathological conditions in the oral cavity, both during treatment and after its conclusion. This case report described oral assessment before radiotherapy on a patient with HNC and briefly reviewed radiotherapy oral sequelae.

Case Report: A 56-year-old female was referred to the oral medicine clinic at Cipto Mangunkusumo National Hospital for evaluation and elimination of oral infection foci prior to radiotherapy for HNC. The patient underwent a thorough oral examination, where we noted poor oral hygiene with several necrotic dental roots, teeth requiring extractions, multiple dental caries, and ill-fitting denture with denture stomatitis. A treatment plan was generated, and the patient received proper dental management and was informed about the possibility of oral complications related to radiotherapy.

Conclusion: In patients with HNC, radiotherapy can induce various pathological conditions within the oral cavity, potentially decreasing the patient's quality of life and compromising treatment outcomes. However, those conditions can be mitigated or

* Corresponding Author's Email: a.irmagita@gmail.com.

prevented by oral precautions, elimination of infection sources, and maintenance of good oral hygiene.

Keywords: Head and Neck Cancer (HNC), radiotherapy, oral infection, oral health

1. INTRODUCTION

The oral cavity can be a site of pathological manifestations of many diseases and their treatments. One example is the head and neck cancer (HNC). In 2012, the WHO GLOBOCAN analysis estimated that there were approximately one million new adult cases of HNC worldwide. This estimate combined malignancies of the lip, oral cavity, esophagus, nasopharynx, larynx.

It was also noted that less developed countries have higher incidence of HNC [1]. Head and neck cancer can arise from various cervicofacial tissues, with approximately 90% of HNC cases were classified as squamous cell carcinoma and referred to as head and neck squamous cell carcinoma (HNSCC) [2, 3]. Head and neck squamous cell carcinoma is often used interchangeably with HNC, and for simplicity, HNC will be used throughout the remainder of this paper.

There are many risk factors associated with the onset of HNC, of which the most well-known are smoking and alcohol [4-6]. Betel quid chewing and smokeless tobacco are the prominent risk factors in several parts of the world, especially in the South and Southeast Asia [7, 8]. Dietary factors like consumption of salted fish are also a potential etiological factor related to nasopharyngeal cancer. Head and neck cancer is also associated with viral infections, specifically the Human Papilloma Virus and Epstein–Barr Virus, which may alter the clinical profile of these diseases and are therefore considered as distinct entities [6, 9, 10].

The main treatment modalities for HNC are surgery, radiotherapy and chemotherapy. Surgery is usually the first-line treatment, but limited only to small and accessible tumor masses [3]. For advanced stage disease, radiotherapy, chemotherapy, or a combination thereof may be indicated, based on cancer staging [2]. Head and neck cancer treatment by radiotherapy can induce pathological conditions within the oral cavity such as salivary hypofunction, xerostomia, dysgeusia, osteoradionecrosis, secondary infections, and oral mucositis, both during treatment and after its conclusion, thus dental clearance before radiotherapy is indicated to minimize the side effects [11, 12].

Dentists, especially oral medicine specialists, have a role in providing care for patients with HNC before their treatment. In this case report, we presented a patient with HNC who was referred to our clinic as a part of a pre-radiotherapy assessment. We also reviewed potential adverse effects related to HNC therapy, specifically radiotherapy.

2. Case Report

A 56-year-old female was referred to the oral medicine clinic at Cipto Mangunkusumo Hospital in Jakarta, Indonesia, for evaluation and elimination of oral infection foci prior to radiotherapy for HNC. The patient has consented that her condition was included for publication of this case report. Prior to this visit, she has been treated with six rounds of chemotherapy at another hospital; however there were no improvement. Around one year previously, the patient detected a small lump, in the size of a glass bead, on the right side of her neck. This lump eventually grew bigger, extending towards the posterior side of her right ear, eventually forming an open wound on the surface of her skin. On this visit, the patient was diagnosed with HNC, stage T4N0M0. Two weeks prior, the patient complained of difficulty in opening her mouth, rotating her head, chewing and swallowing solid food. She had an ill-fitting removable partial anterior maxillary denture which she only took off and cleaned while brushing her teeth in the morning and in the afternoon. The patient denied dry mouth, mouth soreness or gum bleeding. The patient never smoked, but her husband and children smoked at home.

We were unable to perform a complete extra-oral examination since there was a large tumor mass that limited examination of the right submandibular and cervical lymph nodes. No abnormalities were found upon examination of other head and neck lymph nodes. Her lips were desquamated with a lower lip deviation and a dry patch of skin close to the right commissure and right chin. The denture-bearing area of the mucosa had an asymptomatic, slight patch of erythema near the left central incisive until the first left premolar (Figure 1). The patient had poor oral hygiene with subgingival and supragingival calculus, as well as debris and dental staining.

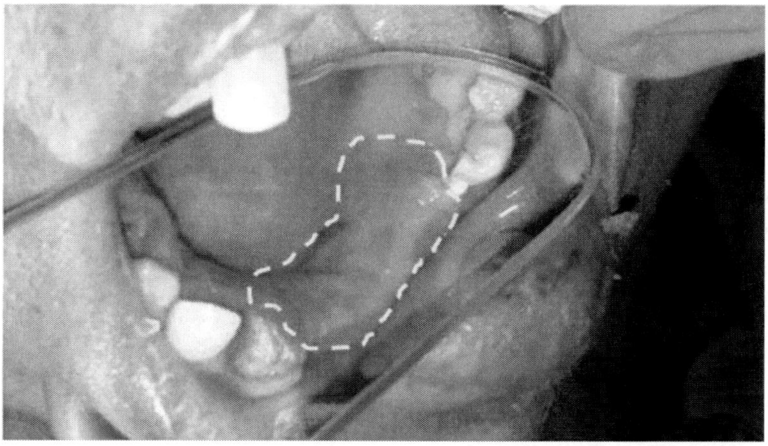

Figure 1. Area of mild erythema (marked with yellow dash line) on the mucosa underneath the partial removable denture of the maxilla as seen by a reflector. Desquamated lower lip is also visible.

Teeth examination, including panoramic radiography, revealed several gangrenous dental roots related to 14, 15, and 43. We also noted carious teeth with pulpal involvement in 25 and 26; cavities in 13, 34, and 44; and mobility of the anterior mandibular teeth. Only teeth 12, 11, 27, and 28 were healthy.

On the basis of these findings, we diagnosed the patient with chronic generalized gingivitis, localized periodontitis, gangrenous dental roots, gangrenous teeth, and dental caries. The patient's recent blood work was within normal limits; therefore no issue to undergo dental treatments. Elimination of the oral infections, consisting of calculus removal and extractions of gangrenous roots and the associated teeth, were prioritized and followed by carious teeth restoration. After she completed radiotherapy, we recommended the fabrication of a new removable denture to replace all of the missing teeth. The patch of erythematous mucosa underneath the patient's denture was diagnosed as denture stomatitis, so 0.2% chlorhexidine oral rinse was prescribed with the instruction to swish-and-spit twice a day for 1 min. We also instructed the patient to rinse after tooth brushing in the morning and before sleeping and to refrain from eating, drinking or gargling for 30 min after rinsing with chlorhexidine. The patient was also instructed to remove her denture during radiotherapy and sleeping. Denture sanitization was performed by submerging the denture in chlorhexidine solution for 20 min every day. Unfortunately, the patient failed to return to oral medicine clinic for further follow up of denture stomatitis after she finished her dental treatments.

3. Discussion

The majority of pre-radiotherapy patients is known to have poor oral hygiene. This requires clinicians to provide comprehensive oral health education, dental scaling, periodontal therapy to remove calculus, teeth extractions, and preventive measures such as topical fluoride or chlorhexidine application to maintain or improve oral hygiene. Plaque control is best achieved by brushing with a soft toothbrush or alternatively, by using mouthwash if tooth brushing causes oral pain. The use of antiseptic mouthwashes, like chlorhexidine gluconate 0.2%, are recommended before radiotherapy to help with periodontal health and remove plaque. In addition to being used as a mouthwash, these solutions can also be applied to gauze and used as oral swab [13, 14]. In this patient, denture stomatitis was most likely caused by the patient's poor oral and denture hygiene (infrequent denture cleaning and overnight denture use). We prescribed 0.2% chlorhexidine gluconate and instructed the patient to use it as an oral rinse. The oral rinse is expected to have beneficial effects on patient's oral hygiene, also this solution has mild antifungal property that may help to alleviate denture stomatitis. The solution can also be used to clean the denture, since denture's porous surface can harbor pathogens. Previous reported study showed the growth of fungal colonies in the oral cavity during radiotherapy, secondary to diminished saliva production. Thus, oral hygiene improvement is an important effort before starting radiotherapy [15]. Additionally, the patient was advised to avoid using the denture until the completion of radiotherapy [16].

Our patient had several necrotic dental roots and teeth that required extractions. Studies have shown that approximately half of patients who undergo radiotherapy require at least one tooth extraction [16, 17]. Pre-radiotherapy extractions are important countermeasures against sepsis from dental foci (e.g., caries, periodontal disease, and periapical lesions) that occur as a result of cancer therapy-related immunosuppression [18]. Ben-David et al. proposed useful criteria when considering teeth extractions in patients undergoing radiotherapy, recommending extractions for teeth with poor prognosis [19]. Extractions should be completed at least 2 weeks before radiotherapy to allow proper wound healing and ideally, these extractions should be performed within one week of initial assessment, so as not to delay the initiation of radiotherapy [16, 17, 20].

Osteoradionecrosis, the most fatal side effect of radiotherapy, is defined as the presence of exposed devitalized irradiated bone without local tumor involvement, with failure to heal within 3 to 6 months. However, the incidence of osteoradionecrosis has been decreasing because of better radiation dose distribution, improved oral care, and the use of oral prophylaxes [19].

Since dental extractions are often associated with osteoradionecrosis, Eliyas et al. tried to elucidate whether pre-radiotherapy tooth extraction reduced late oral complications following radiotherapy. They concluded that there was not a sufficient evidence to support these extraction [21]. Nevertheless, Buglione et al. published a consensus in 2016 that stated that post-radiotherapy extractions tend to induce osteoradionecrosis and that poor oral hygiene before radiotherapy is an osteoradionecrosis risk factor [22]. So, it can be concluded that performing oral precautions before radiotherapy is recommended for preventing oral problems during the post-radiotherapy period.

There are several treatment modalities for HNC. Surgery is usually considered as the first-line treatment for HNC. However, primary radiotherapy, with or without chemotherapy, may be indicated (a) to minimize cosmetic or functional impairments in patients with early HNC;(b) in patients who are not surgical candidates; (c) in patients with co-morbidities or poor systemic conditions; (d) in patients with recurrent disease where additional surgery cannot be performed; and (e) according to the patient's wish [23].

MacCarthy et al. reported that there has been an increase in the number of patients referred to dental professionals for complete oral assessments before radiotherapy [17]. Aside from elimination of oral infection, we should understand the oral effects of radiotherapy to anticipate necessary management strategies and also to ensure that the course of radiotherapy can be completed successfully and without interruption, particularly since HNC is in close proximity to, or may involve, the oral cavity [13].

Patients typically receive a total radiation dose of 60 – 70 Gy, divided into small doses of 2 Gy per day [16, 24, 25]. Over the course of treatment, radiotherapy can cause toxicity in the oral cavity by the same mechanism by which radiotherapy is used to treat cancer. Xerostomia is the most common complaint of patients receiving radiotherapy, followed by mucositis, candidiasis, caries caused by radiotherapy, and osteoradionecrosis [16]. Other complaints include periodontal disease, functional and sensory changes and tissue fibrosis [11]. On the basis of the onset of oral symptoms, relative to the start of radiotherapy, symptoms can be classified as immediate or late effects. Immediate effects are those likely to occur during radiotherapy and include symptoms like dysgeusia, xerostomia, oral infection and oral mucositis. Late effects of radiotherapy may include osteoradionecrosis and hyposalivation.

Salivary gland hypofunction is an additional devastating complication experienced by post-radiotherapy patients. Clinically, patients perceive discomfort secondary to oral dryness. This can be accompanied by insufficient saliva production due to radiotherapy-related effects on the salivary glands [26]. Gland hypofunction reduces not only the quantity of saliva but also the quality. Saliva is essential for preventing caries and periodontal disease, preserving the balance of oral microflora, and promoting oral mucosal health since saliva contains immunoglobulins and electrolytes. Although saliva substitutes can assist with restoring oral lubrication, they lacked other crucial properties in natural saliva. Optimal oral hygiene is therefore important to compensate salivary function [16, 26].

Patients undergoing radiotherapy are also at higher risk of radiation caries due to hyposalivation, consumption of dietary sugars, and increased cariogenic oral flora. Caries can develop as early as three months after radiotherapy [11]. For this reason, dental restoration should be performed as soon as possible before the start of radiotherapy to slow or stop the progression of dental caries. However, complex restorative work should be postponed until after radiotherapy as to not delay potentially life-saving cancer treatments [16]. Finally, although our patient had not received radiotherapy at the time of presentation, she has already showed signs of limited range of motion, which was likely due to the pressure of the tumor mass.

This condition may worsen because of the fibrosis-inducing effects of radiotherapy. Many patients undergoing radiotherapy will develop mandibular hypomobility, including diminished temporomandibular joint movement [27]. Oral radiotherapy-related fibrosis can continue to worsen and eventually interfere with speech production and swallowing, potentially leading to communication and nutritional deficits [13].

Conclusion

Patients who receive radiotherapy for HNC may experience various oral complications which can also occur after treatment. However, those complications can be limited or prevented by exercising comprehensive oral precautions, eliminating sources of infection, and optimizing oral hygiene. Aside from caring for patients' dental and oral complications, dentists are advised to encourage proper oral hygiene and give lifestyle changes recommendations to improve patient's quality of life.

References

[1] Ferlay, J., Soerjomataram, I., Dikshit, R., Eser, S., Mathers, C., Rebelo, M. et al. (2015). Cancer incidence and mortality worldwide: sources, methods and major patterns in GLOBOCAN 2012. *Int. J. Cancer,* 136(5):E359 - 386.

[2] Marur, S., Forastiere, A. A. (2016). Head and Neck Squamous Cell Carcinoma: Update on Epidemiology, Diagnosis, and Treatment. *Mayo Clin. Proc.,* 91(3):386 - 396.

[3] Feller, L., Lemmer, J. (2012). Oral Squamous Cell Carcinoma: Epidemiology, Clinical Presentation and Treatment. *J. Cancer Ther.,* 03(04):263 - 268.

[4] Maasland, D. H., van den Brandt, P. A., Kremer, B., Goldbohm, R. A., Schouten, L. J. (2014). Alcohol consumption, cigarette smoking and the risk of subtypes of head-neck cancer: results from the Netherlands Cohort Study. *BMC Cancer,* 14(1):187.

[5] Koyanagi, Y. N., Matsuo, K., Ito, H., Wakai, K., Nagata, C., Nakayama, T. et al. (2016). Cigarette smoking and the risk of head and neck cancer in the Japanese population: a systematic review and meta-analysis. *Jpn. J. Clin. Oncol.,* 46(6):580 - 95.

[6] Jayalie, V. F., Paramitha, M. S., Jessica, Liu C. A., Ramadianto, A. S., Trimartani, et al. (2016). Profile of Nasopharyngeal Carcinoma in Dr. Cipto Mangunkusumo National Hospital. *eJKI,* 2016;4(3):156 - 162.

[7] Joshi, P., Dutta, S., Chaturvedi, P., Nair, S. (2014). Head and neck cancers in developing countries. *Rambam Maimonides Med. J.,* 5(2):e0009.

[8] Wyss, A. B., Hashibe, M., Lee, Y.-C. A., Chuang, S.-C., Muscat, J., Chen, C. et al. (2016). Smokeless Tobacco Use and the Risk of Head and Neck Cancer: Pooled Analysis of US Studies in the INHANCE Consortium. *Am. J. Epidemiol.,* 184(10):703 - 716.

[9] Adham, M., Stoker, S. D., Wildeman, M. A., Rachmadi, L., Gondhowiardjo, S., Atmakusumah, D. et al. (2014). Current status of cancer care for young patients with nasopharyngeal carcinoma in Jakarta, Indonesia. *PLoS One,* 9(7):6 - 7.

[10] Young, D., Xiao, C. C., Murphy, B., Moore, M., Fakhry, C., Day, T. A. (2015). Increase in head and neck cancer in younger patients due to human papillomavirus (HPV). *Oral Oncol.,* 51(8):727 - 730.

[11] Sroussi, H. Y., Epstein, J. B., Bensadoun, R.-J., Saunders, D. P., Lalla, R. V., Migliorati, C. A. et al. (2017). Common oral complications of head and neck cancer radiation therapy: mucositis, infections, saliva change, fibrosis, sensory dysfunctions, dental caries, periodontal disease, and osteoradionecrosis. *Cancer Med.,* 6(12):2918 - 2931.

[12] Yap, A. (2017). Oral Health Equals Total Health: A Brief Review. *J. Dent. Indones.,* 24(2):59 - 62.

[13] Jawad, H., Hodson, N. A., Nixon, P. J. (2015). A review of dental treatment of head and neck cancer patients, before, during and after radiotherapy: part 1. *Br. Dent. J.,* 218(2):65 - 68.

[14] Jawad, H., Hodson, N. A., Nixon, P. J. (2015). A review of dental treatment of head and neck cancer patients, before, during and after radiotherapy: part 2. *Br. Dent. J.,* 218(2):69 - 74.

[15] Suryawanshi, H., Ganvir, S. M., Hazarey, V. K., Wanjare, V. S. (2012). Oropharyngeal candidosis relative frequency in radiotherapy patient for head and neck cancer. *J. Oral Maxillofac. Pathol.,* 16(1):31 - 37.

[16] Beech, N., Robinson, S., Porceddu, S., Batstone, M. (2014). Dental management of patients irradiated for head and neck cancer. *Aust. Dent. J.,* 59(1):20 - 28.

[17] MacCarthy, D. (2017). An audit of the baseline dental status and treatment need of individuals referred to Dublin Dental University Hospital for a pre-radiotherapy dental and oral assessment. *Irish Dent. Assoc.,* 63(5):269 - 276.

[18] Mirabile, A., Numico, G., Russi, E. G., Bossi, P., Crippa, F., Bacigalupo, A. et al. (2015). Sepsis in head and neck cancer patients treated with chemotherapy and radiation: Literature review and consensus. *Crit. Rev. Oncol. Hematol.,* 95(2):191 - 213.

[19] Ben-David, M. A., Diamante, M., Radawski, J. D., Vineberg, K. A., Stroup, C., Murdoch-Kinch, C.-A. et al. (2007). Lack of osteoradionecrosis of the mandible after intensity-modulated radiotherapy for head and neck cancer: likely contributions of both dental care and improved dose distributions. *Int. J. Radiat. Oncol. Biol. Phys.,* 68(2):396 - 402.

[20] Devi, S., Singh, N. Dental care during and after radiotherapy in head and neck cancer. (2014). *Natl. J. Maxillofac. Surg.,* 5(2):117 - 125.

[21] Eliyas, S., Al-Khayatt, A., Porter, R. W., Briggs, P. (2013). Dental extractions prior to radiotherapy to the jaws for reducing post-radiotherapy dental complications (Review). *Cochrane Database Syst. Rev.,* (2):CD008857.

[22] Buglione, M., Cavagnini, R., Di Rosario, F., Sottocornola, L., Maddalo, M., Vassalli, L. et al. (2016). Oral toxicity management in head and neck cancer

patients treated with chemotherapy and radiation: Dental pathologies and osteoradionecrosis (Part 1) literature review and consensus statement. *Crit. Rev. Oncol. Hematol.,* 97:131 - 142.

[23] Huang, S.-H., O'Sullivan, B. (2013). Oral cancer: Current role of radiotherapy and chemotherapy. *Med. Oral Patol. Oral Cir. Bucal.,* 18(2):e233 - 240.

[24] Castelli, J., Simon, A., Louvel, G., Henry, O., Chajon, E., Nassef, M. et al. (2015). Impact of head and neck cancer adaptive radiotherapy to spare the parotid glands and decrease the risk of xerostomia. *Radiat. Oncol.,* 10(1):6.

[25] Sonis, S. T. (20110). Oral mucositis. *Anticancer Drugs,* 22(7):607 - 612.

[26] Da Silva Deboni, A. L., Giordani, A. J., Lopes, N. N. F., Dias, R. S., Segreto, R. A., Jensen, S. B. et al. (2012). Long-term oral effects in patients treated with radiochemotherapy for head and neck cancer. *Support Care Cancer,* 20(11):2903 - 2911.

[27] Tolentino, E. de S., Centurion, B. S., Ferreira, L. H. C., Souza, A. P. de, Damante, J. H., Rubira-Bullen, I. R. F. (2011). Oral adverse effects of head and neck radiotherapy: literature review and suggestion of a clinical oral care guideline for irradiated patients. *J. Appl. Oral Sci.,* 19(5):448 - 454.

In: Clinical Reports in Dentistry
Editor: Lisa R. Amir

ISBN: 978-1-53617-328-4

Chapter 7

Angular Cheilitis and Recurrent Aphthous Stomatitis as Detection of Hematinic Deficiencies: Two Case Studies

Yuli F. Ossa[1] and Febrina Rahmayanti[2,*]
[1]Oral Medicine Residency Program, Faculty of Dentistry,
Universitas Indonesia, Jakarta, Indonesia
[2]Department of Oral Medicine, Faculty of Dentistry,
Universitas Indonesia, Jakarta, Indonesia

Abstract

Introduction: This case report aimed to describe the oral lesions indicating hematinic deficiency.

Case report: The first case is a 20-year-old female patient with chief complaints of ulceration at the corner of her mouth. Laboratory examination revealed low haemogloblin, hematocrit, erythrocyte index, and RDW-CV levels. After clinical examination, she was diagnosed with angular cheilitis, related to iron deficiency anemia. She was prescribed 0.2% chlorhexidine gluconate mouthwash and multi-vitamins. The second case is 21-year-old male patient complaining of oral discomfort. Clinical examination revealed multiple ulcers in the oral mucosa. The working diagnosis was recurrent aphthous stomatitis and laboratory examination was conducted. Based on clinical and complete blood count, the patient was diagnosed recurrent aphthous stomatitis-related iron deficiency. He was prescribed 0.2% chlorhexidine gluconate mouthwash and multi-vitamins.

Conclusion: Recurrent aphthous stomatitis and angular cheilitis are common oral lesions that indicate signs of hematinic deficiency. The dentists must carry out subjective and objective examinations along with appropriate investigations to detect the presence of systemic factors of underlying diseases for adequate case management.

* Corresponding Author's Email: febrina_r.@ui.ac.id.

Keywords: recurrent aphthous stomatitis, angular cheilitis, hematinic deficiencies

1. Introduction

Recurrent aphthous stomatitis is the most common oral lesion, and characterized by an oval or round ulcerated lesion with a yellowish-white base, surrounded by halo erythematous and may involve keratinized or non-keratinized mucosa. Angular cheilitis is a clinical condition that occurring at the corner of the mouth, characterized by maceration, fissured erythematous, bloody crust, and sometimes pruritus. The exact cause of recurrent aphthous stomatitis and angular cheilitis are unknown, but there are a number of predisposing factors that can contribute to these conditions, such as hematinic and nutrient [1, 2]. Hematinic is a nutrient essential to the process of hematopoiesis. The main component of hematinics are iron, folid acid, and B_{12}; deficiencies in these components can cause anemia [3]. Anemia is characterized by decreasing levels of haemoglobin, and affects one-third of the world's population, half of which are iron deficient. The World Health Organization (WHO) defined anemia as a condition of haemoglobin concentration levels <13mg/dL in men and <12mg/dL in women [4, 9]. In Indonesia, the number of anemic patients based on the Riset Kesehatan Dasar (Riskesdas) in 2013 in women was 23.9% and men 18.5% [4].

Iron deficiency anemia is the most common type of anemia affecting 2 billion of the world's population. According to WHO, in Southeast Asia, 50% of women of childbearing age have concerns of iron deficiency anemia [5]. Iron deficiency anemia can be caused by poor iron intake, impaired iron absorption, or chronic bleeding conditions [5, 6]. Overall, 20% of women are likely to have iron deficiency anemia related to menstruation or childbirth, compared to only 2% in men, generally associated with gastrointestinal diseases [7].

Patients with iron deficiency anemia have clinical features of fatigue, weakness, dizziness, lethargy, slowed breath, postural hypotension, and pallor [1, 5]. Oral manifestations of iron deficiency anemia are atrophic glossitis, burning sensation, angular cheilitis, and recurrent aphthous stomatitis [8]. This case report described two cases of oral lesions, angular cheilitis and recurrent aphthous stomatitis, as signs of hematinic deficiencies.

Patients who often experience these oral lesions do not realize that there is a link between oral lesions and systemic conditions. Whereas, abnormalities in the oral cavity including abnormalities in the soft tissues can be a manifestation of systemic condition, one of which is hematological conditions. The role of dentists is very important to be able to provide education to patients regarding these conditions.

2. Case Report

2.1. First Case

A 20-year-old female patient came to dental hospital of Dentistry Faculty Universitas of Indonesia (RSKGM FKG UI) with complaints of soreness and bleeding at the corner of her mouth starting two days prior. The wound caused pain when the patient opened her mouth to speak. The patient had the same condition two months prior, but the wound healed without any treatment. The wound appeared just before the menstrual period. The patient also had a history of recurrent aphthous stomatitis and occurs at different sites each time. The recurrent aphthous stomatitis also appears prior to the menstrual period and also when the patient has a lot of activities.

The history of recurrent aphthous stomatitis lasted for 4 to 5 days without being treated with medication. The patient consumed vitamin C to accelerate the healing process. Her menstrual period was irregular, and could last up to 14 days or more. Patient often experienced dizziness, and got tired quickly, especially when she has many. On family history, her mother has similar symptoms. Patient has a history of allergies and gastritis.

On extra-oral examination, there was an erythemathous fissure at right corner of her mouth, bleed and pain. The conjunctiva pale. Intra-oral examination, labial mucosa and gingival was pale, with mild atrophy at dorsal aspect of the tongue (Figure 1A, B). The patient was referred for a complete blood count (CBC). The lesion was treated with 0.2% chlorhexidine gluconate mouthwash on the ulcer for 2 to 3 min at the lesion site 3 times a day.

The patient was instructed not to touch the lesion. Patient was educated to maintain oral hygiene by brushing teeth twice a day, and consume fruits and vegetables. CBC showed decreased haemoglobin, 6.9g/dL (normal: 11.7 – 15.5g/dL); hematocrit, 26.6% (normal: 35% – 47%); MCV, 57.2fl (normal: 80 – 110fl); MCH, 14.8pg (normal: 26 – 34pg); MCHC, 25.9g/dL (normal: 32 – 36g/dL); eosinophils, 1% (normal: 2% – 4%), and monocytes, 1% (normal: 2% – 8%), and increased of RDW-CV, 19.6% (normal: 11.5% – 14.5%).

Laboratory results showed a condition of microcytic hypochrome anemia because decreased of haemoglobin, MCV,MCH, and MCHC levels. Based on clinical and laboratory examinations, the patient was diagnosed with angular cheilitis related to iron deficiency anemia. The patient was referred to an internal medicine specialist, where she was treated with multivitamin capsules that consisted of calcium carbonate, folic acid, iron, vitamin B_{12}, vitamin C, and cholacalciferol. The patient came back for follow up after 2 weeks and the lesion has healed.

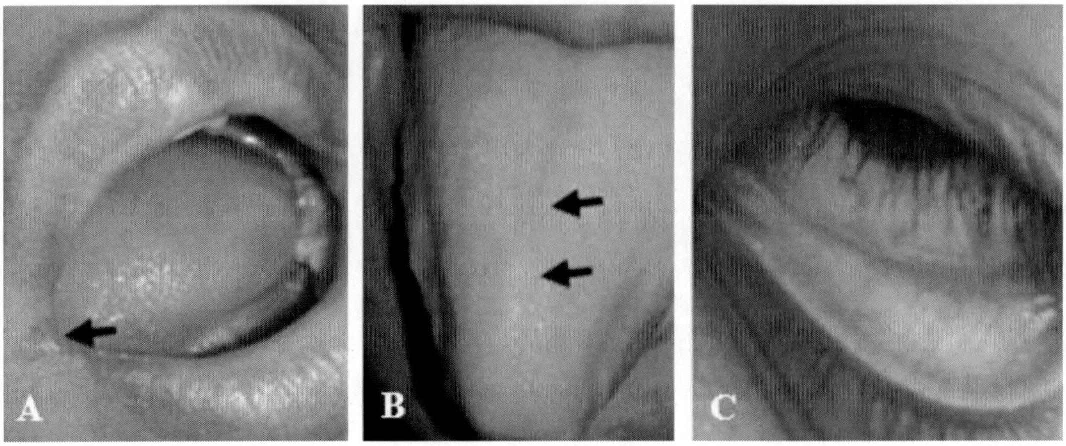

Figure 1. Erythematous fissure at the corners of the mouth (black arrow) (A); Mild papillary atrophy at the dorsum of tongue (black arrow) (B); Pale conjuntiva (C).

2.2. Second Case

A 21-year-old male patient came to RSKGM FKG UI with complaints of a canker sore on his lower left lip. The lesion manifested after the patient noticed decreased endurance. He had histories of lesions every month in different locations. Ulceration usually occurs when a patient experiences stress due to work or thesis examinations, and also when his body condition was weak.

Patient had a history of gastritis experienced since high school, and he had undergone appendectomy 2 years ago. On intra-oral examination, there was yellowish-white based irregular major ulcer (12mm in diameter) with halo erythematous on lower labial mucosa looks. There was a small ulcer 5mm in diameter with irregular halo erythematous on the tips of the tongue. There was single ulcer at the lateral aspect of the tongue, in region 46, with halo erythematous 5mm in diameter (Figure 2A-C). As a result of these ulcerated lesions, the patient complained of difficulty speaking due to the pain that arises each time the patient opened his mouth. The CBC showed decreased levels of MCV, 76.5fl; MCH, 25.8pg; neutrophils, 48% (normal: 50% – 70%); and normal level of haemoglobin, 14.8g/dL.

The patient was diagnosed with recurrent aphthous stomatitis related iron deficiency. The patient was educated about lesions found in the oral cavity and was advised to consume vegetables and fruits, to drink two liters of water a day, and improve oral health by brushing teeth twice a day.

The lesions were treated with 0.2% chlorhexidine gluconate mouthwash on the ulcer for 2 – 3min, 3 times a day. Patient was also given Surbex® Z once a day for a week.

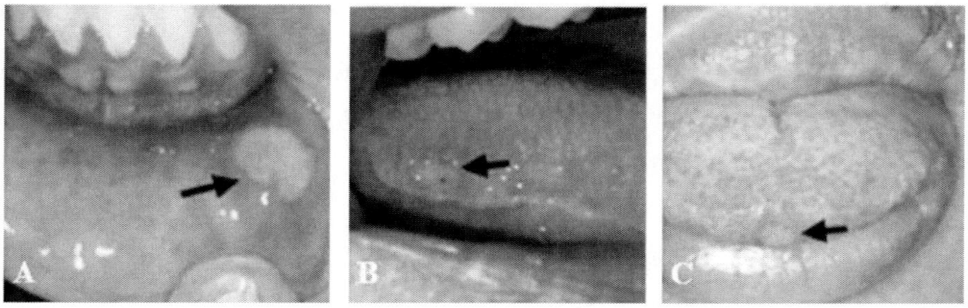

Figure 2. Ulceration in the lower left labial mucosa of region 23 (black arrow) (A); Ulceration on the right lateral edge tongue of the region 16 (black arrow) (B); Ulceration on anterior dorsal of the tongue, region 11 (black arrow) (C).

Three weeks after his initial visit, the patient came back to our clinic. The ulceration has healed, but there was new ulcer in a different location. There was a small ulcer with yellowish-white based, irregular and halo erythematous on the tips of the tongue (5mm in diameter). There was a small ulcer with white based, irregular on the right lateral of the tongue (5mm in diameter) (Figure 3A-C). The patient was instructed to continue chlorhexidine and multivitamins that had been given. The patient was educated to keep up the oral hygiene, and increased consumption of water, fruits and vegetables.

3. Discussion

The changes in the oral cavity associated with hematinic deficiencies have long been known, and may be related to anemia symptoms. To assess anemia, a CBC can be performed to assess hemoglobin, hematocrit, erytrocyte index (MCV, MCH, MCHC) and RDW-CV levels [13]. According to WHO, anemia is defined as hemoglobin level < 13g/dL in men and < 12g/dL in women [7]. Based on levels of ertrocyte index, anemia can be divided into microcytosis (MCV < 80fl), normocytosis (MCV, 80 – 100fl), or macrocytosis (MCV > 100fl).

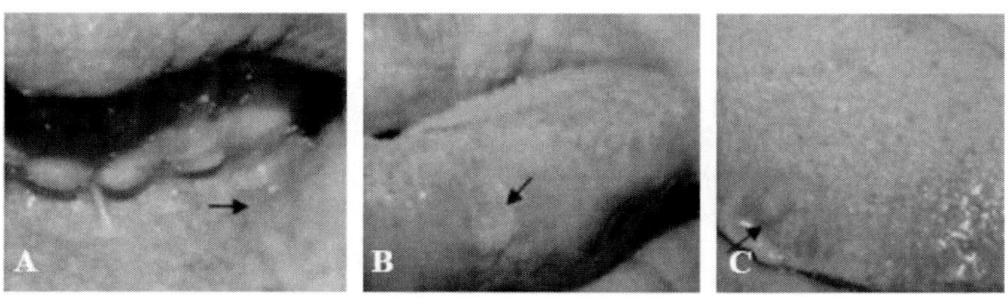

Figure 3. Lesion on healing (black arrow) (A); Ulcer on the tips of the tongue (black arrow) (B); Ulcer on right lateral edge of the tongue (black arrow) (C).

Microcytosis is associated with iron deficiency condition, and can be accompanied with or without anemia symptoms [13]. Sign and symptoms of anemia include weakness, fatigue, dizziness, pale, difficulty concentrating, tachycardia, and postural hypotension. The changes in oral mucosa can be angular cheilitis, recurrent aphthous stomatitis, glossitis, burning sensations, and/or atrophy of the papillae. The first patient presenting with angular cheilitis and mild atrophy of papillae and also had the sign of anemia, and CBC showed lower levels of hemogloblin, MCV, MCH, and MCHC. The same conditions were reported in the study of Shin-Yu Lu (2004) and Yan-Che Wu et al. (2014) [7, 13]. The second patient with recurrent aphthous stomatitis and CBC showed lower levels of MCV and MCH. The microcytosis condition related was to iron deficiency, and the same condition also reported in the study of Shin-Yu Lu (2016) [8].

Angular cheilitis is a clinical diagnosis of a lesion that affects the corner of the mouth, the vermillion, lip commissures which may be unilateral or bilateral. Characteristics of these lesions are maceration, erythema, and crust. The corner of the mouth often appears wrinkled and sometimes a deep fissure forms that bleeds [2, 17, 18]. In our case report, unilateral angular cheilitis was located in the right corner of the mouth. According to Ohman, et al. (1986), the angular cheilitis in this patient was categorized to type II [16]. That is, a lesion with one fissure limited to angle of the mouth. The angular cheilitis was also found to be related to iron deficiency anemia. Angular cheilitis has been associated with *Staphylococcus*, *Candida*, or *Streptococcus* infections. It can have multifactorial predispositions, such as microbiological changes, haematological deficiencies and loss of vertical dimension [2, 16, 18]. In this patient, there was no decrease in vertical dimension but there was evidence of hematinic deficiencies. The cause of anemia in this patient may be affected by genetic conditions, as the patient's mother had a history of anemia. In addition, iron intake in the form of vegetables (spinach, soybeans), boiled eggs, and red meat were rarely consumed by patient [14].

Angular cheilitis was treated with 0.2% chlorhexidine gluconate mouthwash on the wound. Chlorhexidine gluconate has bactericidal or bacteriostatic properties against a wide range of gram negative and gram positive bacteria, yeasts, dermatophyte fungi and lipophilic viruses [17]. The patient was given a multivitamin containing iron, folic acid, vitamin C, and vitamin D3. These multivitamin administrations aim to reduce the symptoms of anemia, accelerate wound healing, and improve nutrition for the patient [14]. Hematinic is a nutrient needed to help hematopoiesis. The main components of hematinics are iron, folic acid, and B_{12}; deficiency of these components can cause anemia [3]. Patients with anemic conditions are characterized by decreased haemogloblin levels, thus reducing their ability to carry oxygen throughout the body [10]. Decreased oxygen level in the oral mucosa can cause atrophy of the oral mucosa. In addition, iron also plays an important role in the normal function of the epithelial cells of oral cavity. If iron deficiency occurs, the oral epithelial cells will quickly develop atrophy or produce immature epithelial layers [14].

Iron has vital function for organs such as the hemoglobin synthesis process and oxygen transport throughout the body [9, 15]. The total amount of iron absorbed by the body in a healthy individual is 1 – 2mg, which can compensate for the daily iron loss of 1mg in men and 1.5 – 2mg in women during the menstrual period [8, 9]. Iron deficiency is due to inadequate iron intake, inhibited absorption, or due to chronic blood loss such as menstruation. In addition, conditions such as pregnancy, vegetarian diet, consumption of acid-reducing drugs, peptic ulcers, chronic bleeding caused by colon cancer, uterine cancer, gastrointestinal polyps and hemorrhoids can also cause iron deficiency [8, 9, 15].

In women of childbearing age, chronic blood loss on the menstrual period is the most common cause of iron deficiency anemia. Conversely, gastrointestinal diseases are the main cause of iron deficiency anemia on male patients [8, 9]. In this case report, a 20-year-old female patient with an abnormally long menstrual period ($\geq$ 14 days) was also a predisposing factor for anemia in this patient. For the 21-year-old male patient, his history of gastritis since high school was a predisposing factor for iron deficiency. In the second patient, CBC showed normal levels of haemogloblin, but there was a decrease in MCV and MCH levels, which indicate an iron deficiency. The iron deficiency can be accompanied with or without anemia and may progress to anemia [8, 15]. One cause of iron deficiency is due to lack of iron consumption [9, 19]. In this case report, the male patient rarely consumes vegetables and fruits. Also, the recurrent aphthous stomatitis arises when patient in a stress condition. The patient was facing the final examination of his thesis. The patient was treated with 0.2% chlorhexidine gluconate mouthwash on the ulcer and was instructed to take Surbex® Z multivitamin. Surbex® Z contains vitamin E, C, B_9, B_2, B_3, B_6, B_{12}, panthotheric acid, and zinc. Multivitamin therapy provides nutrition for the body, accelerates the healing process, and zinc can help the formation of new epithelial cells [14].

Recurrent aphthous stomatitis is the most common lesion in the oral cavity with the definite cause still unknown. There are several factors that can trigger lesions, including genetic factors, stress, local trauma, vitamin and micronutrient deficiencies, certain food allergies, hormonal changes, and some systemic diseases (celiac disease, Chron's disease and ulcerative collitis) [1, 7, 11, 19]. Recurrent aphthous stomatitis is characterized by oval or round lesions, with a yellowish-white base and halo erythematous [1, 11, 13]. Risk factors of iron deficiency anemia include chronic bleeding, malabsorption, lack of vitamin C intake, and consumption of coffee or tea [14]. Iron deficiency can reduce the effectiveness of the immune system against the infections due to cellular immunity disorders, decreased bactericidal activity of polymorphoneuclear leukocytes, inadequate antibody response, and abnormalities of epithelial cells [8, 9]. Iron deficiency causes decreased activity of enzymes in mitochondria. This is due to a decrease supply of oxygen and nutrients into the cell, such that it can inhibit differentiation and epithelial formation. The process makes the oral mucosa thinner because the epithelial keratinization disappears, and the resulting epithelium becomes irritable [13]. In first patient, iron deficiencies were associated with reduced iron intake and related to chronic bleeding. Whereas in the second patient, the iron deficiency related to less iron intake.

Symptoms of anemia cannot be determined only from haemoglobin level, because of differences in tolerance between individuals. Healthy young individuals often do not complain of symptoms until the haemoglobin level drops dramatically [13]. When haemoglobin, MCV or MCH levels decrease and patient is unaware of the symptoms of anemia or even in the pre-anemic stage, oral mucosa changes can be an important indicator for the earliest symptoms of hematinic deficiencies. CBC is required to support the diagnosis.

CONCLUSION

Recurrent aphthous stomatitis and angular cheilitis are oral lesions that can indicate signs of hematinic deficiencies. The dentists must carry out subjective and objective examinations comprehensively along with appropriate investigations to detect the presence of systemic factors of underlying disease and additional investigations should have been done to establish the cause of microcytis anemic such that adequate case management can be carried out.

REFERENCES

[1] Chavan, M. et al. (2012). Recurrent aphthous stomatitis: a review. *J. Oral Pathol. Med.*, 41:577 - 583.

[2] Zaidan, T. F. (2008). Angular cheilitis and iron deficiency anemia. *Mustansiria Dent. J.*, 5:37 - 41.

[3] Bao, Z. X., Shi, J., Yang, X. W., Liu, L. X. (2018). Hematinic deficiencies in patients with recurrent aphthous stomatitis variation by gender and age. *Medicina Oral Patologia Oral Y Cirugia Bucal*, 23:e161 - e167.

[4] Kementerian Kesehatan Republik Indonesia; Riset Kesehatan Dasar (Riskesdas) (2013). *Badan Penelitian dan Pengembangan Kesehatan Kementerian Kesehatan,* RI. Jakarta.

[5] Soofi, S. et al. (2017). Prevalence and possible factors associated with anaemia, and vitamin B12 and folate deficiencies in women of reproductive age in Pakistan; Analysis of national-level secondary survey data. *Br. Med. J. Open*, 7:e018007.

[6] Wu Yang-Che et al. (2014). Oral manifestation and blood profile in patient with iron deficiency anemia. *J. Formosan. Med. Assoc.*, 113:83 - 87.

[7] Lu Shin-Yu. (2016). Perception of iron deficiency from oral mucosa alterations that show a high prevalence of *Candida* infection. *J. Formosan. Medic. Assoc.*, 115:619 - 627.

[8] Ibanez, G. B. et al. (2016). Iron deficiency anaemia: review article. *Revista Médica de Hospital General de México*, 79:88 - 97.

[9] Vinall, C., Stassen, L. F. A. (2007). Dental management of the anaemic patient. *J. Irish Dent. Assoc.*, 53:191 - 195.

[10] Slebioda, Z., Szponar, E., Kowalska, A. (2014). Etiopathogenesis of recurrent apthous stomatitis and the role of immunologic aspect; Literature review. *Archivum Immunologiae et Therapiae Experimentalis*, 62:205 - 215.

[11] Akintoye, S. O., Greenberg, M. S. (2014). Recurrent apthous stomatitis. *Dent. Clin. North America*, 58: 281 - 297.

[12] Lu Shin-Yu, Wu Hong-Cheng. (2004). Initial diagnosis of anemia from sore mouth and improved classification of anemias by MCV and RDW in 30 patients. *Oral Sur. Oral Med. Oral Pathol. Oral Radiol. Endod.,* 98:679 - 678.

[13] Tolkachjov, S. N., Bruce, A. J. (2017). Oral manifestation of nutritional disorders. *Clin. Dermatol.*, 35(5): 441 - 452.

[14] Camaschella, C. (2017). New Insights into iron deficiency and iron deficiency anemia. *Blood Review*, 31:225 - 233.

[15] Cross, D., Eide, M. L., Kotinas, A. (2010). The clinical features of angular cheilitis occuring during orthodontic treatment: a multi-centre observational study. *J. Orthodon.*, 37:80 - 86.

[16] Oza, N., Doshi, J. J. (2017). Angular cheilitis; A clinical and microbial study. *Ind. J. Dent. Res.*, 28:661 - 665.

[17] Sethi, G., Kumar, K. (2018). A comparative evaluation of efficacy of 0.2% chlorhexidine with a herbal mouthwash as preprocedural mouthrinse in the reduction of aerosol contamination produced by ultrasonic scaler. *Acta Sci. Dent. Sci.*, 2.7: 02 - 06.

[18] Mandasari, M., Astuti, A. K., Rahmayanti, F. (2018). A case on inconspicuous recurrent herpes labialis mimicking unilateral cheilitis. *J. Dent. Indones.*, 25(3):171 - 174.

[19] Wulandari, E. A. T., Setyawati, T. (2008). Tata laksana sar minor untuk mengurangi rekurensi dan keparahan (laporan kasus). [Minor sar management to reduce recurrence and severity (case report).] *J. Dent. Indones.*, 15(2):147 - 154.

In: Clinical Reports in Dentistry
Editor: Lisa R. Amir

ISBN: 978-1-53617-328-4

Chapter 8

PFAPA SYNDROME: A CASE REPORT

***Hsiao-Chun Chou*[1] *and Yu-Feng Huang*[1,2,*]**
[1]Chung Shan Medical University Hospital,
Department of Stomatology, Taichung City, Taiwan
[2]Chung Shan Medical University, College of Oral Medicine,
Taichung City, Taiwan

ABSTRACT

Introduction: PFAPA syndrome is characterized by periodic fever, aphthous stomatitis, pharyngitis and cervical adenitis. It usually happens to children younger than 5 years of age.

Case report: Herein, we present a case of 14-year-old Taiwanese male who had been suffering from periodic oral aphthous ulcerations and high fever almost every month since he was 1 year old. At the time of examination, yellowish crusts on upper and lower vermillions noted with pain, along with several ruptured vesicles over soft palate and pharyngeal area were seen. Multiple oral aphthous ulcers were noted throughout oral mucosa, including tongue border, buccal mucosa and labial mucosa. Under thorough history taking and medical records, we excluded other diseases, including cyclic neutropenia. A diagnosis of PFAPA syndrome with impetigo on upper and lower vermillion and herpangina was rendered. The patient was treated with supporting treatment on the first week until herpangina resolved, followed by oral prednisolone (5mg, 3 times per day for 5 days) and topical triamcinolone rinse (4mg in 20ml water, topical rinse, 4 times daily for 7 days) and the patient responded well. Thereafter we recommended ranitidine therapy (150mg, once per day for 3 months) as prophylaxis for the recurrent aphthous stomatitis. The patient was doing well without recurrence of aphthous ulcers. The patient is currently under close follow up and ranitidine therapy would be indicated if the symptoms recurred.

Conclusion: Through this case, we want to prove that typical PFAPA syndrome could be easily diagnosed through careful examination of patient's history and clinical features.

---

* Corresponding Author's Email: whuang@csmu.edu.tw.

Keywords: PFAPA, oral aphthous ulcers

1. Introduction

Recurrent aphthous stomatitis (RAS) is the most common ulcerative disease of the oral mucosa, showing painful oval-to-round, shallow ulceration with well-defined erythematous border and whitish-grey pseudomembrane. Oral symptom usually dissolves in 10 - 14 days [1]. There is no single definitive factor that causes RAS, many investigators agreed that RAS is epithelial destruction by cytotoxicity of T-cell mediated response. There are several systemic diseases which oral manifestation may be confused with RAS, including Behçet disease, HIV- related ulcerations and PFAPA, clinical examination along with detailed history taking are required for diagnosis of these diseases.

PFAPA syndrome, well known as Marshall syndrome, abbreviated for periodic fever, aphthous stomatitis, pharyngitis and cervical adenitis, was first introduced by Marshall et al. in 1987 in 12 children who were otherwise healthy [2]. The first onset of the syndrome usually happens before 5 years old, with a male predominance. PFAPA usually presents high fever above 39°C with a regular pattern of 26-36 days, each episode lasts about 5 days. The syndrome is self-limited while the patient is healthy and symptom-free between attacks [3]. The diagnosis of PFAPA requires exclusion of other syndrome with periodic fever and oral manifestation or suspected infection, intermittent fever syndromes including Familial Mediterranean fever (FMF), Hyper IgD syndrome (HIDS) and Cyclic neutropenia. Apart from detailed history taking and clinical examination, serology and blood cultures provide important information for differential diagnosis [4]. Treatments of PFAPA accepted by clinicians nowadays includes steroid therapy and cimetidine or even aggressive treatment such as tonsillectomy. Literatures suggested steroid therapy of prednisolone 1-2 mg/kg given as a single dose, the symptom of fever usually resolves dramatically afterwards.

Variation of therapy including increase the dosage up to 7 days. However, steroid may cause growth abnormalities of children, besides although patients responded well to steroid therapy, it did not prevent subsequent cycles. Cimetidine as a sort of H_2 antagonist, also owns the property of immunomodulation to inhibit T-cell activation. Suggested dosage of cimetidine is 150mg once or twice daily or 20-40mg/kg/day for 6 months [4]. Thomas et al. reported that 43% of patients are responsive to cimetidine, from somewhat effective to very effective [5]. They also reported that among 11 patients who had tonsillectomy, febrile episodes had totally resolved in 7 patients (64%). Nevertheless, due to limited information of etiology of the disease, tonsillectomy was not recommended for management of PFAPA if there are no other indications for tonsillectomy [5].

2. Case Report

A 14 year-old male came to our hospital for recurrent aphthous stomatitis occurring every month. After detailed history taking, the patient's parent stated that he had suffered from enterovirus infection when he was about 1 year-old, and had periodic fever along with sore throat and multiple ulcerations in oral cavity almost every month since then. Tracing back the patient's medical history, he was sent to Pediatric department of our hospital from local clinic when he was 1 year old due to fever, skin rash, herpangina and acute pharyngitis. He was then admitted for further evaluation and supportive treatment, fever up to 39.5°C was recorded, and the diagnosis was Hand-foot-mouth disease and Roseola infantum. He had then been discharged after symptoms resolved. However, 36 days later, he was admitted again because of intermittent fever for 2 days and multiple ulcerations in oral cavity. The patient had laboratory tests including CBC and C-protein reaction levels (CRP), the result was normal except that CRP level was slightly elevated (3.62mg/dl). He was discharged 3 days later while condition became stable. After that, he had periodic fever and oral ulcerations almost every month according to the patient's parent.

He was completely symptom-free between the attacks. His parents had taken him to different pediatricians for help in these years, but the doctors only diagnosed him with recurrent aphthous stomatitis or Herpes stomatitis. However, the episodes of attack remained almost every month, so they decided to come to our Oral Pathology department for help. At examination, multiple aphthous stomatitis were noted at right anterior border of tongue, bilateral buccal mucosa and lower lip (Figure 1 A, B). In addition, multiple vesicles with ruptured ulcerations were seen at soft palate and pharyngeal mucosa, suggestive of herpangina (Figure 1C). Yellowish crusts were observed on both upper and lower vermillion with pain, suggestive of impetigo (Figure 1D).

Based on clinical findings and the patient's history, a diagnosis of PFAPA syndrome was rendered.The patient was prescribed with Panadol (500mg/tab, tid) for 4 days along with well hydration and well rest as supportive treatments, along with Gentamycin ointment application on lip. Four days later, the yellowish crusts on vermillions had disappeared, and the vesicles on soft palate had healed, with only aphthous stomatitis remained visible at buccal mucosa, right border of tongue and lower lip. Thus, oral prednisolone (5mg/tab, tid) was prescribed for 5 days along with topical triamcinolone solution rinse (4mg in 20ml water, qid). A week later, the ulcerations had been cleared out. After explanation to the patient and his parent, ranitidine therapy (150mg/tab, bid) for 3 months as prophylaxis of recurrent aphthous stomatitis was suggested. The patient is currently being followed up routinely.

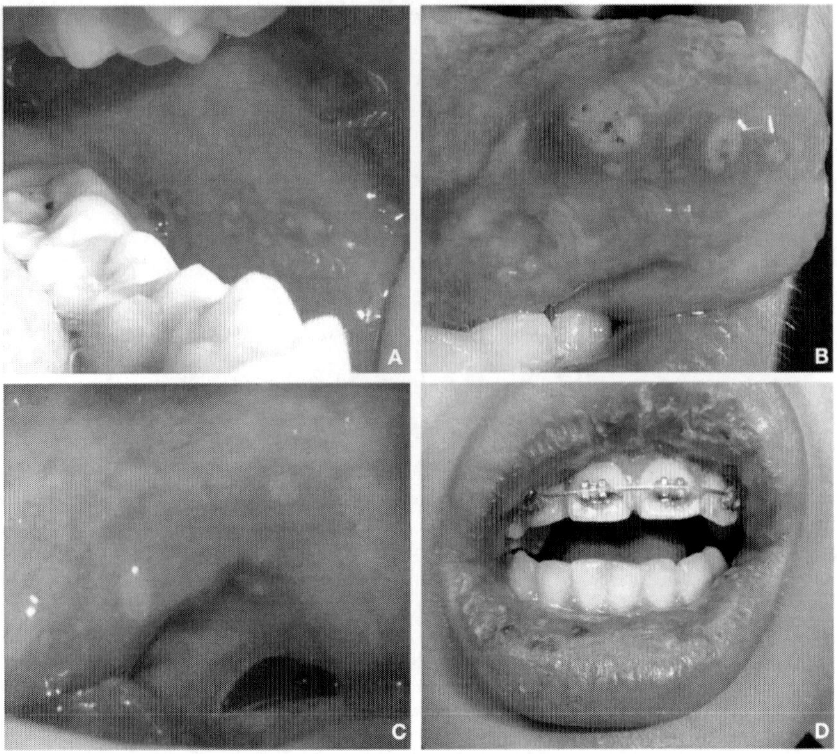

Figure 1. Ulcerations on left buccal mucosa (A); ulcerations on right tongue tip (B); vesicles over soft palate and pharyngeal area, swelling and redness of the area was also noted(C); yellowish crusts were observed on both upper and lower vermillion with pain, suggestive of impetigo (D).

3. Discussion

Fever is a common sign of infection in children, usually revealed respiratory infection. However, periodic fever may indicate more complex situation involving auto-inflammatory diseases, when the immune system were triggered through abnormal antigen-independent activation, which may cause difficulties for clinicians when it comes to diagnosis of the disease. Thomas et al. defined the diagnostic criteria of PFAPA in 1999 as regular recurring fever with early age of onset below 5 years of age, no respiratory infection, and possess at least one of the following signs: pharyngitis, aphthous stomatitis and cervical adenitis [5]. Exclusion of cyclic neutropenia should be done. The patient is completely asymptomatic between the episodes and is healthy other than the symptoms and under normal development.

Differential diagnosis of PFAPA includes other syndrome with periodic fever and oral symptoms mentioned above. Cyclic neutropenia shows periodic fever the interval of 21-24 days; aphthous ulcerations, pharyngitis, lymphadenopathy, malaise and pyogenic infections; premature bone loss may also been observed. Clinical features of cyclic neutropenia resembles those of PFAPA's, thus is differentiated from PFAPA by CBC while blood neutrophil count is under 500/mm^3 during each cycle. Cyclic neutropenia can also be distinguished from PFAPA by that the shorter intervals of cycles than PFAPA, much more severe stomatitis in oral cavity, and it is unlikely for cyclic neutropenia to resolve after application of prednisolone [5-7]. According to the record of our patient at 1 year of age, all the laboratory data including neutrophil count were normal except for CRP that was slightly higher, additionally the ulcerations in his oral cavity was less serious, he can be identified as having PFAPA syndrome.

The patient received supportive treatment in the first week for herpangina. One week later, the vesicles have cleared and oral prednisolone (5mg/tab, tid) was prescribed along with topical triamcinolone solution rinse for 7 days for aphthous stomatitis. The patient responded well and the oral ulcers have cleared without side effects. Thereafter, we recommended a ranitidine therapy as prophylaxis for recurrent aphthous stomatitis [8]. Both cimetidine and ranitidine are H_2 antagonist used to inhibit the secretion of gastric acid and pepsin, and they both possess immunomodulating features, interfering with the generation and expression of suppressor cell function *in vivo* [9]. The chemical structure of ranitidine was similar to cimetidine but shows less drug interactions with other medications. A pilot study was previously conducted to evaluate the degree of pain and discomfort of 15 patients with visual analog scale after a 3 months course of ranitidine therapy, and the level of discomfort reduced after ranitidine therapy that was statistically significant [8]. This patient is currently under monthly follow up.

Conclusion

Our case showed three kinds of common diseases a dentist should have recognized: herpangina, impetigo and PFAPA. However, none of previous doctors had been aware of the classic signs and symptoms of the disease, and proper treatment has been postponed until now, which dramatically affect the patient's quality of life.

There are plenty of systemic diseases that present oral manifestations, and as a dentist, we need to evaluate and examine oral cavity of every patient thoroughly, in additionally record medical and dental history carefully to avoid misdiagnosis resulting in delayed treatment of the diseases.

References

[1] Akintoye, S. O., Greenberg, M. S. (2014). Recurrent Aphthous Stomatitis. *Dent. Clin. N Am.,* 58: 281 - 297.

[2] Marshall, G. S., Edwards, K. M., Butler, J., Lawton, A. R. (1987). Syndrome of periodic fever, pharyngitis, and aphthous stomatitis. *J. Pediatr.,* 110: 43 - 46.

[3] Femiano, F., Lanza, A., Buonaiuto, C., Gombos, F., Cirillo, N. (2008). Oral Aphthous-like lesions, PFAPA syndrome: a review. *J. Oral Pathol. Med.,* 37: 319 - 323.

[4] Pinto, A., Lindemeyer, R. G., Sollecito, T. P. (2006). The PFAPA syndrome in oral medicine: Differential diagnosis and treatment. *Oral Surg. Oral Med. Oral Pathol. Oral Radiol. Endod.,* 102: 35 - 39.

[5] Thomas, K. T., Feder, H. M. Jr., Lawton, A. R., Edwards, K. M. (1999). Periodic fever syndrome in children. *J. Pediatr.,* 135: 15 - 21.

[6] Feder, H. M., Salazar, J. C. (2010). A clinical review of 105 patients with PFAPA (a periodic fever syndrome). *Acta Pædiatrica,* 99: 178 - 184.

[7] Wright, D. G., Dale, D. C., Fauci, A. S., Wolff, S. M. (1981). Human cyclic neutropenia: Clinical review and long-term follow-up of patients. *Med.,* 60: 1 - 13.

[8] Peng, C. Y., Lee, Y. H., Yang, H. W., Huang, Y. F. (2015). A novel treatment for recurrent aphthous stomatitis: A preliminary report. *Taiwan J. Oral Maxillifac. Surg.,* 26: 1 - 7.

[9] Griswold, D., Alessi, S., Badger, A. et al. (1984). Inhibition of T suppressor cell expression by histamine type 2 (H2) receptor antagonists. *J. Immunol.,* 132: 3054 - 3057.

SECTION 2: ORAL SURGERY AND PROSTHODONTICS

In: Clinical Reports in Dentistry
Editor: Lisa R. Amir

ISBN: 978-1-53617-328-4

Chapter 9

IMPACT OF CONE-BEAM COMPUTED TOMOGRAPHY ON IMPLANT PLANNING AND PREVENTION OF NERVE INJURIES: A CASE REPORT

Mieke Sari[1] and Benny S. Latief[2,*]

[1]Oral Maxillofacial Surgery Residency Program,
Faculty of Dentistry, Universitas Indonesia, Jakarta, Indonesia
[2]Department of Oral Maxillofacial Surgery, Faculty of Dentistry,
Universitas Indonesia, Jakarta, Indonesia

ABSTRACT

Introduction: The mandibular canal is a crucial anatomical indicator for implant planning in the posterior mandibular region. Implant positioning near the mandibular canal may result in damage to the inferior alveolar nerve, leading to paresthesia of the lower lip and chin.

Case report: A 38-year-old man with no relevant medical history presented to Pondok Indah Hospital for the replacement of his missing mandibular teeth, which had been removed 1 year prior to presentation. The patient wanted to have the missing dentition restored using a dental implant. We placed dental implants at the 1st, 2nd and 3rd right mandibular molars. The risk of damage to the trigeminal nerve branches is known as a complication of implant treatment in the posterior mandibular region. CBCT provides three-dimensional (3D) images with a moderate radiation dose, and numerous studies have reported its value in diagnosing spatial associations between anatomical structures.

Conclusion: The present report highlight the use of CBCT for assessing the distance between anatomical structures. CBCT is regarded as a credible and precise tool.

Keywords: dental implants, mandibular canal, cone-beam computed tomography

* Corresponding Author's Email: bennylatief@gmail.com.

1. Introduction

The mandibular canal is a crucial anatomical landmark for implant planning in the posterior mandibular region. Implant positioning near the mandibular canal may result in damage to the inferior alveolar nerve, leading to paresthesia of the lower lip and chin [1]. The risk of damage to the trigeminal nerve branches (inferior alveolar, lingual, and mental nerves) is a known complication of implant treatment in the posterior mandibular region. Previous studies shows the percentage of inferior alveolar nerve injuries caused by dental implant surgery is multifarious, ranging from 0% – 44% [2, 3].

Errors in the treatment planning and evaluation, bone preparation, the use of vasoconstrictors with local anesthesia, are the most frequent causes of injury to the mandibular division of the trigeminal nerve related to dental implant placement. Panoramic radiography is typically used as the primary imaging technique to evaluate the height of the vertical dimension from the crest of the mandibular alveolar ridge to the superior angle of the inferior alveolar canal. Cone-beam computed tomography (CBCT) is an important feature in the examination of such patients. Leading imaging modalities, such as panoramic radiography and CBCT, support the localization of the inferior alveolar canal. Typically, panoramic images cannot identify the location of the mandibular canal. The effectiveness of CBCT in identifying the mandibular canal has been reported in many studies.

The aptitude of CBCT and panoramic radiography in identifying the mandibular canal was reported by Angelopoulos et al. who demonstrated that CBCT has significantly better visualization than panoramic radiography [4].

2. Case Report

A 38-year-old man with no relevant medical history presented to Pondok Indah Hospital for the replacement of his missing mandibular teeth, which had been removed 1 year prior to presentation (Figure 1A). CBCT examination showed 2 mm distance of the apical root of the adjacent teeth with the mandibular canal (Figure 2). The patient wanted to have the missing dentition restored using a dental implant. We placed dental implants at the 1st, 2nd, and 3rd right mandibular molars (Straumann Dental Implant; length, 10mm; diameter, 4.1mm)(Figure 1B). No further signs of paresthesia of the lower lip, chin, and mental muscle region were noted after a 6-month observation period.

3. Discussion

Substitution of a tooth with a dental implant may be indicated in cases of periodontal disease, dental caries, tooth loss as a result of trauma, and congenitally missing teeth.

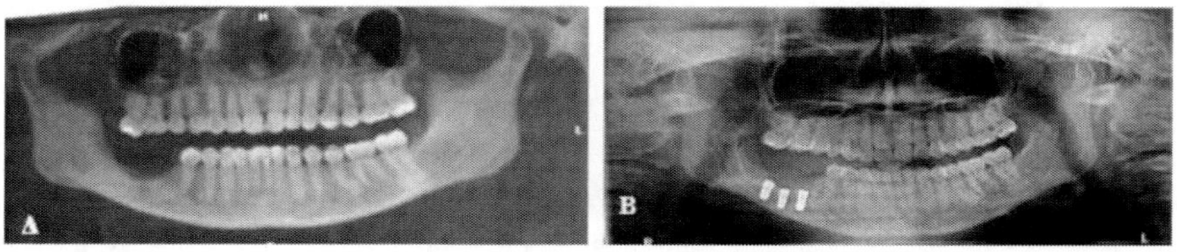

Figure 1. Preoperative panoramic image (A); Postoperative panoramic image (B).

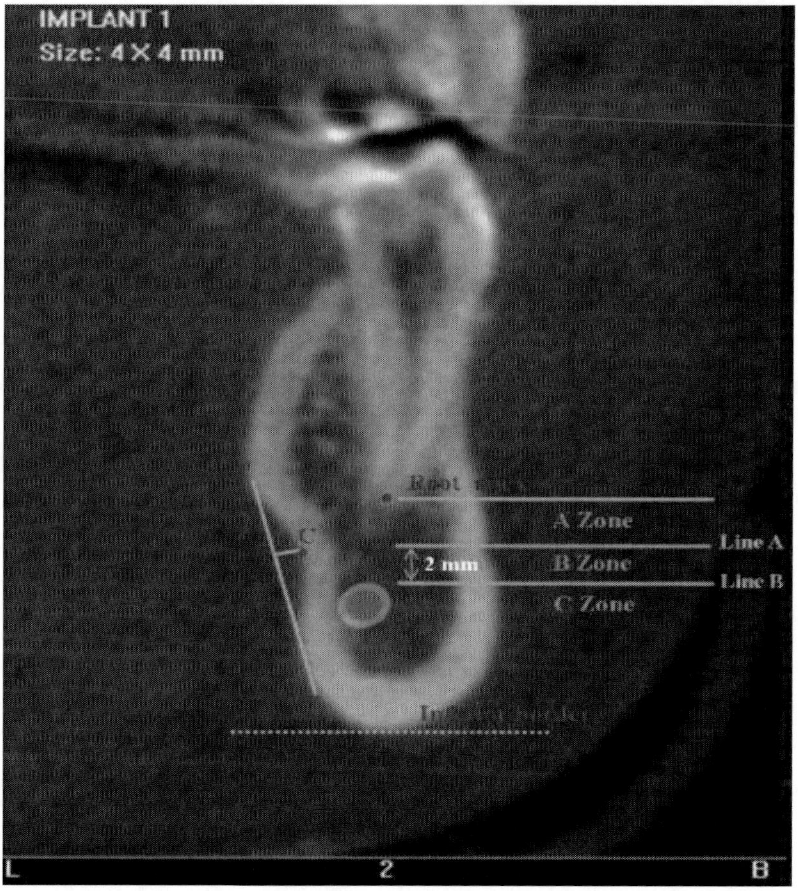

Figure 2. Cross-sectional view of the lingual concavity ridge type. Line A represents a reference 2mm superior to the inferior alveolar nerve. Line B represents the superior border of the inferior alveolar canal.

In such cases, a dental implant is used to replace the missing tooth space when it is surrounded by healthy teeth or an intact prosthetic reconstruction of the neighboring teeth. Appropriate preoperative surgical planning leads to successful dental implant placement. The risk of damage to the trigeminal nerve branches (inferior alveolar, lingual, and mental nerves) is known as a complication of implant treatment in the posterior mandibular region. The trigeminal nerve branches provide sensation to the lower lip and chin and innervate the associated dentition. The infratemporal fossa (ITF) contains some muscles of mastication, inferior alveolar nerves, chorda tympani nerves, lingual nerves, and the maxillary artery. The inferior alveolar and lingual nerves generally pass between the lateral and medial pterygoid muscles to their terminal sites. However, the mandibular nerve is fixed between the mandibular foramen and foramen ovale and can be compressed as a result of both its course and its association with the surrounding structures, particularly when passing between the medial and lateral pterygoid muscles. Contraction of the pterygoid muscles may compress both the inferior alveolar and lingual nerves.

The varying anatomy of the posterior mandible and diverse positioning of the inferior alveolar nerve can pose a challenge for successful implant placement. Previous studies have attempted to quantify the adjacency of root apices to the mandibular canal, and some studies showed that the closest root was the distal root of the second molar. CBCT provides three-dimensional (3D) images with a moderate radiation dose, and numerous studies have reported its value in diagnosing spatial associations between anatomical structures [2-4]. Recent studies have approved the use of CBCT for assessing the distance between anatomical structures; CBCT is regarded as a credible and precise tool. The mental foramen in the edentulous mandible may be located at the crest of the alveolar ridge and may be traumatized by incision and flap elevation. Typically, panoramic radiography cannot visualize the entire course of the mandibular canal. The etiology of inferior alveolar nerve injury is commonly associated with insufficient planning of dental implant placement. Nerve injury can occur as a result of either miscalculating the nerve position from preoperative radiographic assessment during implant bed preparation or implant placement too apically into the nerve canal. CBCT can be utilized as part of treatment planning to not only plan for the location, implant size, and vector placement but also to identify and prevent mandibular canal injury.

If bone grafting is necessary for appropriate implant site development, CBCT is an important modality for evaluating ridge topography and 3D proximity to vital anatomical structures. Moreover, CBCT images are superior to those obtained using other two-dimensional imaging modalities. CBCT can accurately assess the thickness of cortical bone, such as the buccal/facial and lingual/palatal cortical plates, nasal cavity floor, and the medial and lateral walls of the maxillary sinuses, thereby aiding clinicians in identifying these important anatomical features to avoid potentially serious complications.

Conclusion

CBCT accurately predicts the dental implant size and the need for bone grafting. It should be reserved for cases in which guided surgery is planned because such cases involve a greater risk of injury to vital structures. Surgeons should continuously re-evaluate the necessity for 3D imaging as radiation exposure from CBCT decreases.

REFERENCES

[1] Benavides, E., Rios, H. F., Ganz, S. D., An, C. H., Resnik, R., Reardon, G. T., Feldman, S. J., Mah, J. K., Hatcher, D., Kim, M. J., Sohn, D. S. Use of cone beam tomography in implant dentistry: The International Congress of Oral Implantologists consensus report. *Implant Dent.,* 2012; 21: 78 - 86.

[2] De Oliviera-Santos, C., Souza, P. H. C., de Azambuja Berti-Couto, S., Stinkens, L., Moyaert, K., Rubira-Bullen, I. R., Jacobs, R. Assessment of variations of the mandibular canal through cone beam computed tomography. *Clin. Oral Investig.,* 2012. 16:387 - 393.

[3] Lin, M. H., Mau, L. P., Cochran, D. L., Shieh, Y. S., Huang, P. H., Huang, R. Y. Risk assessment of inferior alveolar nerve injury for immediate implant placement in the posterior mandible: A virtual implant placement study. *J. Dent.,* 2014; 42:263 - 270.

[4] Tepper, G., Hofschneider, U. B., Gahleitner, A., Ulm, C. Computed tomography diagnosis and localization of bone canals in mandibular region for prevention of bleeding complications during implant surgery. *Int. J. Oral Maxillofac. Implants,* 2001; 16:68 - 72.

In: Clinical Reports in Dentistry
Editor: Lisa R. Amir

ISBN: 978-1-53617-328-4

Chapter 10

Lateral Sinus Lift Procedure for Placement of Dental Implant in a Thin Maxillary Alveolar Bone: A Case Report

***Putri K. Santi*[1,*] *and Benny S. Latief*[2]**

[1]Oral and Maxillofacial Surgery Residency Program,
Faculty of Dentistry, Universitas Indonesia, Jakarta, Indonesia
[2]Department of Oral and Maxillofacial Surgery, Faculty of Dentistry,
Universitas Indonesia, Jakarta, Indonesia

Abstract

Introduction: The use of dental implants has gained popularity over the past few decades. However, sufficient vertical dimensions are a pre-requisite to warrant the success of these implants. Vertical bone defects including ridge resorption and sinus pneumatization frequently occur in the posterior maxillary region. Lateral sinus lift is one of the most extensively used augmentation procedures. The technique allows for the placement of an implant on the dorsal side of the maxilla where the quality of the alveolar bone is often poor due to the maxillary sinus. Herein we describe a case of vertical ridge augmentation using lateral sinus lift with simultaneous implant placement in the posterior maxillary region.

Case Report: A 52-year-old male with missing teeth (16 and 17) in the maxillary posterior region reported to our clinic. The height of alveolar ridge in the area was measured at 2.1 mm. Two threaded implants (width, 4.1 mm; length, 10 mm) were placed immediately after performing the lateral sinus lift and were surrounded with bone graft material.

Conclusion: Lateral sinus lift appears to be a useful pre-prosthetic surgical procedure for vertical augmentation of atrophied alveolar ridges with low sinus floors.

Keywords: alveolar ridge augmentation, vertical ridge augmentation, lateral sinus lifting

---

* Corresponding Author's Email: drg.putrikumala@gmail.com.

1. Introduction

The use of dental implants has gained immense popularity since the beginning of the era of modern dentistry. In addition to the restoration of chewing functions and aesthetics in partially edentulous patients, implants have proved extremely beneficial for the treatment and management of completely edentulous patients [1, 2]. Alveolar bone resorption along with sinus enlargement results in low bone altitude in some patients [3]. Pneumatization of the maxillary sinus causes a decrease in the vertical dimension of the alveolar bone, which can also be caused by tooth loss or periodontal disease. The thickness of the alveolar bone may be reduced to a few millimeters and remains so in areas that have been edentulous for extended periods of time [4-7]. Treatment using dental implants is feasible after judging the condition of the bone regarding both quantity and quality.

However, the presence of low amounts of alveolar bone can complicate the installation of these implants. This is most commonly observed in the posterior maxillary region where alveolar bone resorption and sinus pneumatization are exacerbated by poor bone quality. Maxillary sinus floor elevation is the treatment of choice for restoring the vertical dimension in these areas [1, 8].

Lateral sinus lift is one of the most extensively used vertical bone augmentation procedures because it enables implantation in the posterior maxilla, where the quality of the bone is generally poor [9]. Several studies have reported high survival rates of dental implants following the augmentation of the maxillary sinus [3]. Tatum et al. were the first to report that alveolar bone height can be augmented by lateral sinus lift and bone graft administration.

Since then, different types of techniques and grafting materials are used for the augmentation of alveolar bone height [4]. Several studies have shown that primary stability of simultaneous implants can be achieved when the remaining thickness of the alveolar bone (vertical dimension) is >5 mm. However, in cases wherein the residual thickness is <5 mm, a delayed two-stage approach has been recommended for improving the success of the implants [3]. The purpose of maxillary sinus augmentation is the restoration of the height of the alveolar ridge in the posterior region of the maxilla for the successful placement of the dental implant. The current paper presented a case wherein lateral sinus lift was performed followed by simultaneous implantation in the maxillary posterior region (residual alveolar bone thickness, <3 mm).

2. Case Report

A 52-year-old man reported to our clinic with the chief complaint of missing upper posterior teeth. History of the present illness revealed missing of the first and second upper right permanent molars due to caries. The patient did not have any other medical or family history of medical conditions. He was a non-smoker and appeared to be systemically healthy. Clinical examination revealed missing teeth (16 and 17), while panoramic radiography findings indicated that the bone height in the region was 2.1 mm (Figure 1). Subsequently, one-stage surgery was planned. The surgical procedure was explained to the patient and written informed consent was obtained.

The surgery was performed under general anesthesia. An incision was made on the alveolar ridge of the edentulous area. A window was created in the bone on the lateral and buccal sides of the teeth (16 and 17) using a round diamond bur with a large diameter until the sinus membrane was identified (Figure 2A,B). The buccal bone window was pushed into the sinus during membrane elevation. Sinus elevators with small heads and blunt surfaces were used for raising the sinus membrane. For the placement of bone graft material, the maxillary sinus membrane was reflected or separated from the sinus wall carefully to create a space for the graft.

After ensuring that no perforations had occurred within the sinus membrane, the space between the membrane and the sinus wall in the 16 and 17 regions was filled with a mixture of blood and particulate bovine bone graft (Bio-Oss, Switzerland)(Figure 2C). Two implants (Roxolid® SLA® active; Straumann), 4.1 mm in diameter and 10 mm in length were placed directly into the space that was filled with the bone graft material (Figure 2D). The mucoperiosteal flaps were approximated and sutures (Vicryl 4-0, Johnson & Johnson Medical, USA) were placed (Figure 2E).

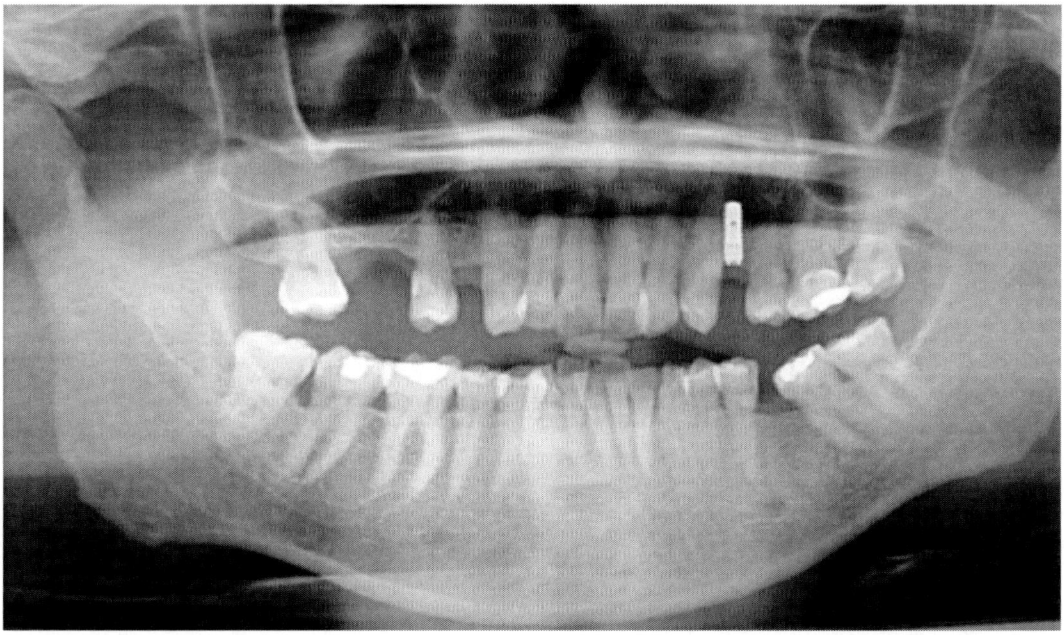

Figure 1. Panoramic radiograph showing bone loss in the region of tooth numbers 16 and 17.

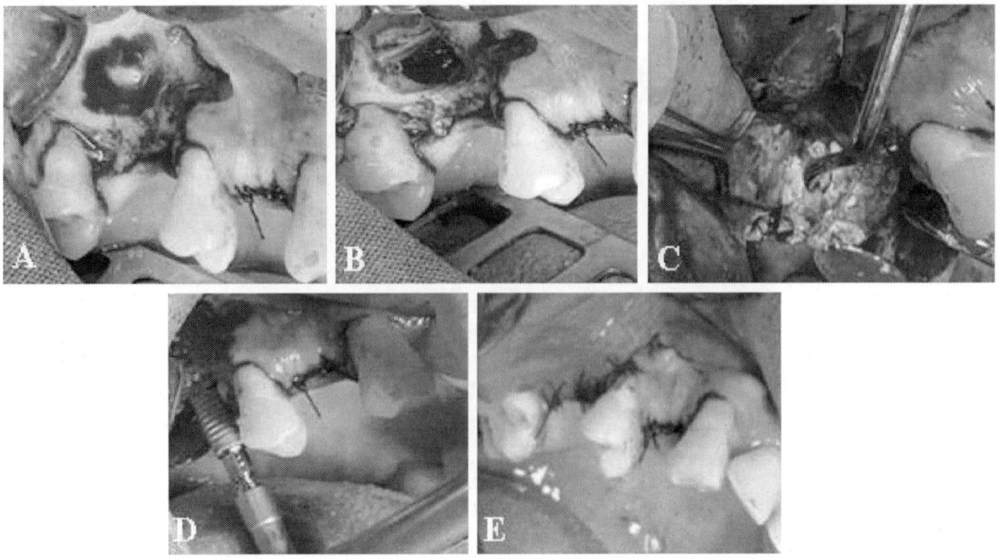

Figure 2. The procedure of surgery; Outlining of buccal window (A, B); Placement of graft material (C); Placement of implants (D); Primary approximation of mucoperiosteal flaps (E).

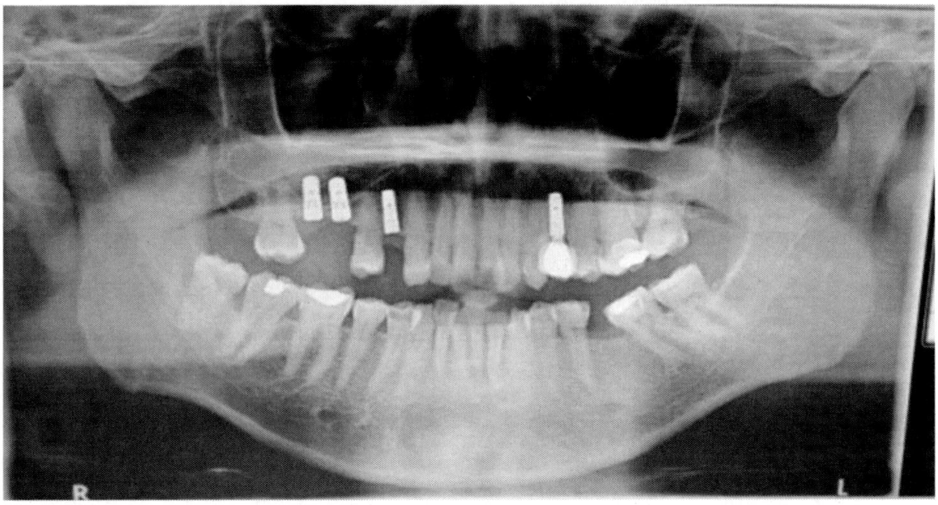

Figure 3. Panoramic image after implant placement.

Following treatment, the patient was advised to maintain oral hygiene using dental floss, toothbrush and chlorhexidine mouthwash and was instructed to visit the clinic at regular intervals.

Panoramic radiograph obtained immediately after sinus augmentation and implant placement shows the new osseous height achieved after the procedure (Figure 3). Based on the findings of present study, the protocol was developed for alveolar bone augmentation of the maxillary sinus (Table 1).

Table 1. Protocol for alveolar bone augmentation of the maxillary sinus

Height of Residual Alveolar Ridge	Technique	Time
<3 mm	one-stage procedure	lateral sinus lift followed by implant installation and loading within nine months
3-5 mm	one-stage procedure	lateral sinus lift followed by implant installation and loading within six months
>5 mm	one-stage procedure	lateral sinus lift followed by implant installation and loading within three months

3. DISCUSSION

Presently, dental implants are one of the most viable options available for the treatment of tooth loss. Implant placement becomes easy when the alveolar bone condition is adequate in its quantity and quality. However, bone resorption of the alveolar ridge necessitates an increase in bone volume before implant installation [10]. Osseointegration is crucial during the installation of dental implants and is influenced by the primary stability of the dental arch. The posterior maxillary region is the most challenging area for obtaining primary stability owing to its low bone density when compared with other areas in the jaw, thus resulting in decreased contact between the bone and the implant. During the process of mastication, the posterior maxillary region resists occlusal forces that are five times higher than those in the anterior region. Therefore, good bone condition in this region in terms of density and volume is a prerequisite for dental implants to function properly. Some studies have recommended the use of implants that are 4.0 mm or higher in diameter with a length of at least 10 mm to increase the primary stability and strength of the region [4].

The three methods of alveolar bone augmentation suggested by Tolstunov (2016) are as follows: lateral sinus augmentation followed by later implant placement; lateral sinus augmentation and implant placement in one-stage surgery; and lateral sinus augmentation and simultaneous implant placement using the osteotome technique. When the vertical dimension was <3 mm, lateral sinus augmentation was performed, followed by implant placement six months later, which was then followed by restoration of the implants within a period of four months. According to Kurtzman (2017), when the residual thickness of the alveolar bone is <5 mm, a delayed two-stage approach should be used for improved implant success [3]. In another study, delayed dental implant installation (after more than eight months) in a region with very thin alveolar bone (<3 mm) demonstrated a higher success rate when compared with implants placed after 4-8 months (97% vs. 84%, respectively) [11].

In the present case study, the remaining height of the alveolar bone was 2.1 mm. A one-stage procedure was performed, wherein the lateral sinus was lifted followed by simultaneous implant installation. Integration and restoration of the implants were planned to be completed nine months later. In the study by Jensen and Iacono (1996), no statistically significant difference between simultaneous and delayed placement of implants was noted [11]. Thus, based on the findings of present study and by adapting the guidelines proposed by Tolstunov, a protocol for alveolar bone augmentation of the maxillary sinus has been presented (Table 1). Lateral sinus lift for atrophic maxillae in the posterior region is gaining popularity as a well-established, predictable, and accepted procedure. In cases where the alveolar bone in edentulous posterior maxillary regions is thin, a one-stage procedure can be performed. In such cases, the protocol suggested in this case report for alveolar bone augmentation of the maxillary sinus may prove useful.

CONCLUSION

Lateral sinus lift for atrophic maxillae in the posterior region is gaining popularity as a well-established, predictable, and accepted procedure. In cases where the alveolar bone in edentulous posterior maxillary regions is thin, a one-stage procedure can be performed. In such cases, the protocol suggested in this case report for alveolar bone augmentation of the maxillary sinus may prove useful.

REFERENCES

[1] Helmy MA. (2017). Maxillary Sinus Lifting: Review of the Two Main Approaches. *Glob. J. Oto.*, 8(4):555745. doi:10.19080/GJO. 2017.08.555745.

[2] Esposito M, Grusovin MG, Rees J, et al. (2010). Effectiveness of sinus lift procedures for dental implant rehabilitation: a Cochrane systematic. *Eur. J. Oral Implantol.*, 3(1):7-26.

[3] Kurtzman GM. (2013). Lateral Sinus Augmentation: A Simplified Safer Approach. *Int. J. Oral Implantol. Clin. Res.*, 4(2):83-89. doi:10. 5005/JP-Journals-1012-1098.

[4] Tolstunov L. (2016). Implant diagnosis and treatment planning for the posterior edentulous maxilla. Vertical alveolar ridge augmentation in implant dentistry: a surgical manual. *J. Oral Implantol.*, 42(6):518.

[5] Pawar SK, Pawar HS, Sapra N, Ghangas P, Sangwan R. (2017). Maxillary Sinus Floor Elevation Techniques with Recent Advances: A Literature Review. *Asian Pac. J. Health Sci.*, 4(1):112-129. doi:10. 21276/apjhs.2017.4.1.20.

[6] Tarun Kumar AB, Anand U. (2015). Maxillary sinus augmentation. *J. Int. Clin. Dent. Res. Organ*, 7:81-93. doi:10.4103/2231-0754. 172935.

[7] Velázquez-cayón R, Torres-lagares D, Pérez-dorao B. (2012). Hydrodynamic ultrasonic maxillary sinus lift: Review of a new technique and presentation of a clinical case. *Med. Oral Patol. Oral Cir. Bucal*, 17(2):271-275. doi:10.4317/ medoral.17430.

[8] Balaji SM. (2013). Direct vs Indirect sinus lift in maxillary dental implants. *Ann. Maxillofac Surg.*, 3(2):148-153. doi:10.4103/2231-0746.119228.

[9] Pandit A, Chopra S. (2016). Maxillary Sinus Floor Elevation: Review of Anatomy and Lateral Sinus Lift Technique. *IOSR Journal of Dental and Medical Sciences*, 15(1):29-33. doi:10.9790/0853-15142933.

[10] Hu XL, Zhou X, Li JH, Lin Y. (2015). A New Technique for Minimally Invasive Maxillary Lateral Sinus Augmentation: a Case Report. *Chin. J. Dent. Res.*, 18(4):241-246. doi:10.3290/j.cjdr.a 35149.

[11] Jensen OT, Iacono VJ. (1998). Report of the Sinus Consensus Conference of 1996. *Int. J. Oral Maxillofac. Implants*, 13:11-45.

In: Clinical Reports in Dentistry
Editor: Lisa R. Amir
ISBN: 978-1-53617-328-4

Chapter 11

TREATMENT OF BILATERAL TEMPOROMANDIBULAR JOINT ANKYLOSIS WITH INTERPOSITIONAL TEMPORAL MUSCLE GRAFT ARTHROPLASTY: A CASE REPORT

Addys Rino[1], Wenny Yulvie[2] and Iwan Tofani[3,*]
[1]Oral and Maxillofacial Surgery Residency Program,
Faculty of Dentistry, Universitas Indonesia, Jakarta, Indonesia
[2]Division of Oral Maxillofacial and Surgery, Department of Dentistry,
Rumah Sakit Cipto Mangunkusumo, Jakarta, Indonesia
[3]Department of Oral and Maxillofacial Surgery, Faculty of Dentistry,
Universitas Indonesia, Jakarta, Indonesia

ABSTRACT

Introduction: Temporomandibular joint ankylosis (TMJA) is characterized by a limited range of motion of the mandible and is mainly caused by untreated trauma, TMJ surgery, or other diseases such as rheumatoid arthritis. Treatment of choice for TMJA is surgery with the following techniques: (1) gap arthroplasty, (2) interpositional muscle graft arthroplasty, and (3) total TMJ replacement with an autogenous or alloplastic graft. The primary objective of TMJA treatment is to restore joint function and prevent reankylosis. *Case Report:* A 13-year-old female was referred to our hospital with the chief complaint of having had difficulty in mouth opening over the past year. The patient had a history of a bicycle accident 2 years before presentation, during which she hit the sidewalk and suffered an open wound in the chin area without loss of consciousness. The wound was subsequently sutured at a hospital, and she was discharged without any medications. We performed bilateral interpositional temporal muscle graft arthroplasty. The patient showed uneventful postoperative healing with a 3-cm interincisal opening. *Conclusion:* Interpositional temporal muscle graft arthroplasty is suitable for the

* Corresponding Author's Email: iwan.tofani@yahoo.com.

treatment of bilateral temporomandibular joint ankylosis provided that regular physiotherapy and close follow-up are continued.

Keywords: temporomandibular joint ankylosis, interpositional temporal muscle graft arthroplasty, gap arthroplasty, rheumatoid arthritis

1. Introduction

Temporomandibular joint ankylosis (TMJA), characterized by restricted motion range of mouth opening, is a condition in which the mandibular condyle is fused to the glenoid fossa by bone or fibrous tissue. The most common etiology of TMJA is trauma, in particular condylar fracture. TMJA can induce distressing conditions such as impaired speech, difficulty in chewing, poor oral hygiene, facial disfigurement, and psychological stress, in addition to compromising the airway [1].

Surgery is the treatment of choice for TMJA with techniques comprising the following: (1) gap arthroplasty, (2) interpositional muscle graft arthroplasty and (3) reconstruction of the articulation following resection of the ankylotic mass with an autogenous or alloplastic graft [2]. The aims of the surgery included improvement in aesthetics, functionality and psychological stress and prevention of reankylosis. Following the surgery, other significant complementary treatment was physiotherapy in the form of intensive mouth-opening exercises [3]. Surgery for TMJA is commonly recommended immediately following diagnosis of the condition. The present case report presented the management of bilateral TMJA with interpositional temporal muscle graft arthroplasty.

2. Case Report

A 13-year-old female was referred to the Department of Oral and Maxillofacial Surgery at Rumah Sakit Cipto Mangunkusumo (Central Jakarta, Indonesia) for evaluation and treatment of bilateral TMJA. She had a history of bicycle accident 2 years prior to presentation, during which she hit the sidewalk. The patient suffered an open wound in the chin area but had no loss of consciousness, and she was brought to the emergency department in Serang City. The patient was subsequently sutured and discharged without any medications. A month prior to her referral, the patient had visited Serang General Hospital with the chief complaint of having had difficulty in mouth opening over the past year. Previous hypertension, diabetes mellitus and allergies were denied.

Extra-oral examination revealed no facial asymmetry, swelling, pain in the tragus area, or crepitation; the inter-incisal opening was 5 mm (Figure 1). Intra-oral examination revealed absence of malocclusion. CT examination showed irregularities and bilateral sclerotic fossa temporomandibular and mandibular condyles in addition to ankylosis in the temporomandibular joint (Figures 2A-C). We diagnosed the patient with bilateral temporomandibular joint ankylosis and planned to perform interpositional temporal muscle graft arthroplasty as a definitive treatment.

Inter-positional temporal muscle graft arthroplasty was initiated under general anesthesia. Access to the temporomandibular joint was designed using Al-Kayat's approach (Figure 3A)[4]. Local anesthesia was injected into the subcutaneous layer throughout the design, and a skin incision was performed along the incision design through the cutaneous, subcutaneous, and superficial fascia layers to the level of the temporal fascia. Blunt dissection was performed downward to a point approximately 2 cm above the zygomatic arch. Beginning at the root of the zygomatic arch, an incision running at a 45° angle upward and forward was performed through the temporal fascia (Figure 3B). Later, the periosteum of the zygomatic arch was securely incised, and the zygomatic arch bone was exposed. At this point, a small branch of the superficial temporal artery was encountered and safely ligated. Below the zygomatic arch, the ankylotic joint was exposed. Osteotomy was performed using a round bur and osteotome to create a 10-mm gap between the superior and inferior parts of the ankylotic joint (Figure 3C) Injury to the surrounding tissues was carefully avoided. Later, the contralateral ankylotic joint was performed using the same gap arthroplasty procedure. Mouth opening was checked, and a 30 mm intra-operative inter-incisal opening was achieved (Figure 3D).

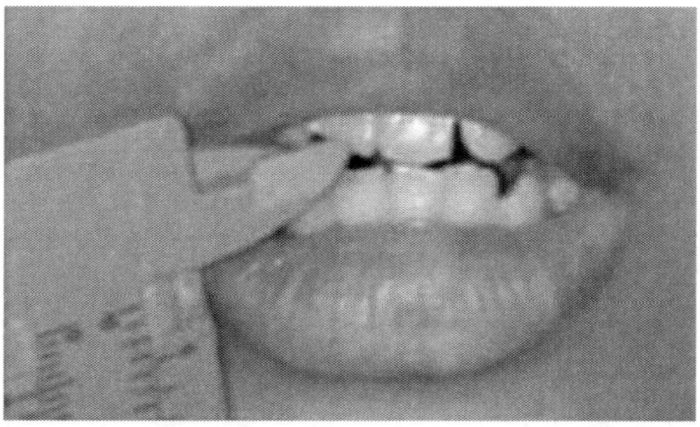

Figure 1. Preoperative mouth opening.

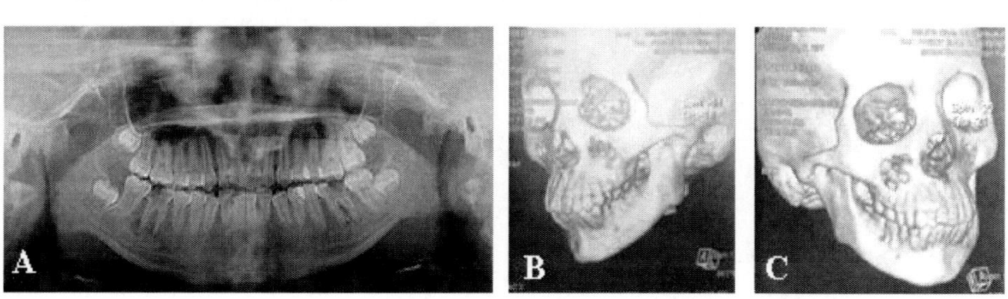

Figure 2. Panoramic imaging (A); CT imaging of the left (B) and right sides of the jaw (C).

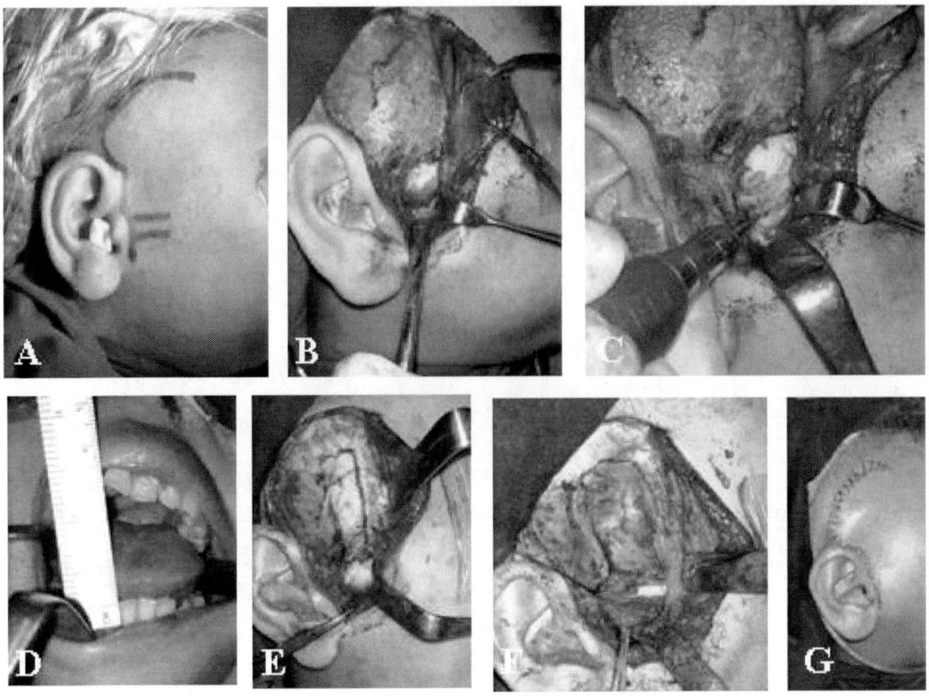

Figure 3. Design for Al-Kayat's approach (A); Exposure of the ankylosing joint. (B); Osteotomy of the ankylosing joint (C); Achievement of a 30-mm intraoperative interincisal opening (D); Design of the temporal muscle graft incision (E); Suture of the graft to the remaining surrounding muscle (F); Final suture (G).

To prevent re-ankylosis of the joints, temporal muscle graft arthroplasty was performed. Parallel incisions were made through the temporalis muscle (Figure 3E). Commencing from the top edge of the temporalis muscle, the flap was pull downward through the medial part of the zygomatic arch covering the glenoid fossa. The flap was subsequently sutured to the surrounding muscle, followed by verification that the muscle remained on top of the remaining condylar bone during mandibular function (Figure 3F). A bone-supported screw was placed, and rubber inter-maxillary fixation was assigned for occlusal guidance. A vacuum drain was left to prevent formation of dead space, and the incision was sutured in a layer-wise manner (Figure 3G). The postoperative facial nerve function was examined, and no facial paralysis was discovered. The post-operative inter-incisal opening was 20 mm, and the patient was given a mouth-opening physical therapy with ice cream sticks to increase the inter-incisal opening.

3. DISCUSSION

The etiology of TMJA varies from trauma (79%), infection (11.8%), birth trauma (forceps during delivery; 2.7%), to unknown cause (6.5%) [5]. Furthermore, the predisposition for TMJA is 47.62% in males and 52.38% in females [6]. In the present case, the patient was a 13-year-old female with an etiology of untreated trauma prior to TMJA. Duan et al. (2015) reported that disc displacement with sagittal fractures of the condyle indicate a high risk of ankyloses [7]. Another study by Xiang et al. (2014) indicated that fractures of the condylar head are more prone to postoperative ankylosis of the TMJ, and the risk factors appear to include the surgical technique used (miniplate fixation, wire fixation, and fragment removal), damage to the disc and persisting fractured fragment [8]. Pathological changes in TMJA described by Duan et al. (2015) involve not only the joint space but also the bone marrow showing osteoarthritis- and enthesopathy-like histopathological changes [7].

The main objectives of the treatment for TMJA are to improve aesthetics, functionality, psychological stress and to prevent re-ankylosis. Zhi et al. (2009) reported that joint reconstruction with inter-positional arthroplasty using the remaining disc, costochondral graft, or temporalis superficial fascia flap was effective in preventing recurrence and improving joint function [6]. Danda et al. (2009) concluded that there is no significant difference in the outcome between patients treated with inter-positional arthroplasty and those treated with gap arthroplasty [9]. Ma et al. (2015) stated in their meta-analysis research that inter-positional arthroplasty and gap arthroplasty showed no significant difference in terms of re-ankylosis incidence, but inter-positional arthroplasty resulted in a significantly larger inter-incisal opening. Moreover, prevention of re-ankylosis is recommended in the following way: (a) complete resection of the ankylosis; (b) use of appropriate inter-positional materials; (c) early mobilization; (d) inter-maxillary fixation is not recommended; (e) regular physiotherapy; (f) good cooperation and close follow-up [1]. De Roo et al. (2016) stated in their meta-analysis that the largest absolute increase in mouth opening is observed with reconstruction arthroplasty as compared with any other surgical technique [10].

Conclusion

Inter-positional temporal muscle graft arthroplasty as a treatment for TMJA is recommended provided that regular physiotherapy and close follow-up continues.

Acknowledgments

We thank Dr. drg. Pradono, SpBM who provided great insight and expertise and drg. Saifuddin Suhri for assistance in the operating room. We would also like to thank Dr. drg. Menik Priaminiarti, SpRKG for comments that greatly improved the manuscript.

REFERENCES

[1] Ma J, Liang L, Jiang H, Gu B. (2015). Gap arthroplasty versus interpositional arthroplasty for temporomandibular joint ankylosis: A meta-analysis. *PLoS One*, 10(5):1-12. https://www.ncbi.nlm.nih.gov/ pubmed/26010224.

[2] Yan YB, Liang SX, Shen J, Zhang JC, Zhang Y. (2014). Current concepts in the pathogenesis of traumatic temporomandibular joint ankylosis. *Head Face Med.*, 10(1):35-47. https://www.ncbi.nlm.nih. gov/pmc/articles/PMC4158390/.

[3] Cho JW, Park JH, Kim JW, Kim SJ. (2016). The sequential management of recurrent temporomandibular joint ankylosis in a growing child: a case report. *Maxillofac. Plast. Reconstr. Surg.*, 38(1):39-45. https://www.ncbi.nlm.nih.gov /pubmed/27774442.

[4] Al-Kayat A, Bramley P. (1979). A modified pre-auricular approach to the temporomandibular joint and malar arch. *Br. J. Oral Maxillofac. Surg.*, 17(2):91-103.

[5] Bhatt K, Roychoudhury A, Bhutia O, Pandey RM. (2014). Functional outcomes of gap and interposition arthroplasty in the treatment of temporomandibular joint ankylosis. *J. Oral Maxillofac. Surg*, 72(12):2434-9.

[6] Zhi K, Ren W, Zhou H, Gao L, Zhao L, Hou C, et al. (2009). Management of temporomandibular joint ankylosis: 11 years' clinical experience. *Oral Surg. Oral Med. Oral Pathol. Oral Radiol. Endod.*, 108(5):687-692. https://www.ncbi.nlm. nih.gov/pubmed/19782 622.

[7] Duan D, Li J, Xiao E, He L, Yan Y, Chen Y, et al. (2015). Histopathological features of hypertrophic bone mass of temporomandibular joint ankylosis (TMJA): An explanation of pathogenesis of TMJA. *J. Craniomaxillofac. Surg.*, 43(6):926-933. https://www.ncbi.nlm.nih.gov/pubmed/26026887.

[8] Xiang GL, Long X, Deng MH, Han QC, Meng QG, Li B. (2014). A retrospective study of temporomandibular joint ankylosis secondary to surgical treatment of mandibular condylar fractures. *Br. J. Oral Maxillofac. Surg.*, 52(3):270-274. https://www.ncbi.nlm.nih.gov/pub med/24485809.

[9] Danda AK, Ramkumar S, Chinnaswami R. (2009). Comparison of gap arthroplasty with and without a temporalis muscle flap for the treatment of ankylosis. *J. Oral Maxillofac. Surg.*, 67(7):1425-1431. https://www.ncbi.nlm.nih.gov/pubmed/1953 1413.

[10] De Roo N, Van Doorne L, Troch A, Vermeersch H, Brusselaers N. (2016). Quantifying the outcome of surgical treatment of temporomandibular joint ankylosis: A systematic review and meta-analysis. *J. Craniomaxillofac. Surg.*, 44(1):6-15. https://www.ncbi. nlm.nih.gov/pubmed/26433770.

In: Clinical Reports in Dentistry
Editor: Lisa R. Amir ISBN: 978-1-53617-328-4

Chapter 12

MAXILLARY TUBEROSITY TRIANGLE PHENOMENON IN IMPACTED UPPER THIRD MOLAR: A CASE REPORT

Tri H. Prasetyo[1,*] and Benny S. Latief[2]
[1]Oral and Maxillofacial Surgery Residency Program,
Faculty of Dentistry, Universitas Indonesia, Jakarta, Indonesia
[2]Department of Oral and Maxillofacial Surgery, Faculty of Dentistry,
Universitas Indonesia, Jakarta, Indonesia

ABSTRACT

Introduction: We reported a case of odontectomy of a Class C or grade 4 impacted upper left third molar (M3) that was surgically removed using alternative classification and technique.

Case Report: A 20-year-old woman presented with the chief complaint of pain in the upper left posterior jaw. Clinical examination showed a normal appearance without eruption of upper M3. Panoramic radiograph showed impacted 28 and 18 teeth at the apex region of 27 and 17. Odontectomy was performed in 15 minutes under general anesthesia. The incision was extended from the maxillary tuberosity to the mesial cervicobuccal region of teeth #28 and #16 and continued with a curved oblique buccal incision to the mucobuccal fold. The impacted upper M3 was clearly identified by the presence of bulging on the buccal maxillary bone. Finally, odontectomy and wound closure were performed.

Conclusion: An impacted upper M3 may be treated easily by understanding the surrounding anatomic structures. Oral surgery experts can also apply suitable surgical techniques to ease the odontectomy.

Keywords: maxillary tuberosity, maxillary sinus, impacted upper third molar, odontectomy

* Corresponding Author's Email: bennylatief@gmail.com.

1. INTRODUCTION

An impacted upper third molar (M3) is common in young patients of 20 – 29 years old. Clinical symptoms, such as pain or discomfort, may cause the patient to seek help. These cases require precision during surgical removal (odontectomy) by the oral surgery experts [1, 2].

The position of impacted upper third molars can be classified to Class A, B and C based on the vertical level of the adjacent upper second molar from the occlusal plane up to the apex. Furthermore, angulation was also described in this classification method (Figure 1).

Based on the investigator experience, an imaginary dimension was noted, known as the maxillary tuberosity triangle. This is an anatomic structure affecting the position of the impacted upper M3 and is formed by the maxillary sinus wall, the upper M3 and the maxillary tuberosity (Figure 2, 3). The maxillary tuberosity triangle influences the level of difficulty and the alternative techniques to perform M3 odontectomy [3,4].

Odontectomy of the upper M3 is generally performed by incising the buccal gingiva in a straight oblique manner starting from the middle cervical line of the upper M2 up to the mucobuccal fold of the upper M1 region.

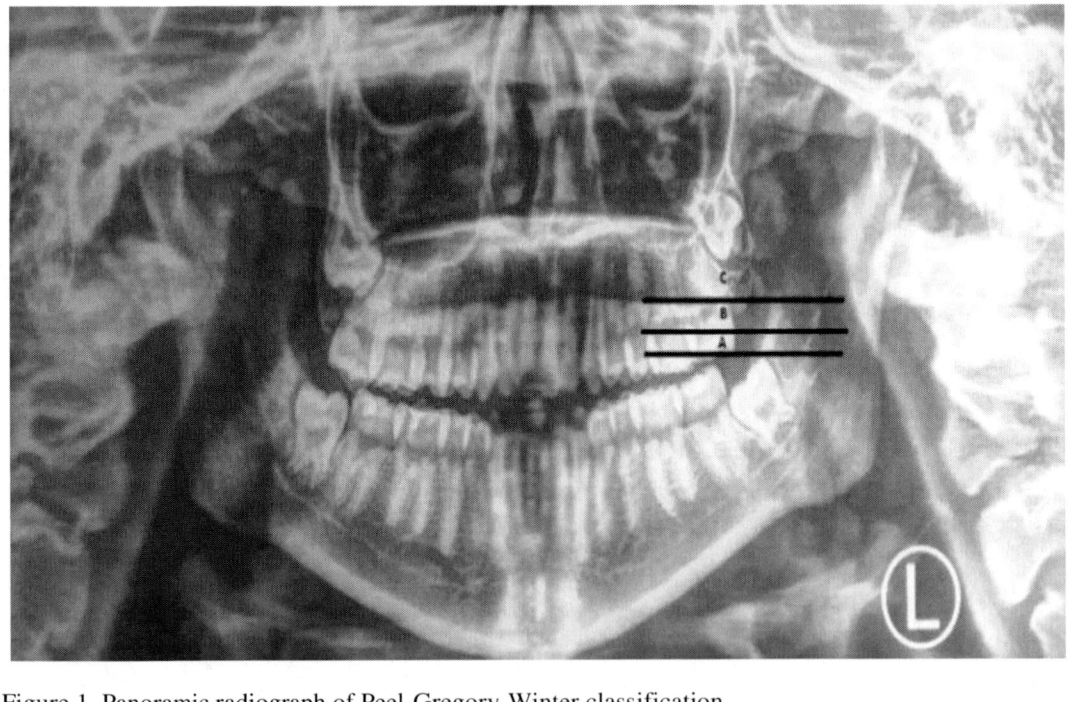

Figure 1. Panoramic radiograph of Peel-Gregory-Winter classification.

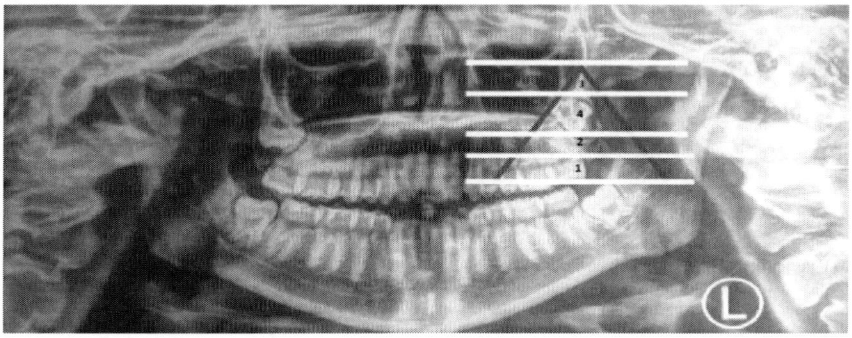

Figure 2. Alternative classification.

Additionally, a crest incision is made on the maxillary tuberosity region. A mucoperiosteal flap then is raised based on these incisions. An alternative technique is to perform a curved oblique incision and shift it mesially, which increases visibility to access the location of an impacted upper M3, Class C (Peel–Gregory–Winter classification). The zone in the peak of the triangle is not the most difficult position and it is especially easier to locate an impacted upper M3 due to the push force of the expanding maxillary sinus out to the buccal bone caused by the impacted tooth [2,4].

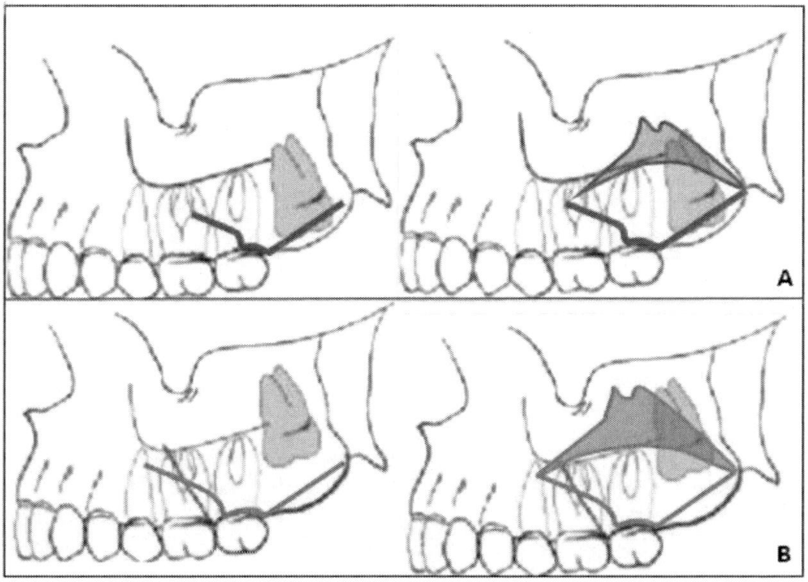

Figure 3. Envelope flap raised for lower position of the impacted M3 (A); Triangular flap designed for higher position of the impacted M3 (B).

2. Case Report

A 20-year-old woman presented to the Jakarta Hospital, Indonesia with the chief complaint of pain in the upper left posterior jaw that she could not locate exactly. Clinical examination showed a normal appearance. A panoramic radiograph showed 28 impacted tooth at the apex level of 27 tooth and 18 impacted tooth at the apex level of 17 tooth. Based on the Peel–Gregory–Winter classification, these impactions were considered as Class C (Figure 1). Alternatively, in the maxillary tuberosity triangle, the difficulty with odontectomy was categorized into the fourth zone (Figure 2). Both classes were categorized as the most difficult.

Odontectomy was performed with the patient under general anesthesia to eliminate intraoperative difficulty, as the patient still felt pain while under local anesthesia, as well as to achieve operative visibility easily. The vasoconstrictor was injected at the mucobuccal fold of the upper M3 region. Using a No. 15 blade, the incision extended from the maxillary tuberosity to the distal upper M1 and continued with a curved oblique incision to the mucobuccal fold of the upper M1 region. A flap was raised with a raspatorium and the impacted M3 was located by the presence of bulging (Figure 3). Using a No. 8 round bur (straight handpiece, 35.000 RPM) with normal saline irrigation, the bone surrounding the buccal side of the impacted tooth was reduced.

Odontectomy was performed using an elevator and the wound was irrigated with povidone iodine and sterile normal saline and closed with 3 - 0 absorbable suture. The same procedure was performed for 18 tooth (Figure 4).

One week postoperatively, the patient demonstrated healing gingiva and had no pain or swelling. The sutures were removed and the site was irrigated with povidone iodine and sterile normal saline. This procedure was performed within 15 minutes from the start of the incision until wound closure.

3. Discussion

Development of anatomic structures around the maxillary M3s, such as the maxillary sinus and maxillary tuberosity contributes to their eruption into the mouth [1].

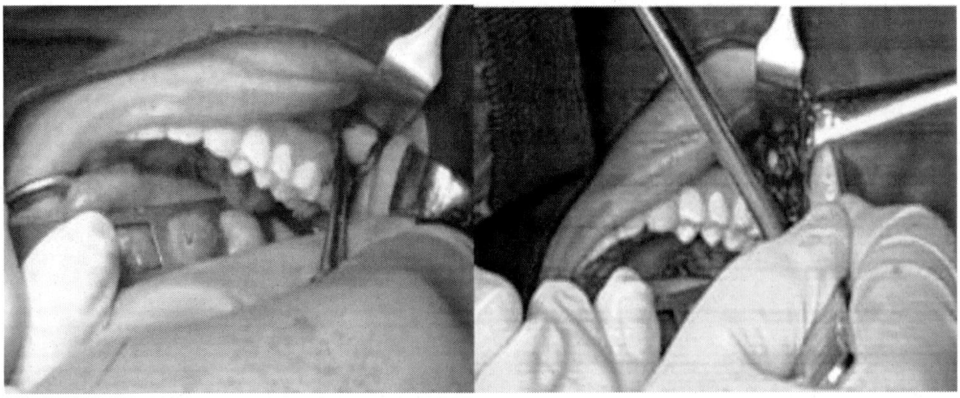

Figure 4. Incision designed to raise a buccal gingival flap in upper M3 odontectomy.

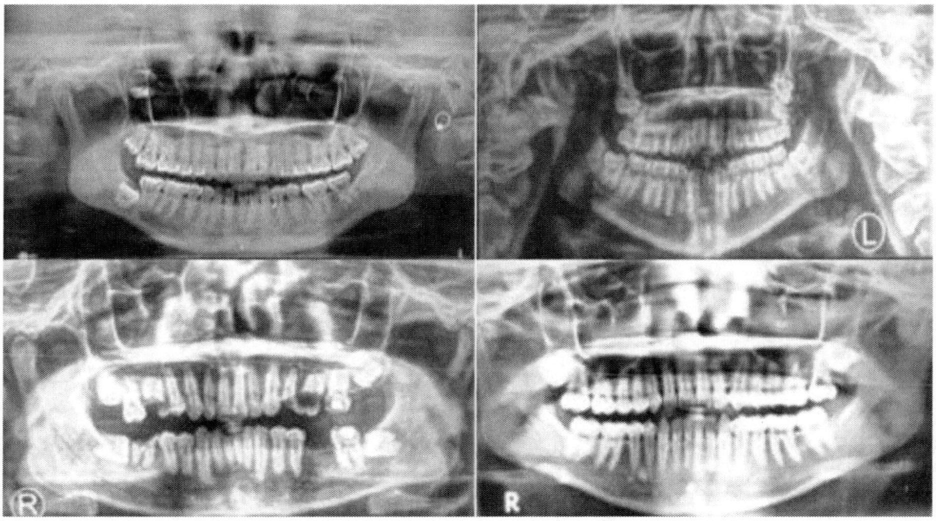

Figure 5. Panoramic radiograph appearance of the impacted upper and lower M3.

The maxillary sinus grows and evolves from ridges and furrows, beginning at the embryonal age of 8 weeks and continuing to adulthood. During its development, the maxillary sinus forms an air-filled cavity in a process of pneumatization.

The maxillary sinus wall is lined with mucoperiosteum, which facilitates pneumatization in the development of the sinus cavity. The cavity thus formed will push the anatomic structures around it, such as the zygomatic bone and maxilla, so that there is an increase in the dimension of the surrounding anatomic structures. The maxillary sinus cavity develops rapidly until the age of 14 years and then its development decreases until the age of 20 years [1, 2].

The growth of the upper M3 begins at the age of 7 years and normal eruption may occur between the ages of 19 and 21 years. Eruption of the upper M3 is often inhibited due to several factors resulting from the process of human evolution since the Neolithic era, in which the jaw function became more developed and due to the interdental friction that occurs as a result of the human diet and harder-textured foods compared to modern diets and refined food, so there is no mesiodistal dimensional deficiency of teeth before eruption of the upper M3 [2, 5]. The maxillary tuberosity is located at the posteroinferior maxilla, which is located in the distal upper M3. The maxillary tuberosity borders with the maxillary sinus in the caudal aspect and the distal side is adjacent to the pterygopalatine fissure and the pyramidal process of the palatine bone. The maxillary tuberosity shifts position according to the maxillary posterior teeth growth. Initially, the maxillary tuberosity is in the distal M1 of the upper jaw at the age of 6 years. Then, at 20 years, it shifts to the distal M3 of the upper jaw. It can be explained that late eruption of the posterior upper teeth of the upper jaw will lead to growth of the maxilla under normal size. The maxillary tuberosity growth slightly depends on the growth of the suture maturation, periosteal growth and maxillary sinus pneumatization. The peak of the maxillary tuberosity growth occurs upon eruption of the upper M2 and decreases gradually just before eruption of the upper M2 (between ages 8 – 11 years) [1, 5].

Cortical bone lining of the maxillary tuberosity continuity can be seen clearly on a panoramic radiograph. The radiopaque lining of the maxillary tuberosity shows continuity of the cortical bone surrounding the impacted upper M3 (Figure 5).

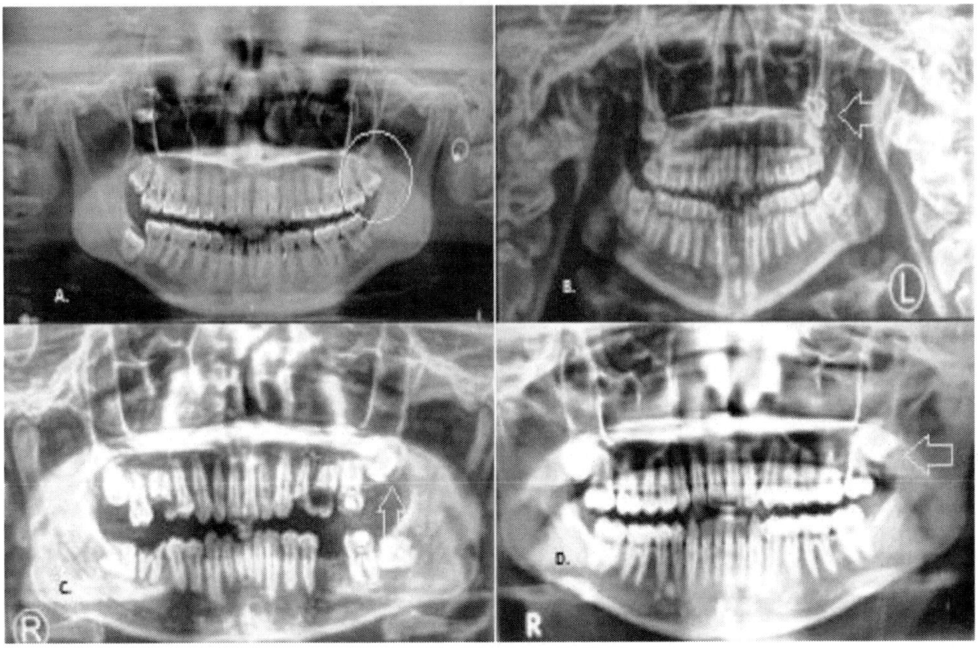

Figure 6. Panoramic X-ray shows white lining feature (yellow line). Note the continuity of the line.

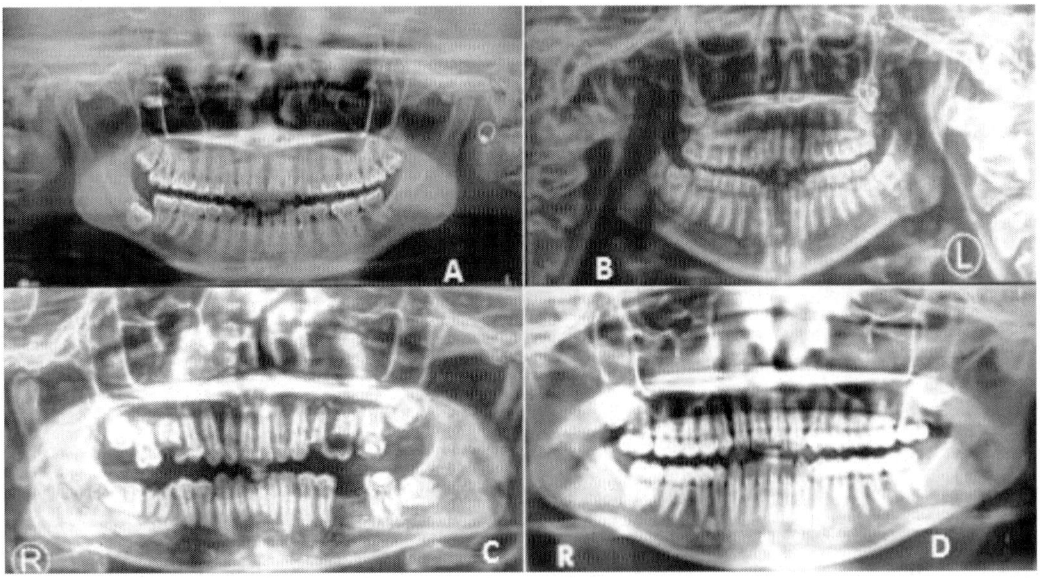

Figure 7. Peel–Gregory–Winter classification. (A) Class A. (B–D) Class C.

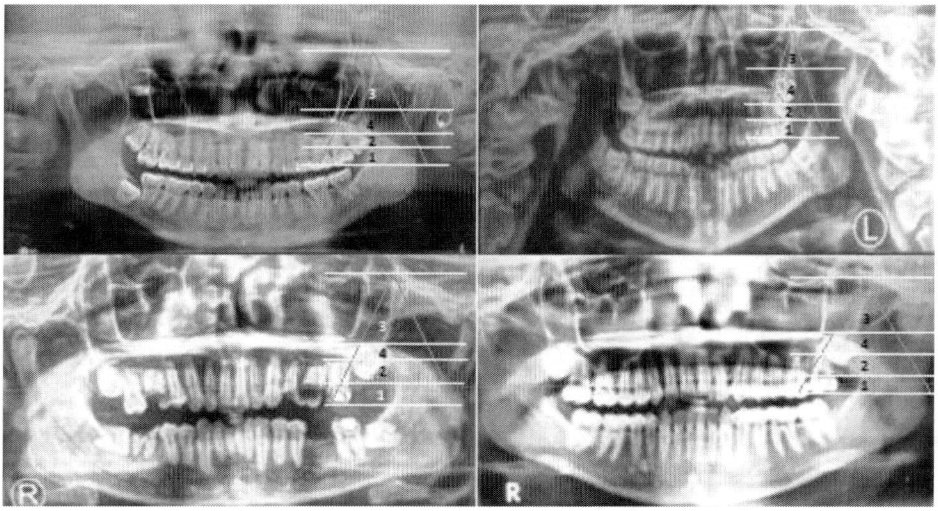

Figure 8. Zones of the impacted upper M3 in alternative classification.

Discontinuity of this lining implicates the lower level of difficulty to locate an impacted upper M3. The opposite condition is when an intact continuity is seen, implying a higher level of difficulty when performing odontectomy (Figure 6) [1]. An impacted upper M3 occurs frequently in oral surgery. In 2014, Pillai et al. studied 1,100 panoramic radiographs and found 2,210 (56.52%) impacted M3s, of which 20.81% were impacted upper M3s [3]. An impacted upper M3 is caused by various factors that inhibit tooth eruption, such as the smaller upper jaw arches compared to the upper tooth arch. The various positions of these impacted teeth require certain skills by the oral surgeon when performing odontectomy. The position of the impacted upper M3 can be estimated with a simple diagnostic procedure such as a panoramic radiograph (Figure 7) [4]. In fact, impacted upper M3s are always surrounded by three anatomic structures (the distal buccal wall of the maxillary sinus, the maxillary tuberosity and the impacted upper M3 itself), called the maxillary tuberosity triangle. We formulated the concept of a triangle made from three connected lines representing the maxillary sinus, the maxillary tuberosity and the upper M3. Then, five horizontal lines divide the triangle into four zones (Figure 3) as follows: (a) at the region of the triangle base; (b) above the line of the cervical erupted upper M1 or M2; (c) at the region above the maxillary tuberosity; and (d) between the horizontals line of the maxillary tuberosity and the impacted upper M3 apex (Figure 8).

Variation of the impacted upper M3 position requires the ability and experience of an oral surgeon in performing odontectomy [2]. Identification of the impacted upper M3 inside the maxillary bone should be performed carefully before grinding the maxillary bone using a bur to obtain proper access in odontectomy more efficiently. Growth of the maxillary sinus, eruption period of the upper M3, and growth of the maxillary tuberosity in the deficient the jaw arch will push the impacted upper M3 towards the buccal aspect of the maxillary bone. The maxillary tuberosity triangle will show a mark as a bulging or bone irregularity surrounding the impacted upper M3, which will help identifying the location of the deeply embedded upper M3 intra-operatively. In a study that included 8139 patients, Kauto et al. reported that odontectomy was performed at the age of 20 – 29 years in 2824 (34%) patients, 38% of whom had an impacted upper M3 [6]. This corresponded to the eruption period of the upper M3 in the maxillary tuberosity triangle and allowed sufficient time for emergence of clinical signs of the impacted M3 to settle on the distal buccal alveolar process of the maxilla. It also facilitated the identification of the location of the impacted tooth by the oral surgeons, even at a high position and when it was totally embedded inside the maxillary bone [1, 2].

Attention should be paid to the surgical technique (i.e., oblique incision) to raise a gingival buccal flap for achieving visibility of the surgical area. The higher the impacted upper M3 position, the more anterior incision must be made due to increased intra-operative visibility. In 2018, Emanueli et al. performed surgical removal of an impacted upper M3 [5]. We performed odontectomy for a class C or grade 3 impaction to identify the location of the impacted upper M3. In this case, it is useful to understand the maxillary tuberosity triangle phenomenon when performing odontectomy for an impacted upper M3 without additional instruments. Experience in performing the surgical removal of impacted teeth and understanding the alternative classification and technique could shortened the duration of operation.

Conclusion

Treating an impacted upper M3 could be challenging in cases of Class C or grade 3 and 4 impactions. By understanding the growth of surrounding anatomical structures that form particular signs, an oral surgeon can apply a suitable surgical technique to shorten the operative time for odontectomy.

References

[1] Killey, H. C, Kay, L. W. (1975). The maxillary sinus and its dental implications. In: *The Maxillary Sinus and Its Dental Implications.* Wright, Bristol.

[2] Adreasen, J. O., Ptersen, J. K. L. D. M. (1997). Textbook and Color Atlas of Tooth Impactions. 1st ed. Missouri: Mosby.

[3] Emanuelli, E., D. Borsetto, G. Brunello, S. S. (2018). Endoscopy-assisted removal through combined lower and middle meatotomies of an ectopic upper third molar in the sinus associated with a dentigerous cyst. *Oral Maxillofac. Surg. Cases,* 4:23 - 31.

[4] Aravindaksha, P. S. (2015). *Atlas of Oral and Maxillofacial Surgery.* Elsevier Health Sciences, London.

[5] Dan Vardimon, A., Shoshani, K., Shpack, N., Reimann, S., Bourauel, C., Brosh, T. (2010). Incremental growth of the maxillary tuberosity from 6 to 20 years-A cross-sectional study. *Arch. Oral Biol.,* 55(9): 655 - 662. doi:10.1016/j.archoralbio. 2010.05.012.

[6] Kautto, A., Vehkalahti, M. M., Ventä, I. (2018). Age of patient at the extraction of the third molar. *Int. J. Oral Maxillofac. Surg.,* 47(7): 947 - 951. doi:10.1016/j.ijom. 2018.03.020.

In: Clinical Reports in Dentistry
Editor: Lisa R. Amir

ISBN: 978-1-53617-328-4

Chapter 13

MANAGEMENT OF SCHNEIDERIAN MEMBRANE PERFORATION USING COLLAGEN MEMBRANE: A CASE REPORT

***Ken Ayu Miranthy*[1] *and Benny S. Latief*[2,*]**
[1]Oral and Maxillofacial Surgery Residency Program, Faculty of Dentistry, Universitas Indonesia, Jakarta, Indonesia
[2]Department of Oral and Maxillofacial Surgery, Faculty of Dentistry, Universitas Indonesia, Jakarta, Indonesia

ABSTRACT

Introduction: Dental implants are widely used for replacing teeth loss. Sinus augmentation is one of the procedures used to obtain increased vertical height for dental implant placement when the proportional bone height is not achieved. The most common complication during this procedure is *Scheneiderian* membrane perforation, which can be managed using collagen membranes.

Case report: A case of *Schneiderian* membrane perforation that occurred during a sinus augmentation procedure and was subsequently managed using a collagen membrane. A 51-year-old female patient with missing teeth numbers 14, 15, 16, 17 and with an alveolar height less than 3 cm. The *Schneiderian* membrane perforation was managed using tissue additives and a collagen membrane followed by bone graft particulate and dental implant placement.

Conclusion: The treatment of *Schneiderian* membrane perforation can be effectively managed using collagen membrane.

Keywords: Schneiderian membrane perforation, collagen membrane, sinus lift

---

* Corresponding Author's Email: bennylatief@gmail.com.

1. Introduction

These days, dental procedures for mouth rehabilitation using dental implants in edentulous areas with challenging anatomical sinus maxillaries are not avoidable. Thus, it is essential to develop standardized, predictable, and safe procedures to gain optimum results. Sinus augmentation is known to be one of the most suitable techniques for obtaining favorable height and width to place dental implants.

The primary goal of this technique is to improve bone volumes where there is a lack thereof for implant placement because of alveolar ridge atrophy or sinus expansion. The most common site of insufficient vertical dimension bone volume is the posterior maxilla. Sinus augmentation in conjunction with implant placement is the most common procedure for treatment of this area, followed by immediate bone graft. Sinus augmentation with implant placement has a high success rate, falling in the range of 98.6% – 93.5% after 3 – 5 years of use [1].

Several categories of complications arise during sinus augmentation, including intra-operative, early post-operative, and late post-operative complications. Even though these complications are very infrequent, one of the most common intra-operative complications is *Schneiderian* membrane perforation, with an incidence perforation approximately 10% – 60% of cases [1,2]. *Schneiderian* membrane perforation may occur because of an iatrogenic and challenging anatomy such as the presence of septum, sinus pathology, previous entrance into the sinus, or overfilling at the time of graft placement [2]. The perforation of the *Schneiderian* membrane has some impacts, such as impairment of the functional homeostasis of the antral cavity, which could affect the outcome of surgery caused by bacterial contamination of the graft [3]. Therefore, several techniques have been developed to manage such complications.

Perforation of the *Schneiderian* membrane is typically managed using graft material. Various techniques have been advocated for management of *Schneiderian* membrane perforation during sinus augmentation. The first technique discovered for the management of these perforations is known as the Loma Linda pouch, which was further developed as the modified pouch technique [3]. This technique is performed by covering the perforated membrane with collagen, simulating the natural membrane, with the graft material itself then covered by folding the membrane. The purpose of this study was to report the management of *Schneiderian* membrane perforation using soaked collagen membranes and xenograft material followed by implant placement.

2. Case Report

A 51-year-old female patient underwent oral and maxillofacial surgery for the rehabilitation of the edentulous region. Her complaint included dissatisfaction with the esthetic as well as difficulties in mastication and she wanted to replace her posterior teeth with fixed prosthesis, which has been previously lost due to extensive caries. Neither abnormal medical history nor previous systemic illness was found and she did not exhibit habits correlated with poor oral hygiene and never experienced swelling in her jaw due to toothache.

Clinical and radiographic examination revealed the absence of tooth elements left maxillary second permanent premolar, first permanent molar and second permanent molar (#15-#17)(Figure 1). On the basis of radiographic examination, the height of the alveolar crest was less than 3 cm to the base of maxillary sinus. Sinus augmentation was performed to gain an adequate crest height. Infiltration using a mixture of lidocaine and epinephrine 1:80,000 solution was carried out in the vestibular region of 15, 16, 17 and palate region.

A triangular incision with full thickness flap was made along teeth #14-#17 (Figure 2). Subsequently, a rotary instrument was used to reach the *Schneiderian* membrane and a hand instrument smoothly and gently elevated the membrane. The perforation of the *Schneiderian* membrane was identified, and a soaked collagen membrane was used to cover its perforation. This procedure was followed by implant placement and bone graft administration (Figure 3).

3. Discussion

Sinus augmentation is the most commonly performed procedure for preparing the of implants placement in the anthropic maxillary posterior region.

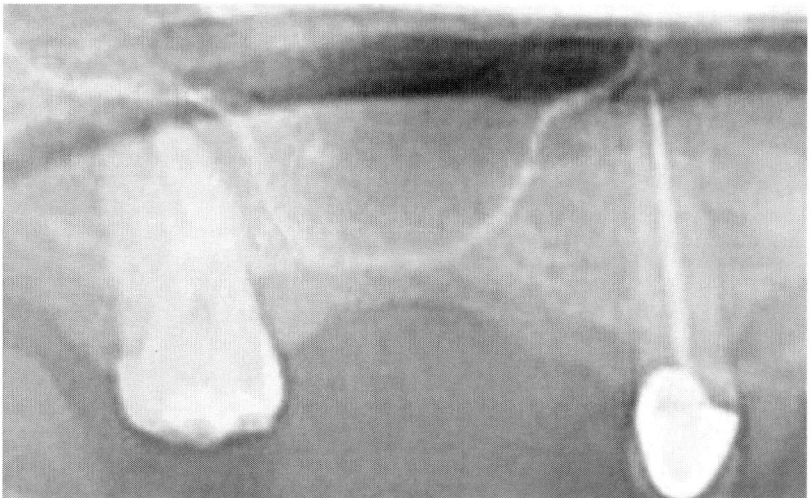

Figure 1. Radiograph before sinus augmentation.

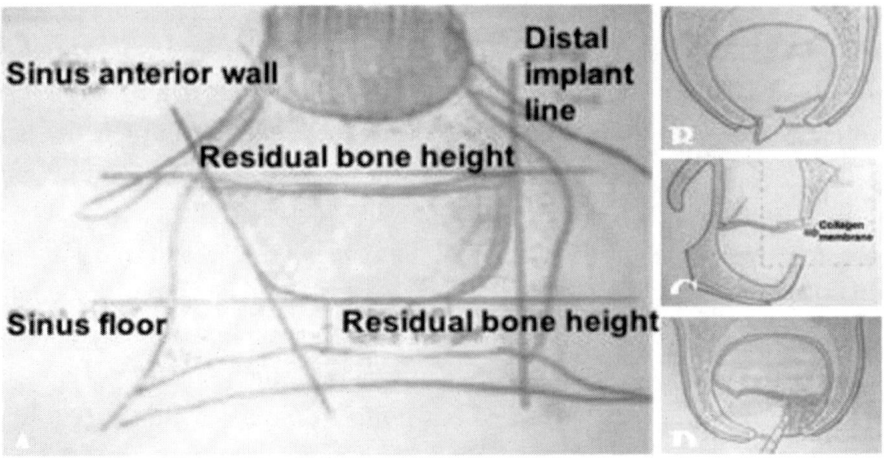

Figure 2. Full thickness flap was made to reveal alveolar bone (A); Management of Schneiderian membrane perforation: Identification of Schneiderian membrane perforation (B); A soaked collagen membrane was used to cover perforation of the Schneiderian membrane (C); Graft material followed with implant placement (D).

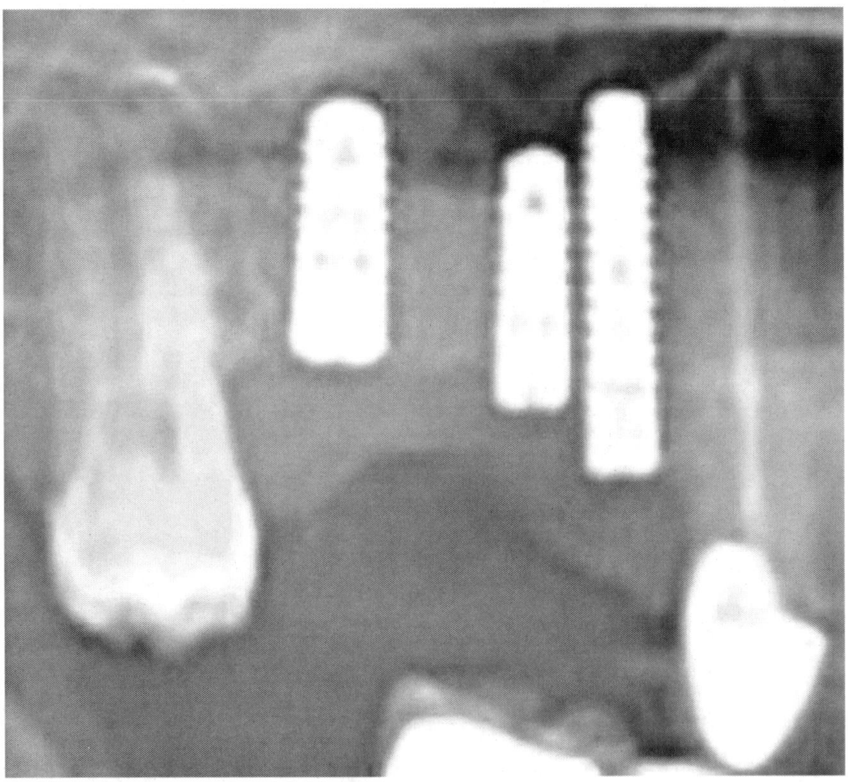

Figure 3. Radiograph control shows the ideal bone height and stability of the achieved implant.

Nevertheless, this technique is not without complications. On the basis of various studies, reported complication rate of this procedure is very low, which encompass those related to systemic disease, infection, prosthetics, anatomy, and surgical procedures [4,5]. The most common intra-operative complications arising from anatomy and surgical procedures are *Schneiderian* membrane perforations, with a prevalence rate of 10%–55% [2]. Barone et al. reported an implant survival rate in sinus augmentation with *Schneiderian* membrane perforation at about 94.3% [6]. In these cases, sinus augmentation with *Schneiderian* membrane perforation resulted in the achievement of desirable height and stability of the implant.

As previously indicated, *Schneiderian* membrane perforation can cause postoperative complications following sinus augmentation. The *Schneiderian* membrane consists of a pseudociliated stratified respiratory epithelium that plays an important role in the protection of the maxillary sinus. During sinus augmentation the *Schneiderian* membrane can be damaged, and as a result there could be communication between sinus maxillary cavity and the graft material.

Losing the biological barrier could contaminate the sinus cavity, which could become more susceptible to infection [5, 7]. On the contrary, Schwartz–Arad et al. reported no correlation between *Schneiderian* membrane perforation or post-operative complications and implant survival rate [7]. Ardekian et al. also reported that *Schneiderian* membrane perforation did not predispose to sinusitis. Along with others, Jensen et al. reported that a small *Schneiderian* membrane perforation showed complete and spontaneous regeneration [4].

There are various maneuvers performed during sinus augmentation that could put the *Schneiderian* membrane at risk of perforation. Flap elevation while placing an elevator on a thin crestal or lateral wall could traumatize the membrane. The preparation of a lateral window using rotary instruments is reported to be a predisposing factor that could lead to membrane perforation [8]. The placement of graft material with excessive pressure could also disrupt the *Schneiderian* membrane. Patil et al. stated that the elevation of the *Schneiderian* membrane with hand instruments in a medial direction and placing the elevator in close proximity to septa could also make the membrane more susceptible to perforation [8,9].

According to the study conducted by Gehrke et al., *Schneiderian* membrane perforation should not be considered as an absolute contraindication for immediate implant placement [9]. Numerous authors advocated *Schneiderian* membrane perforation treatment using membrane collagen followed by graft material. As Patil et al. reported, implant survival rate could reach above 95% by taking into consideration graft material, implant surfaces, and the membrane in the lateral window. Using soaked collagen membrane over the *Schneiderian* membrane overlaid with graft material was found to be successful in this case.

In addition to the collagen membrane and graft material used for the management of *Schneiderian* membrane perforation, the reparation technique should also be taken into account. This technique to repair membrane perforation, first defined as the Loma Linda pouch technique, involves the placement of the collagen membrane over the perforation membrane to surround and isolate the graft material [9].

Conclusion

Sinus augmentation is the most common procedure used to increase the height of the alveolar bone for implant placement. This procedure has a high predictable success rate with minimal complications. However, *Schneiderian* membrane perforation is the most frequent complication during sinus augmentation, occurring in 7%–35% of sinus augmentation procedures. Perforation of the *Schneiderian* membrane often occurs due to a challenging anatomy or operational maneuvers performed during the procedure. Since this could cause postoperative complications, it must be well managed to prevent further issues. There are many solutions advocated by researchers, such as the application of a collagen membrane followed by graft materials, employment of several techniques, and flaps. One technique that is often used to manage *Schneiderian* membrane perforation is the modified pouch technique, in which the graft material is fully covered by a collagen membrane on one side, with the side lateral to the bone walls without the collagen membrane. The purpose of this technique is to allow the graft material to obtain enough vascularization from the blood supply, thereby integrating the graft material faster to the environment with increased bone stimulation.

References

[1] Irinakis, T., Dabuleanu, I., Aldahlawi, S. (2017). Complications during maxillary sinus augmentation associated with interfering septa: a new classification of septa. *Open Dent. J.*, (11):140 - 150.

[2] Nolan, P. J., Freeman, K., Kraut, R. A. (2014). Correlation between Schneiderian membrane perforation and sinus lift graft outcome: a retrospective evaluation of 359 augmented sinus. *J. Oral Maxillofac. Surg.*, (72):47 - 52.

[3] Meleo, D., Mangione, F., Corbi, S., Pacifici, L. (2012). Management of the Schneiderian membrane perforation during the maxillary sinus elevation procedure: a case report. *Annali di Stomatologia*, (III): 24 - 30.

[4] Aredkian, L., Peleg, E., Mactei, E., Peled, M. (2006). The clinical significance of sinus membrane perforation during augmentation of the maxillary sinus. *J. Oral Maxillofac. Surg.*, (64):277 - 282.

[5] Katarani, A., Fotek, P., Wang, H.-W. (2008). Sinus augmentation complications: etiology and treatment. *Implant Dent.*, (III), 339.

[6] Barone, A., Santini, S., Sbordone, L., Cres pi, R., Covani, U. (2006). A clinical study of the outcomes and complications associated with maxillary sinus augmentation. *Int. J. Oral Maxillofac. Implants*, (2):81.

[7] Gehrke, S. A., Taschieri, S., Fabbro, M.-D., Corbela, S. (2012). Repair of a perforated sinus membrane with a subepithelial palatal conjunctive flap: technique report and evaluation. *Inter. J. Dent.*, 1 - 7: 489762.

[8] Patil, P. S., Bhongade, M. L. (2016). Sinus augmentation complications: part-i associated with lateral technique (direct approach): a review. *Journal of Implant and Adv. Clin. Dent.*, (VIII): 6 - 13.

[9] Jensen, J., Sindet-Pedersen, S., Oliver, A. J. (1995). Varying treatment strategies for reconstruction of maxillary atrophy with implants: results in 98 patients. *J. Oral Maxillofac. Surg.*, (2): 210 - 216.

In: Clinical Reports in Dentistry
Editor: Lisa R. Amir
ISBN: 978-1-53617-328-4

Chapter 14

FREE FIBULAR FLAP AND DELTOPECTORAL FLAP FOR RECONSTRUCTION OF DEFECT CAUSED BY ADVANCED SQUAMOUS CELL CARCINOMA OF MANDIBLE

***Yi-Tzu Chen*[1,2,*] *, Pei-Yin Chen*[1] *and Hsueh-Ju Lu*[3,4]**
[1]Department of Oral and Maxillofacial Surgery,
Chung Shan Medical University Hospital, Taichung, Taiwan
[2]School of Dentistry, College of Oral Medicine,
Chung Shan Medical University, Taichung, Taiwan
[3]Division of Medical Oncology, Department of Internal Medicine,
Chung Shan Medical University Hospital, Taichung, Taiwan
[4]School of Medicine, Chung Shan Medical University, Taichung, Taiwan

ABSTRACT

Introduction: Oral squamous cell carcinoma (OSCC) of the mandible is characterized as tumors developing adjacent to the mandibular bone, including the mandibular alveolar ridge, lower buccal sulcus, sublingual sulcus and mandibular retromolar area. The first choice of therapy for most resectable stages is surgical treatment. However, mandibular reconstruction is a challenge associated with postoperative aesthetics and functional outcomes. Although aggressive treatment has improved local and regional tumor control, a number of patients still die of distant metastases.

Case Report: A 72-year-old male was diagnosed with OSCC of the inner mucosa of the lower lip, gingiva, cheek and mandible (cT4aN2bM0 stage IV in July 2017). Owing to an extensive lesion, induction chemotherapy was initially undertaken. Although the original mucosal lesion was nearly resolved after chemotherapy, a progressive bony

* Corresponding Author's Email: chenyitzu0831@gmail.com.

lesion was observed. Accordingly, the patient underwent segmental mandibulectomy, bilateral neck dissection and reconstruction with free fibula flap and *deltopectoral* (DP) *flap*. The final pathology results showed moderately differentiated SCC pyT4aN2bM0 at stage IV. He underwent adjuvant treatment postoperatively. However, bilateral lung metastases occurred when palliative chemotherapy and supportive care were undergoing.

Conclusion: Early operative treatment should be an option for patients suffering from a progressive head and neck tumor, which may help achieve considerably better life expectancy and quality of life for a longer period.

Keywords: squamous cell carcinoma, mandible, virtual surgical planning, double flap, prognostic factors

1. Introduction

The diagnosis, surgical techniques, treatment results and prognosis of carcinoma in mandibular region remain a challenge. The disease may interrupt the innervation of sensory and motor nerves, resulting in serious problems with mastication, swallowing and speech. Surgery is the initial definitive treatment for the majority of oral cancers. However, in poor mandibular reconstruction, the functional, aesthetic and social consequences that may lead to poor quality of life (QoL).

Fibula free flaps are currently the most popular flaps for mandibular reconstruction with the advantages of consistent shape, abundant length, distant location to allow a two-team approach, and low complication rate. It can provide up to 25 cm of dense cortical bone based on the peroneal artery, and skin paddles based on septocutaneous as well as on musculocutaneous peroneal perforators as large as 10x20 cm in the adult. Nowadays various advances in this surgical technique have developed for the reconstruction, and this technique has been shown minimize these consequences and improve the outcomes [1-4].

Adjuvant concurrent chemoradiotherapy (CCRT) improves the outcomes in advanced-stage disease. Generally, the following factors are associated with local control and prognosis in oral cancer patients: clinical and pathological TNM stage, tumor thickness (depth of invasion), nerve invasion, and cervical lymph node status [5,6]. Hoffmannová et al. reported that an increase in tumor size was associated with decreased survival rate [7]. In addition, therapeutic neck dissection significantly reduced survival rate and elevated lymph node relapse. They also noted that >21% of the patients with distant metastases survived 5 years post-operation [8]. Hence, we described a case of advanced-stage oral squamous cell carcinoma (OSCC) involving the mandible, cheek, and inner mucosa of the lower lip. In addition, double-flap reconstruction was performed and a follow-up of the disease progression with a review of the related literature are provided.

2. Case Report

A 72-year-old male visited our outpatient department in July 2017 and complained of pain and swelling in his lower jaw for four months. Related risk factors included smoking and *betel quid chewing* for 30 years. No alcohol consumption or specific systemic disease were reported. Examination revealed a limited opening of the mouth as small as 15 mm, an approximately 70 × 40 mm exophytic indurated mass over the lower left 2nd premolar to the right 1st premolar, severe mobility of all teeth, and extended lower vestibule and anterior mouth floor (Figure 1). Numbness over the left lower lip was also observed, and a non-tender lymph node over the left submandibular area was palpable. This diffuse radiolucent shadow extended from the distal root of his left 1st molar to right 1st premolar and involved the cortical outline of the mandibular canal inferiorly were noted through panoramic radiograph (Figure 2). Furthermore, incisional biopsy revealed a moderately differentiated OSCC. Magnetic resonance imaging showed a large infiltrative contrast-enhancing lesion (approximate size, 74 × 42 mm) predominantly over the left anterior lower buccal gingiva, right anterior lower buccal gingiva, anterior mouth floor and close to the facial skin over the anterior mandibular region, involving the mandibular body. Abdominal ultrasound and chest X-ray were performed to determine metastasis. Whole-body fluorine-18-fluorodeoxyglucose positron emission tomographic/computed tomographic (PET/CT) scan revealed increased glucose metabolism in a lesion of the left anterior lower buccal gingival region including the mandibular body and mouth floor. Multiple level II lymph nodes over the left neck also indicated probability of malignancy. Notably, no definite evidence of distant metastases was observed. The clinical stage cT4aN2bM0 was suggested based on AJCC 7th Edition.

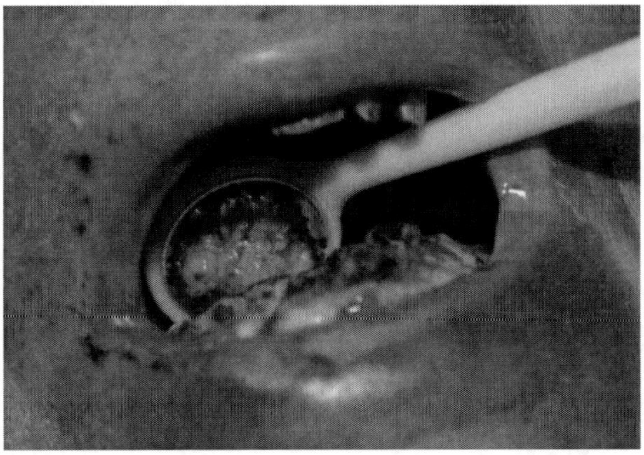

Figure 1. Approximately 70 × 40 mm exophytic indurated mass extended the lower vestibule and anterior mouth floor was noted with limited mouth opening.

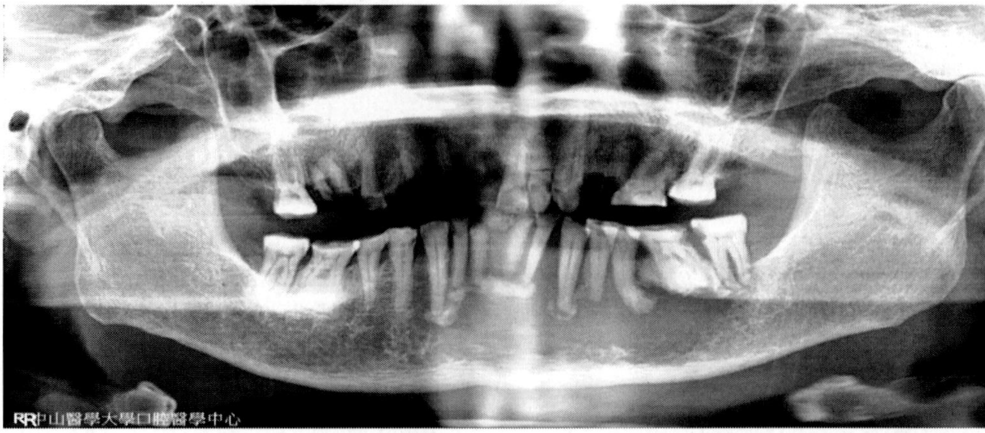

Figure 2. Image of ill-defined bony destruction between the lower left 1st molar to right 1st premolar.

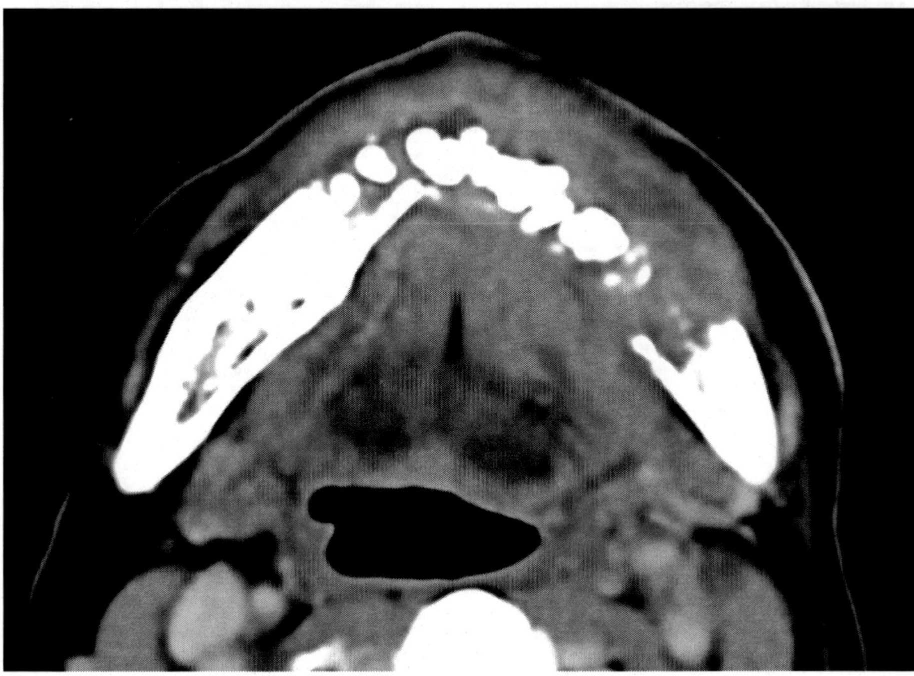

Figure 3. CT scan revealing an extensive and ill-defined bony destruction with perforation of the buccal and lingual cortical plates.

Considering the widespread involvement and borderline respectability, the patient was treated with a modified biweekly TPF regimen comprised of three cycles, with docetaxel 20 mg/m^2 weekly on day 1, 8, repeated every two weeks for three cycles, was adjusted in our daily practice [9].

The patient tolerated induction chemotherapy well without any toxicity. On completion of three cycles, marked reduction of the tumor volume with near-total response was established, but a progressive bony invasion was *observed* (Figure 3). Accordingly, urgent definite surgery was suggested.

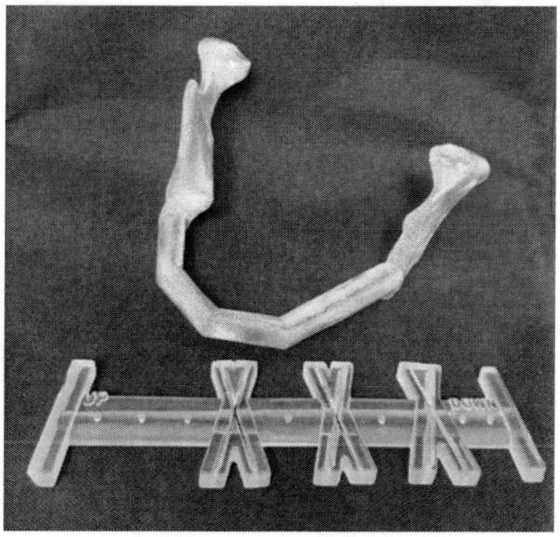

Figure 4. Mandibular defect type displayed as LCL (based on HCL system [10]). Fibular cutting guide was provided with fixation holes for temporary fixation.

Computed tomographic (CT) scan with 1-mm fine slices were used for preoperative 4-segment virtual surgical planning (VSP; Materialize, USA) for bony reconstruction. After a virtual planning session, anatomic resin models (pre- and postoperative) and cutting guides were produced (Figure 4), and a pre-bent 2-mm semi-reconstruction bar was prepared preoperatively (Stryker, USA).

The patient underwent segmental mandibulectomy and bilateral supraomohyoid neck dissection after tracheostomy. Reconstructions were performed by simultaneous transplantation of the right fibula free and regional DP flaps as planned. Further, the peroneal artery was revascularized using end-to-end microsurgical techniques to the left facial artery. The surgical outcomes are presented in Figure 5A. Then, the DP flap was detached from the chest 18 days postoperative. No major per- or postoperative complications were noted, and acceptable functional and aesthetic results were achieved (Figure 5B). Mouth opening was about 20 mm between edentulous ridges because of residual submucosal fibrosis. Laterotrusion bilaterally showed about 3 mm. Subjective satisfaction with eating and chewing was well (Figure 6B). Histopathological examination revealed a moderately differentiated SCC, ypT4aN2b (Figure 7A). The tumor margin was free of invasive carcinoma (<1 mm from the closest base margin and the anterior margin of the buccal gingiva), 3.3 cm away from left margin of mandibular bone, and 3.2 cm away right margin of mandibular bone. Multiple lymph nodes metastasis with extracapsular spread (Figure 7B), perineural invasion and lymphovascular permeation were present.

Due to the age of the patient and poor performance status, adjuvant radiotherapy was indicated for him with a low accumulation of 60 Gy. Disease progression with bilateral lung metastasis was detected in March 2018. Progression-free survival was 7.9 months. Then, palliative chemotherapy was administered with paclitaxel 100 mg/m^2 on days 1, 8; cisplatin 25 mg/m^2 on days 1, 8, repeated every 3 weeks for up to 6 cycles; and cetuximab at an initial dose of 400 mg/m^2, followed by 250 mg/m^2 weekly until disease progression [11]. Until the last follow-up, overall survival was 12.4 months and ongoing. Patient's consent to publish photograph was obtained.

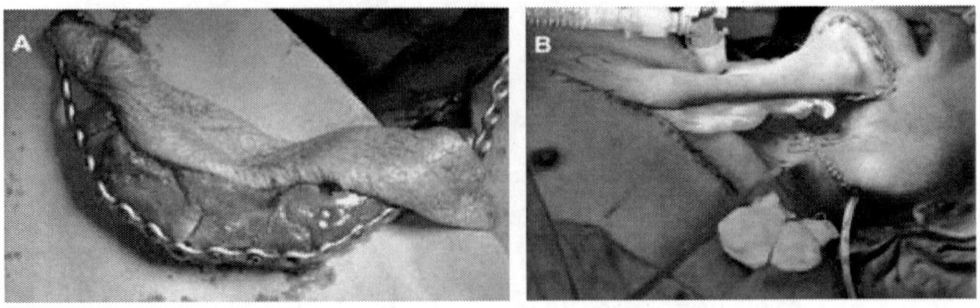

Figure 5. (A) Cutting guides were fixed to the fibula, and following osteotomies, the segment was attached to the pre-bent reconstruction bar. (B) The skin defect caused by the resection was closed with regional DP flap.

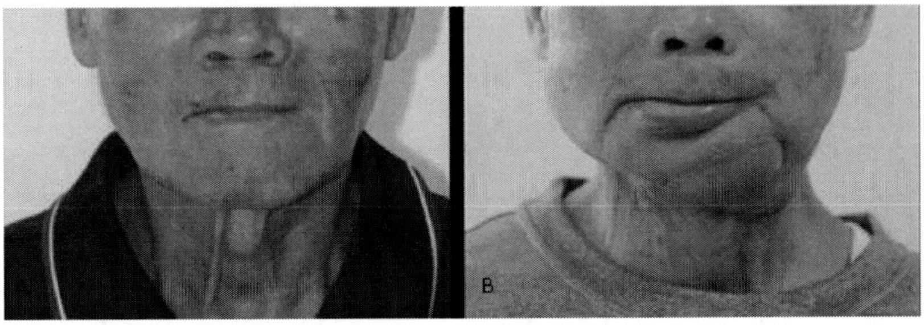

Figure 6. Acceptable symmetric results. (A) Preoperative view; (B) Postoperative 1-month view.

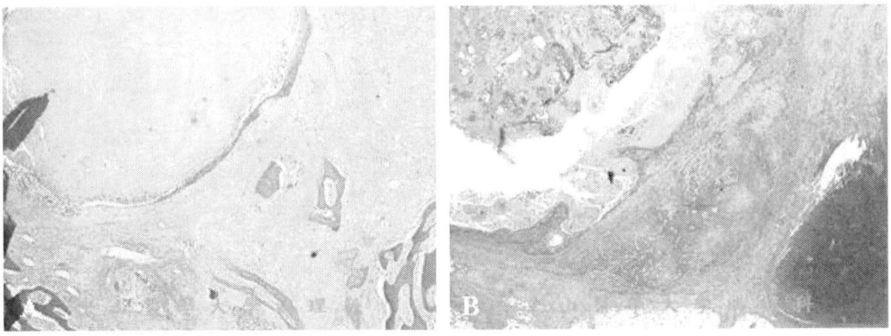

Figure 7. Histopathological examination showing moderately differentiated SCC (A); Histopathological examination showing multiple left lymph node metastasis and extracapsular spread (B).

3. Discussion

OSCC is a multifactorial cancer, and among the most prominent determinant factors for disease progression and prognosis are histopathological features of the primary tumor site [12]. Prevalence of OSCC of mandibular bone involvement ranges from 12% to 56%. However, the treatment results of these lesions are usually poor, with approximately 70%

recurrence rate at the primary site, which ultimately causes death [13, 14]. Moreover, patients with OSCC of the mandibular region who undergo life-saving surgery may still suffer from postoperative facial deformity [15].

We used VSP and medical modeling for mandibular reconstruction. Although this approach is not cost-effective and time-consuming, it is usually suitable in cases involving bone malignancies, which allows easier plate reconstruction [16]. This technique can produce templates for contouring osteotomies, saving operative time and maximizing bone-to-bone contact to promote a strong bony union [17]. Further, it can contribute as a technique involving shorter learning period. However, young surgeons are still encouraged to learn the classic method.

These extensive mandibular defects often involve the mucosa, skin, mandible, and soft tissue. In such patients, surgical reconstruction should be performed with two skin islands to ensure sufficient coverage of the intra- and extra-oral defects, because the application of coverage with one enlarged flap is impossible. Indeed, simultaneous use of double free flap aided reconstruction in large complex defects. It offers the possibility of single stage reconstruction, while reproducing three dimensional anatomical boundaries. However, the increased operation time and technical difficulty are a disadvantage [18]. We selected a combination of fibula free and regional DP flaps to correct the lateral composite mandibular defects resulting from the operation. This decreases operating time and complications about general anesthesia, though no significant differences about surgical complication rate and flap survival condition showed as a systemic review [19]. Adjuvant therapy could be started within 5 weeks. This procedure provided satisfactory reconstruction for extensive head and neck defects and simplified the double free flap method under limited teamwork.

Currently, treatment of advanced-stage OSCC involves a multidisciplinary team approach led by a head and neck surgeon, radiation oncologist and medical oncologist. Although significant progress has been achieved in radical surgical resection with reconstruction and postoperative CCRT, 5-year survival rate has become even lower in patients with locally advanced stages [20]. Restoring oral function after OSCC resection, including speech, swallowing, and appearance, could enhance post-treatment QoL. Mandibular reconstruction is important for most oral functions and maintenance of symmetric temporomandibular joint articulation to allow mouth opening and chewing. In general, a relatively good life expectancy can occur, and QoL can be improved [21].

Conclusion

Patients with advanced-stage OSCC still have poor survival rates. Primary radical surgical management followed by adjuvant therapy remains the optimal therapeutic sequence. However, improving morbidity of various treatment modalities used in oral cancer without compromising survival rate remains a challenge. To ensure proper rehabilitation and nutritional support of patients during postoperative radiochemotherapy, these surgical details should be investigated comprehensively. CAD-CAM indeed is playing important role in reconstruction, especially for mandible. It would increase the ease of the procedure, decrease operation time, and improve precision of fixation. These case highlight the role of free flap combined with regional flap for extensive oromandibular defect, especially in systemic compromised or elderly patient.

REFERENCES

[1] Taylor GI, Miller GD, Ham FJ. (1975). The free vascularized bone graft. A clinical extension of microvascular techniques. *Plast. Reconstruct. Surg.*, 55(5):533-544. Epub 1975/05/01. PubMed PMID: 1096183.

[2] Hidalgo DA. (1989). Fibula free flap: a new method of mandible reconstruction. *Plast. Reconstruct. Surg.*, 84(1):71-79. Epub 1989/07/01. PubMed PMID: 2734406.

[3] Colletti G, Autelitano L, Rabbiosi D, Biglioli F, Chiapasco M, Mandalà M, et al. (2014). Technical refinements in mandibular reconstruction with free fibula flaps: outcome-oriented retrospective review of 99 cases. *Acta Otorhinolaryngolo. Italica*, 34(5):342-348. PubMed PMID: PMC4299154.

[4] Schepers RH, Raghoebar GM, Vissink A, Lahoda LU, Van der Meer WJ, Roodenburg JL, et al. (2013). Fully 3-dimensional digitally planned reconstruction of a mandible with a free vascularized fibula and immediate placement of an implant-supported prosthetic construction. *Head Neck*, 35(4):E109-14. Epub 2011/10/26. doi: 10. 1002/hed.21922. PubMed PMID: 22025326.

[5] Pentenero M, Gandolfo S, Carrozzo M. (2005). Importance of tumor thickness and depth of invasion in nodal involvement and prognosis of oral squamous cell carcinoma: a review of the literature. *Head Neck*, 7(12):1080-1091. Epub 2005/10/22. doi: 10.1002/hed.20275. PubMed PMID: 16240329.

[6] Geum DH, Roh YC, Yoon SY, Kim HG, Lee JH, Song JM, et al. (2013). The impact factors on 5-year survival rate in patients operated with oral cancer. *J. Korean Assoc. Oral Maxillofac. Surg.*, 39(5):207-216. doi: 10.5125/jkaoms.2013.39.5.207. PubMed PMID: PMC3858143.

[7] Hoffmannova J, Foltan R, Vlk M, Sipos M, Horka E, Pavlikova G, et al. (2010). Hemimandibulectomy and therapeutic neck dissection with radiotherapy in the treatment of oral squamous cell carcinoma involving mandible: a critical review of treatment protocol in the years 1994-2004. *Int. J. Oral Maxillofac. Surg.*, 39(6):561-567. Epub 2010/04/27. doi: 10.1016/j.ijom.2010.03.010. PubMed PMID: 20418065.

[8] Hoffmannová J, Foltán R, Vlk M, Šipoš M, Horká E, Pavlíková G, et al. (2010). Hemimandibulectomy and therapeutic neck dissection with radiotherapy in the treatment of oral squamous cell carcinoma involving mandible: a critical review of treatment protocol in the years 1994–2004. *Inter. J. Oral Maxillofac. Surg.*, 39(6):561-567. doi: 10.1016/j.ijom.2010.03.010.

[9] Yi-Sheng Chou, Pen-Yuan Chu, Shyh-Kuan Tai, Tung-Lung Tsai, Yi-Feng Wang, Yen-Bin Hsu, et al. (2010). Induction Chemotherapy with Docetaxel, Cisplatin and 5-Fluorouracil (TPF) in Locally Advanced Head and Neck Cancer: An Asian Single Institute Experience. *J. Cancer Res. Pract., ß*26(2):55-64. doi: 10.6323/JoCRP.2010.26.2.2.

[10] Jewer DD, Boyd JB, Manktelow RT, Zuker RM, Rosen IB, Gullane PJ, et al. (1989). Orofacial and mandibular reconstruction with the iliac crest free flap: a review of 60 cases and a new method of classification. *Plast. Reconstruct. Surg.*, 84(3):391-403; discussion 4-5. Epub 1989/09/01. PubMed PMID: 2762397.

[11] Tahara M, Kiyota N, Yokota T, Hasegawa Y, Muro K, Takahashi S, et al. (2018). Phase II trial of combination treatment with paclitaxel, carboplatin and cetuximab (PCE) as first-line treatment in patients with recurrent and/or metastatic squamous cell carcinoma of the head and neck (CSPOR-HN02). Annals of oncology: *Offic. J. Eur. Soc. Med. Oncol.*, 29(4):1004-1009. Epub 2018/02/07. doi: 10.1093/annonc/mdy040. PubMed PMID: 29408977.

[12] Petti S. (2009). Lifestyle risk factors for oral cancer. *Oral Oncol.*, 45(4):340-350. doi: https://doi.org/10.1016/j.oraloncology.2008.05. 018.

[13] Pandey M, Rao LP, Das SR, Mathews A, Chacko EM, Naik BR. (2007). Patterns of mandibular invasion in oral squamous cell carcinoma of the mandibular region. *World J. Surg. Oncol.*, 5:12-. doi: 10.1186/1477-7819-5-12. PubMed PMID: PMC1803788.

[14] Rao LP, Das SR, Mathews A, Naik BR, Chacko E, Pandey M. (2004). Mandibular invasion in oral squamous cell carcinoma: investigation by clinical examination and orthopantomogram. *Int. J. Oral Maxillofac. Surg.*, 33(5):454-457. Epub 2004/06/09. doi: 10.1016/ j.ijom.2003.10.006. PubMed PMID: 15183408.

[15] Steckler RM, Edgerton MT, Gogel W. (1974). "Andy Gump." *Am. J. Surg.*, 128(4):545-547. Epub 1974/10/01. PubMed PMID: 4609383.

[16] Wilde F, Cornelius C-P, Schramm A. (2014). Computer-Assisted Mandibular Reconstruction using a Patient-Specific Reconstruction Plate Fabricated with Computer-Aided Design and Manufacturing Techniques. *Craniomaxillofac. Trauma Reconstr.*, 7(2):158-166. doi: 10.1055/s-0034-1371356. PubMed PMID: PMC4078148.

[17] Kumar BP, Venkatesh V, Kumar KAJ, Yadav BY, Mohan SR. (2016). Mandibular Reconstruction: Overview. *J. Maxillofac. Oral Surg.*, 15(4):425-441. doi: 10.1007/s12663-015-0766-5. PubMed PMID: PMC5083680.

[18] Chen CL, Zenga J, Roland LT, Pipkorn P. (2018). Complications of double free flap and free flap combined with locoregional flap in head and neck reconstruction: A systematic review. *Head Neck,* 40(3):632-646. Epub 2017/11/16. doi: 10.1002/hed.25005. PubMed PMID: 29140575.

[19] Weitz J, Kreutzer K, Bauer FJ, Wolff KD, Nobis CP, Kesting MR. (2015). Sandwich flaps as a feasible solution for the management of huge mandibular composite tissue defects. *J. Craniomaxillofac. Surg.*, 43(9):1769-1775. Epub 2015/09/04. doi: 10.1016/j.jcms.2015. 07.038. PubMed PMID: 26330301.

[20] Zhong L-P, Zhang C-P, Ren G-X, Guo W, William WN, Sun J, et al. (2013). Randomized Phase III Trial of Induction Chemotherapy With Docetaxel, Cisplatin, and Fluorouracil Followed by Surgery Versus Up-Front Surgery in Locally Advanced Resectable Oral Squamous Cell Carcinoma. *J. Clin. Oncol.,* 1(6):744-751. doi: 10.1200/JCO. 2012.43.8820. PubMed PMID: PMC5569675.

[21] Chinn SB, Myers JN. (2015). Oral Cavity Carcinoma: Current Management, Controversies, and Future Directions. *J. Clin. Oncol.,* 33(29):3269-3276. doi: 10.1200/JCO.2015.61.2929. PubMed PMID: PMC5320919.

In: Clinical Reports in Dentistry
Editor: Lisa R. Amir

ISBN: 978-1-53617-328-4

Chapter 15

MANAGEMENT OF FIBROUS DYSPLASIA OF THE MAXILLA: TWO CASE REPORTS WITH 6-MONTH FOLLOW-UP

Muhammad R. Reksoprodjo[1], Retnowati G. Sudiro[2] and Abdul Latif[3,*]

[1]Oral and Maxillofacial Surgery Residency Program,
Faculty of Dentistry, Universitas Indonesia, Jakarta, Indonesia
[2]Department of Oral and Maxillofacial Surgery,
Tangerang Central Hospital, Tangerang, Indonesia
[3]Department of Oral and Maxillofacial Surgery,
Faculty of Dentistry, Universitas Indonesia, Jakarta, Indonesia

ABSTRACT

Introduction: Fibrous dysplasia is a non-odontogenic bone disease wherein normal bone is replaced by fibrous tissue. The etiology is still unknown but seems to be linked to genetic factors. Patients with this condition typically manifest symptoms by their late teens or early twenties, the primary symptom being facial asymmetry. Herein, we described the management of 2 patients with fibrous dysplasia of the maxilla who underwent excision and surgical contouring, with 6 months of follow-up.

Case report: A 15-year-old male and a 22-year-old female presented to the Department of Oral and Maxillofacial Surgery at Tangerang Central Hospital. Both patients complained of asymptomatic swelling of the left maxilla. For the male, this swelling began 3 years prior to presentation, whereas for the female, there was a 10-year history of swelling. Each patient was bothered by facial asymmetry. On panoramic radiography, both patients exhibited a large radiopaque mass without a distinct border. Both histopathological examinations showed patterns suggestive of fibrous dysplasia and both patients were referred for excision and surgical recontouring.

* Corresponding Author's Email: boblatief06@yahoo.com.

Conclusion: Excision and surgical recontouring are effective in managing patients with fibrous dysplasia; however, extended follow-up is necessary.

Keywords: fibrous dysplasia, maxilla, surgical recontouring

1. Introduction

Fibrous dysplasia (FD) is a developmental tumor-like condition [1]. Among all cases of benign bone disorders, 7% are classified as FD and involve the replacement of normal bone with fibrous tissue [2, 3]. FD can affect single (monostotic) or multiple (polyostotic) bones in the human skeleton [4]. The exact pathogenesis of FD is still unknown, but recent studies indicate that genetic factors may be responsible [5]. FD lesions characteristically "*burn themselves out*" and usually emerge in the late teens or early twenties [6]. FD is most commonly found in the long bones, followed by the jaws (maxilla more often than mandible), base of the skull, and the ribs [4]. The prevalence and incidence estimates are similar among males and females [5, 7].

Treatment planning for FD is based on many factors, such as the patient's age and the location of the lesion [6]. Additionally, not all patients require treatment [8]. The growth of bone affected by FD often stabilizes and occasionally stops once the skeleton is fully matured, after adolescence [2]. When treatment is indicated, the choice is principally surgical, depending on the size and consistency of the lesion. Surgical reduction and recontouring of the dysplasia without complete removal is usually recommended [9]. Long-term clinical and radiographic follow-up is recommended for patients with FD because of its tendency to regrow after surgery [1]. Herein, we report 2 cases of maxillary FD, treated with excision and surgical contouring, with a 6-month follow-up.

2. Case Report

2.1. Case 1

A 15-year-old male patient presented to the Department of Oral and Maxillofacial Surgery at Tangerang Central Hospital. His chief complaint was asymptomatic swelling of the left maxilla, which began 3 years previously. The patient was bothered by his facial asymmetry. There was no history of toothache, pain, fever, or trauma to the region of the lesion. An extra-oral examination revealed a slight facial asymmetry (Figure 1A,B). An intra-oral examination showed an associated swelling, 8 x 6 x 1 cm in size, demarcated from region 22-27 of the left maxilla, with buccal expansion (Figure 1C). The consistency was hard and the color and temperature were the same as that of the surrounding tissue, with no crepitation and no tenderness. The intra-oral examination also revealed caries in teeth 14 and 15 as well as pulp necrosis 36.

A laboratory examination revealed a slightly elevated prothrombin time, with all other values within normal limits. A panoramic radiological examination was performed to help diagnose the lesion. This revealed pulp necrosis of 36, impaction of 27, and a radiopaque hard mass at 22-27 on the left maxilla (Figure 2A). Incision biopsy revealed connective tissue formation, with no sign of malignancy. The working diagnosis was FD. To achieve a final diagnosis, we performed an excision biopsy with jaw recontouring.

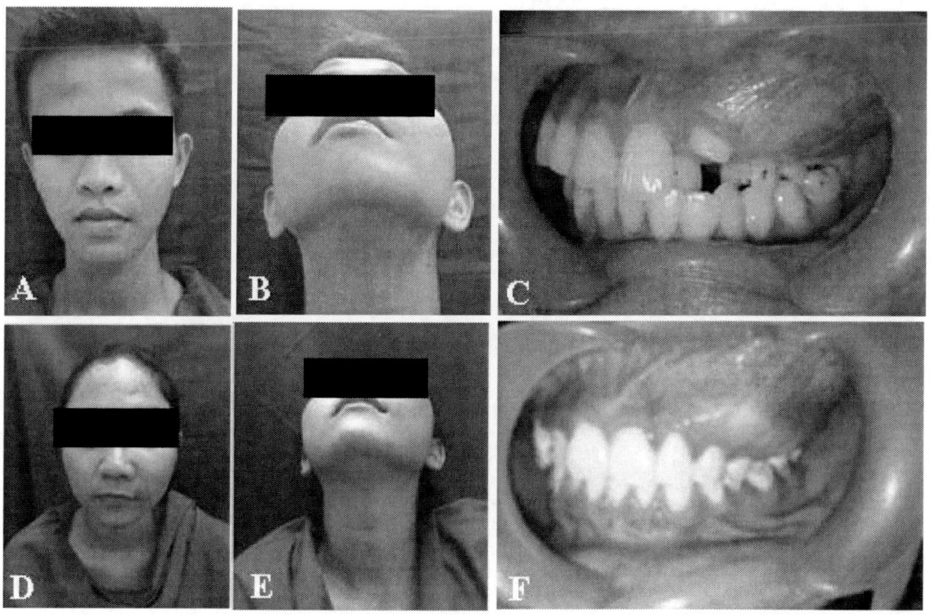

Figure 1. Preoperative extra- and intra-oral views: Case 1 (A-C); Case 2 (D-F).

The treatment planning included extraction of 27 tooth, complete an excision biopsy and recontour the maxilla. The surgery was performed under general anesthesia. Cefotaxime (1 g) was given before surgery as a prophylactic antibiotic. A vertical incision was made in the mesial region 22, followed by a sulcular incision until we reached the distal region of 26 within the left maxilla. The flap was opened using a raspatory until the mass was identified. Before recontouring the mass, we completed an excision using a chisel and mallet (Figure 3A), followed by extracting 27 tooth. The excised mass lesion was separated from the adjacent tissue using Ellis forceps. The mass was then trimmed on the buccal side, using a Fraser bur (Figure 3C). We stored the specimen in 10% liquid formalin and sent it to the Pathological Anatomy Department of Tangerang Hospital for histopathological examination (Figure 3E). The rest of the sharp bone was contoured using the Fraser bur until a good maxillary arch was obtained. The flap was repositioned and sutured using silk 3.0 to prevent bleeding. The final histopathological finding was FD, in agreement with the working diagnosis. The patient returned at 1 week for observation and suture removal, and again at 6 months for follow-up (Figure 4D).

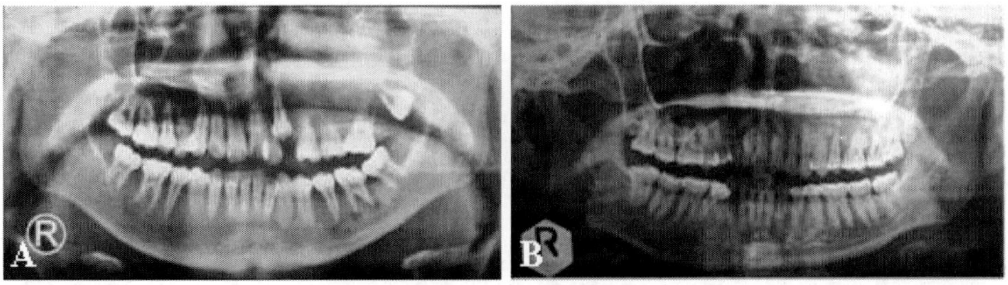

Figure 2. Panoramic radiographs: both have the same irregular "ground-glass" radiopaque appearance on the left maxilla, with an ill-defined border, Case 1 (A); Case 2 (B).

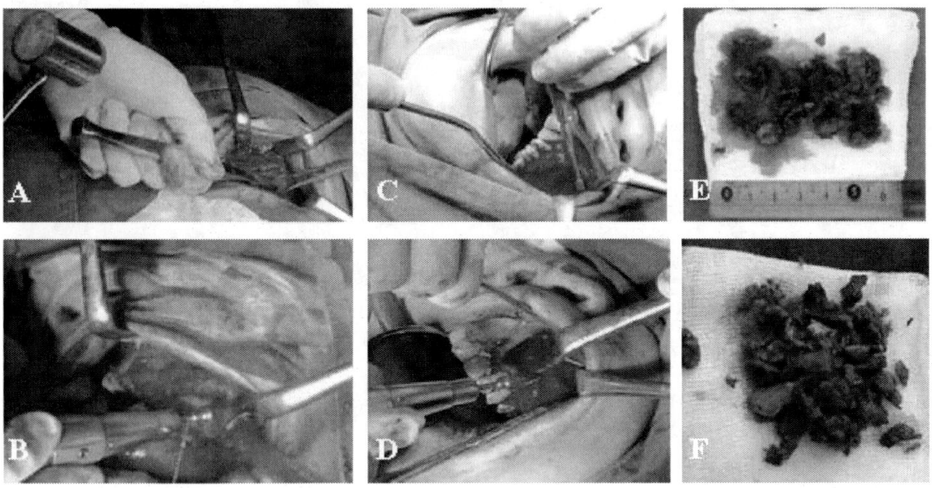

Figure 3. The excision with a chisel mallet (A, B); trimming and recontouring stage using a Frasser bur (C, D); the specimen after excision (E, F).

2.2. Case 2

A 22-year-old female presented to the Department of Oral and Maxillofacial Surgery at Tangerang Central Hospital, complaining of left maxilla swelling that began 10 years ago. Like patient 1, she was bothered by her facial asymmetry. There was no history of toothache, pain, fever, or trauma near the lesion, and no disruption of vision on the left. An extra-oral examination revealed facial asymmetry (Figure 1D and 1E). An intra-oral examination showed a swelling 6x4x2 cm in size, demarcated from region 22-28 of the left maxilla, with buccal expansion (Figure 1F). The lesion was hard, with a color and temperature similar to the surrounding tissue, with no crepitation and no tenderness. An intra-oral examination found no caries.

A laboratory examination revealed slight leukocyte elevation, with all other values within normal limits. A panoramic radiological examination was performed to help diagnose the lesion. This revealed a radiopaque hard mass in the region of 22-28 within the left maxilla (Figure 2B). We performed an incision biopsy to diagnose the lesion, which showed a mixture of trabecular bone tissue pieces surrounded by connective tissue, with no signs of malignancy. The working diagnosis was FD. To arrive at a final diagnosis, we performed an excision biopsy with jaw recontouring under general anesthesia.

Ceftriaxone (2 g) was given before surgery as a prophylactic antibiotic. A vertical incision was made in the mesial region 21, followed by a sulcular incision until we reached the distal region of 26 within the left maxilla. The flap was opened using a raspatory until the mass was identified. The mass involved the zygoma and infraorbital region. Prior to recontouring the mass, an excision was performed using a chisel and mallet (Figure 3B). The excised mass lesion was separated from the adjacent tissue using Ellis forceps. The mass then was trimmed on the buccal side, using a Fraser bur (Figure 3D). We stored the specimen (Figure 3F) in 10% liquid formalin and sent it to the Pathological Anatomy Department of Tangerang Hospital for histopathological examination. The rest of the sharp bone was contoured using the Fraser bur until a good maxillary arch was obtained. The flap was repositioned and sutured using silk 3.0 to prevent bleeding. The final histopathological finding was FD, in agreement with the working diagnosis. The patient returned at 1 week for observation and suture removal, and again at 6 months for follow-up (Figure 4).

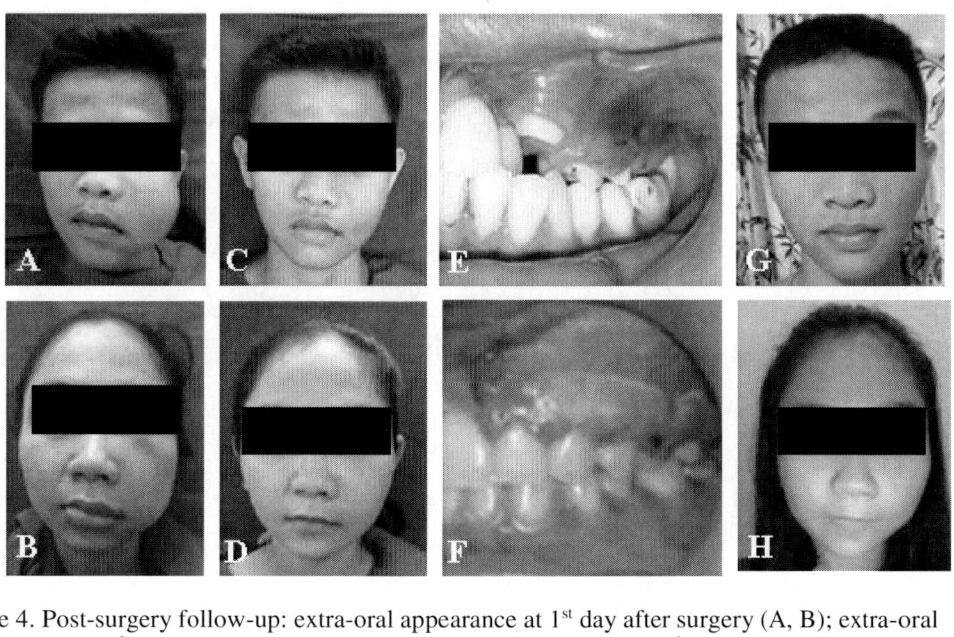

Figure 4. Post-surgery follow-up: extra-oral appearance at 1st day after surgery (A, B); extra-oral appearance at 12th day after surgery (C, D); intra-oral appearance at 12th after surgery (E, F); extra-oral appearance at 6th month after surgery (G, H).

3. Discussion

FD was first described by Von Recklinghausen in 1891 and observed by Lichtenstein in 1938 [1, 2]. This is a rare, non-hereditary, and benign pathological condition where normal medullary bone is replaced by fibrous stroma and immature bone secondary to the abnormal differentiation of osteoblasts [8, 10]. Over time, the fibrous tissue gradually expands and replaces normal bone [11]. Neither patient had any relatives with FD. Both patients reported poor awareness of the initial swelling; however, both felt their lesions slowly enlarge until asymptomatic facial asymmetry developed. FD accounts for 3% of all bone tumors and over 7% of all non-malignant bone tumors [11]. FD usually starts in childhood (typically within the first and second decades of life [6]) and progresses slowly through puberty and adolescence [11].

Some authors report that the lesion's growth tends to stop around puberty; however, other studies report that it can continue to progress after puberty and into adulthood [11, 12, 13]. In this report, our patients presented within the first decade (15-year-old male) and second decade (22-year-old female) of life. Some reports indicate that females are affected more frequently than males, while other reports from Yang et al. noted that males were affected more than females [6, 11]. Many other reports have shown similar prevalence in both males and females [2]. As was the case with our patients, FD affects mostly the younger population, with 75% of patients aged less than 30 years [14]. FD presents most commonly in the long bones, followed by the jaws (maxilla more than mandible), base of the skull and the ribs [4].

Clinically, FD can be classified as *monostotic* when limited to only a single bone and *polyostotic* when more than one bone is involved [7]. The polyostotic form of the disease is involved in the McCune-Albright syndrome and the Jaffe-Lichtenstein syndrome, characterized by *café-au-lait* pigmented skin lesions [1]. Monostotic dysplasia is the most frequent form and occurs in 70-80% of patients, most of whom are 20-30 years old [1,15]. Most cases are unilateral and frequently involve the posterior buccal region [2, 7]. Monostotic lesions tend to cease after skeletal maturation and are typically asymptomatic [2, 7]. Both patients in this report presented with nearly identical unilateral lesions of the posterior buccal region of the left maxilla.

The term *craniofacial FD* can be used if the cranial and facial bones are affected [1]. The most common clinical symptom is a slow-growing and painless swelling that can include facial asymmetry. This may cause a severe deformity that compromises both functional and aesthetic domains [2, 7]. Both our patients 'main complaints involved facial asymmetry. Malocclusion of the teeth and distortion of the facial contour sometimes characterize this lesion [12]. Usually, no tenderness or mobility is noted on palpating the swollen area [9]. Headache, visual and auditory impairments, nasal congestion and/or obstruction, pain, paresthesia, and malocclusion are other common symptoms of FD that can affect the craniofacial region [2, 12]. Orbital and peri-orbital bone involvement produce visual impairments, even causing blindness in severe cases [10]. No visual problems were exhibited by our patients. In its craniofacial form, the maxilla, zygoma, sphenoid, frontal bones, nasal bones, and base of the skull can be involved [6]. In some reports, FD can cause dental complications, such as displacement of the floor of the maxillary sinus [7]. FD has the tendency to become arrested [1]. One of our patients was 22 years old and postpubescent. A previous study suggested that, in patients like case 2, the lesion would not continue to grow, having already reached its "peak." The focus of dysplasia is usually within the alveolar process of the maxilla [16]. Here, dysplasia can cause distension of the bone up to the zygomatic region, thereby contributing to facial deformities [16]. Disease foci often emerge around the canine fossa [9]. Both patients in this report complained of facial deformities, and both lesions involved the zygoma.

FD has a characteristic *ground-glass* appearance, with ill-defined borders, cortical expansion, and tends to blend into the surrounding normal bone [17]. The ground-glass opacification results from a superimposition of poorly calcified bone trabeculae arranged in a disorganized pattern [18]. Within the maxillary region, alteration of the maxillary sinuses should be observed [15]. One theory states that initial lesions are more radiolucent and become more radiopaque over time, as the lesion develops [7]. A computed tomography (CT) examination is recommended to evaluate the extent and shape of the lesions [5]. Neither of our patients underwent CT examinations, but instead received panoramic radiographs that revealed radiopaque lesions, with ill-defined borders that blended with the surrounding tissue within the left maxilla. FD may represent an impairment or developmental arrest of benign fibroosseous proliferation, lacking the ability to fully differentiate [6]. Most cases of FD are believed to be due to a sporadic mutation in the GNAS I gene during embryogenesis [4, 13]. The pathogenesis produces an imbalance between bone formation and destruction [12]. Abnormal bone in the fibrous stroma causes increased bone resorption osteoclast hyperactivity [8].

Biopsy and histopathological examinations are necessary to achieve a definitive diagnosis [10]. A histopathological examination typically reveals fibrous cellular tissue with spindle-shaped cells and immature, trabeculate woven bone [4]. Bundles of collagen fibers characteristically oriented perpendicular to the bony surface can be identified [4]. Trabecular structures are abnormally arranged and appear similar to Chinese letters [10]. In both our patients, histopathological examinations showed bundles of spindle-shaped cellular fibrous tissue, interwoven with trabeculate bone. FD does not resolve spontaneously [8]. Surgical treatment should be limited during the active phase because the lesions are vascular and can bleed quite profusely during surgery [6]. Accordingly, one of our patients (case 1:15 year old male) experienced marked bleeding during surgery, perhaps because he was pubescent, meaning that the lesion was still in the active phase. Following surgery, FD recurs in 25-50% of cases, particularly if surgery is performed at a young age or during the first decade of life [6]. FD tends to stabilize and stop growing when skeletal maturation is reached, usually after adolescence; however, for aesthetic reasons, surgery is often considered necessary [2, 9]. Surgical recontouring and creation of an acceptable bone facial contour, without complete removal, are usually recommended [9]. Since regrowth after surgery appears more common in children and adolescents, surgery should be delayed as long as possible [1, 9]. Both our patients were young, and therefore candidates for treatment delay; however, surgery to treat the facial asymmetry was requested by both patients. The other treatment aim was fracture prevention [15]. Here, there is still no gold standard to treat FD. Some authors prefer a wait-and-see approach, hoping that the lesion will "burn itself out" [16]. In some cases, FD may persist until late adult life [1]. Radiation therapy is contraindicated because of an increased risk of malignant transformation [1]. Teeth proximal to the FD should remain vital, even if the surrounding tissue is affected [3]. In case 2, all teeth remained vital after surgery. Preventing tooth loss should be a treatment aim [3]. For case 1, we extracted a single tooth that was impacted, but the other teeth remained vital throughout the follow-up.

Patients with FD should be evaluated periodically, both clinically and with radiography, due to the lesion's tendency to grow, and potential late development of pain and swelling that may indicate possible malignant changes [7, 9]. Possible relapse or regrowth is very common following surgery, and approximately 20-25% of lesions continue to grow slowly after treatment, regardless of the type of therapy [7, 12]. Surgeons should analyze each case of FD based on gender, age, recurrence, the extent of the lesion, and the involvement of adjacent structures in order to optimize treatment for each patient [12].

It is also very important to explain to the patient the possibility of lesion recurrence or regrowth after surgery so as to underscore the importance of periodic monitoring, including clinical and imaging studies [12]. Both our cases were monitored and followed for a minimum of 6 months after surgery. Here, follow-up revealed no patient complaints and no signs of lesion regrowth.

CONCLUSION

In conclusion, FD of the maxilla is usually accompanied by asymptomatic facial asymmetry, occasionally hampering early diagnosis. Not all cases require treatment, but treatment is indicated if the patient is bothered by facial asymmetry related to the lesion; additionally, patients should be followed and evaluated periodically.

REFERENCES

[1] Nadaf A, Radhika M, Paremala K, Srinath N. (2013). Monostostic fibrous dysplasia with nonspecific cystic degeneration: A case report and review of literature. *Journal of Oral and Maxillofacial Pathology*, 17:274.

[2] Köse T, Dinçer Köse O, Erdem M, Çankaya A. (2016). Monostotic Fibrous Dysplasia Presenting in Maxilla: A Case Report. *J. Istanb. Univ. Fac. Dent.*, 50(2): 38-42.

[3] Kos M, Luczak K, Godzinski J, Klempous J. (2004). Treatment of monostotic fibrous dysplasia with pamidronate. *J. Craniomaxillofac. Surg.*, 32:10-15.

[4] Andersson, L; Kahnberg, KE; Pogrel, MA. (2010). *Oral Maxillofacial Surgery*, Wiley-Blackwell, Oxford.

[5] Saglik Y, Atalar H, Yildiz Y, Basarir K, Erekui S. (2007). Management of fibrous dysplasia A report on 36 cases. *Acta Orthopaedica Belgica*, 73:96-101.

[6] Miloro M, Waite PD, Larsen PE, Ghali GE. (2004). *Peterson's Principles of Oral and Maxillofacial Surgery*, 2nd Ed, BC Decker Inc, Hamilton, London.

[7] Costa E, Peyneau P, Verner F, Almeida S, Ambrosano G. (2017). Monostotic fibrous dysplasia: a case report with cone-beam computed tomography findings. *RGO - Revista Gaúcha de Odontologia*, 65:180-184.

[8] Kutbay NO, Yurekli BS, Baykan EK, Sahin SB, Saygili F. (2015). Characteristics and Treatment Results of 5 Patients with Fibrous Dysplasia and Review of the Literature. *Case Reports Endocrin,* vol. 2015:670809.

[9] Reichart PA, Philipsen HP. (2004). *Odontogenic Tumors and Allied Lesions*, 1st ed. Quintessence.

[10] Hanifi B, Samil KS, Yasar C, Cengiz C, Ercan A, Ramazan D. (2013). Craniofacial fibrous dysplasia. *Clinic Imaging*, 37:1109-1115.

[11] Wu H, Yang L, Li S, Jin X, Xu J, Lu J, Zhang C. (2014). Clinical characteristics of craniomaxillofacial fibrous dysplasia. *J. Craniomaxillofac. Surg*. 42:1450-1455.

[12] Alves N, de Oliveira R, Takehana D, Deana N. (2016). Case Report Recurrent Monostotic Fibrous Dysplasia in the Mandible. *Case Reports in Dentistry*, Vol. 2016:3920850.

[13] Godse AS, Shrotriya SP, Vaid NS. (2009). Fibrous dysplasia of the maxilla. *J. Pediatr. Surg*., 44:849-851.

[14] Fusconi M, Conte M, Pagliarella M, Vincentiis CD, Virgillio AD, Benincasa AT, Alessi S, Gallo A. (2013). Fibrous Dysplasia of the Maxilla: Diagnostic Reliability of the Study Image. Literature Review. *J. Neurolog. Surg.*, 74:364-368.

[15] Bric- Cioranu V, Ibric-Cioranu S, Nicolae V, Raescu M. (2013). Fibrous Dysplasia of Maxillary Bones. 2 Case Reports. *Inter. J. Med. Dent.*, 3:234-237.

[16] Wojcik S, Koszowski R, Drozdowska B, Smieszek-Wilczewska J, Raczkowska-Siostrzonek A. (2016). Maxillary fibrous dysplasia associated with McCune-Albright syndrome. A case study. *De Gruyter Open Med.*, 11:465-470.
[17] Laskin DM, Abubaker AO. (2007). *Decision Making in Oral and Maxillofacial Surgery*, 1st ed. Quintessence.
[18] Neville BW, Damm DD, Allen CM, Chi AC. (200). *Oral and Maxillofacial Pathology*, 2nd ed. Philadelphia: W. S. Saunders.

In: Clinical Reports in Dentistry
Editor: Lisa R. Amir
ISBN: 978-1-53617-328-4

Chapter 16

MANDIBULAR AMELOBLASTOMA IN A YOUNG PATIENT: A CASE REPORT

Yus A. Wibawa[1], Dwi Ariawan[2,*] and Arfan Badeges[3]

[1]Oral and Maxillofacial Surgery Residency Program,
Faculty of Dentistry, Universitas Indonesia, Jakarta, Indonesia
[2]Department of Oral and Maxillofacial Surgery, Faculty of Dentistry,
Universitas Indonesia, Jakarta, Indonesia
[3]Division of Oral and Maxillofacial Surgery, Persahabatan Central Hospital,
East Jakarta, Indonesia

ABSTRACT

Introduction: Ameloblastoma is a slow-growing, epithelial odontogenic benign tumor which is aggressive and locally invasive. It is commonly seen in the posterior lower jaw and is characterized by formation of dental embryonic residual. The etiology of ameloblastoma might be related to odontogenic cyst epithelial layer, dental lamina, enamel organ, stratified squamous epithelium of the oral cavity, or displaced epithelial residual. Many cases of ameloblastoma have been reported to have residual epithelial residues originally degenerated from dentigerous cysts.

Case report: Here we reported the surgical management of ameloblastoma mimicking a dentigerous cyst. A 14-year-old girl complained of experiencing swelling in the lower right jaw for one year. The lesion was hard and cystic with a well-defined border. She had no pain. Color and temperature of the lesion were equal to color and temperature of the surrounding tissue. There was no history of trauma and toothache and no pus or bloody discharge. Initial diagnosis was a dentigerous cyst and the patient underwent surgical enucleation of the mass followed by extraction of the involved teeth under general anesthetic. Histopathological examination of the removed specimen revealed a plexiform ameloblastoma pattern.

* Corresponding Author's Email: dwiariawan75@gmail.com.

Conclusion: Ameloblastoma is a locally malignant tumor requiring enucleation and/or curettage and resection. Long-term follow-up is necessary to rule out recurrent tumor.

Keywords: ameloblastoma, mandible, enucleation

1. INTRODUCTION

Ameloblastoma was formerly introduced by Broca in 1868. In 1934, Churchill coined the term ameloblastoma to replace the term adamantinoma that was identified by Malassez in 1885 [1,2]. Ameloblastoma is a rare, benign, epithelial odontogenic tumor that shows aggressive growth and a high recurrence rate after conservative surgical treatment. Expansion of ameloblastoma cells into the jaw bone destroys the bone and invades the soft tissue outside the bone as well as the intertrabecular spaces of the cancerous bone that are not seen clinically or radiologically [3-5]. Ameloblastoma is derived from the tooth-forming epithelium of the mandible or maxilla. Potential epithelial sources include epithelial enamel, rest of Malassez, and epithelial layer cysts especially dentigerous cysts.

The mandibular jaw is the most common site of ameloblastoma occurrence, rather than the maxilla, with approximately 70% of ameloblastoma cases being reported in the mandibular molar-ramus region (mandible-to-maxilla ratio 5:1). Ameloblastoma represents 1% of all jaw cysts/tumors and 18% of all odontogenic neoplasms [4, 6]. In 2005 the World Health Organization (WHO) classified ameloblastoma into four types: unicystic; multicystic/solid; peripheral; and desmoplastic. Histopathologically, ameloblastoma is classified into six types: follicular; plexiform; acanthomatous; desmoplastic; granular; and basal cells [7].

Ameloblastoma has a tendency to expand and weaken the bone cortex due to the slow growth rate of the lesions, allowing the periosteum to develop a thin bone shell before an enlarged lesion forms. It is painful and produces crepitus when palpated, which is called "egg shell cracking". Pain may occur due to hemorrhage, swelling affecting other structures, tooth avulsion, ulcers, and periodontal disease. Paresthesia is infrequent, with rarely reported cases of perineural invasion [8].

Histologically, ameloblastoma subtypes are plexiform, acanthomatous, follicular, granular, and basal cells. The most common histological type is follicular (64.9%), followed by plexiform (13.0%), and desmoplastic (5.2%), and finally, the rarest type, acanthomatous (3.9%). Radiographically, ameloblastoma appears in the bone as a radiolucency of many sizes and features; sometimes it is a single well-demarcated lesion, although it frequently appears as a multiloculated "soap bubble".

Resorption of the involved teeth can be seen in many cases [2, 6]. Histological examination is necessary to confirm the temporary radiographic diagnosis. We report here the rare distinctive occurrence of ameloblastoma in the right lower jaw of a young girl.

2. Case Report

A 14-year-old girl was referred from the Bekasi General Hospital to the Oral and Maxillofacial Surgery Clinic, the Persahabatan Central Hospital with a dentigerous cyst as the diagnosis. The patient admitted that the peanut-like mass had initially arisen one year previously on the lower right jaw and had gradually increased in size to that of its present state.

The patient had no history of pain, trauma, or any discharge from the swelling. The patient also had no history of cigarette smoking or alcohol use, and no relevant systemic co-morbidities. Results of blood tests were normal. One month before admission to the Bekasi General Hospital, the patient felt uncomfortable with the enlargement of the lesion but had no difficulty swallowing.

Extra-oral examination revealed a diffuse asymmetrical swelling on the right lower jaw that spread into her right cheek to the angle of the mandible. On palpation, there was no tenderness, and the color and temperature were the same as those of the surrounding smooth surface.

The lesion was immobile and hard in consistency, and crepitus was felt over the region of the third molar. No lymph nodes were palpable. Intra-oral examination showed an approximately $4 \times 5 \times 3$cm mass on the right mandible at region 47 to the mandibular angle, with a well-defined border, smooth surface, and color and temperature the same as those of the surrounding tissue (Figure 1A). The mass was non-tender, immobile, and cystic in consistency, with 47 tooth mobility. The unerupted teeth included 18, 28, 23, 38, and 48 teeth (Figure 2C).

A huge unilocular osteolytic lesion extending from her right mandibular second molar to the ramus mandible was noted, with internal radiolucent structures and cortical margins derived from dental crowns around the lesions. Images also showed displacement of 48 tooth to the angle of the mandible with no involvement of the mandibular bone border (Figure 1B). Lesion aspiration demonstrated clear yellowish liquid (Figure 2B). Based on these examinations, dentigerous cyst was the suspected diagnosis. The differential diagnosis included radicular cyst, odontogenic keratocyst, central giant cell granuloma, ameloblastoma, and odontogenic myxoma. Surgery was planned.

Treatment for a dentigerous cyst was enucleation with lifting of unerupted teeth while the patient was under general anesthetic via nasal endotracheal intubation. An aseptic protocol was followed. A crevicular triangular incision was created from mesial 47 to the mandibular ascending ramus. The flap was reflected using a raspatory. The lesion was enucleated along with the unerupted third molar and the second permanent right mandibular molar.

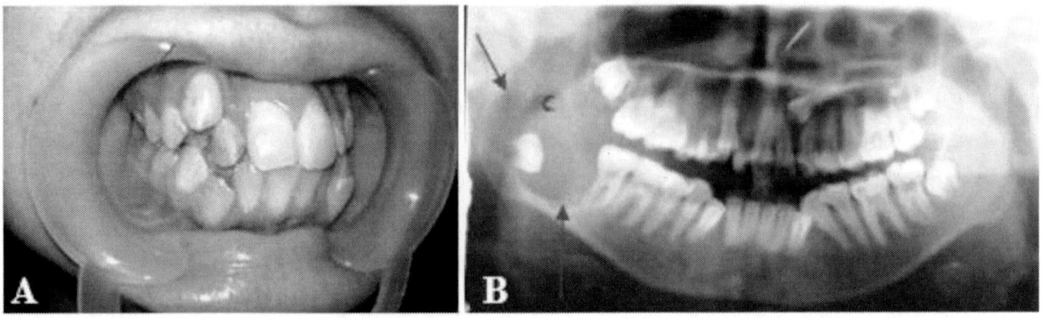

Figure 1. Intra-oral picture shows the mass involving the mandible (A); Orthopantomograph (B).

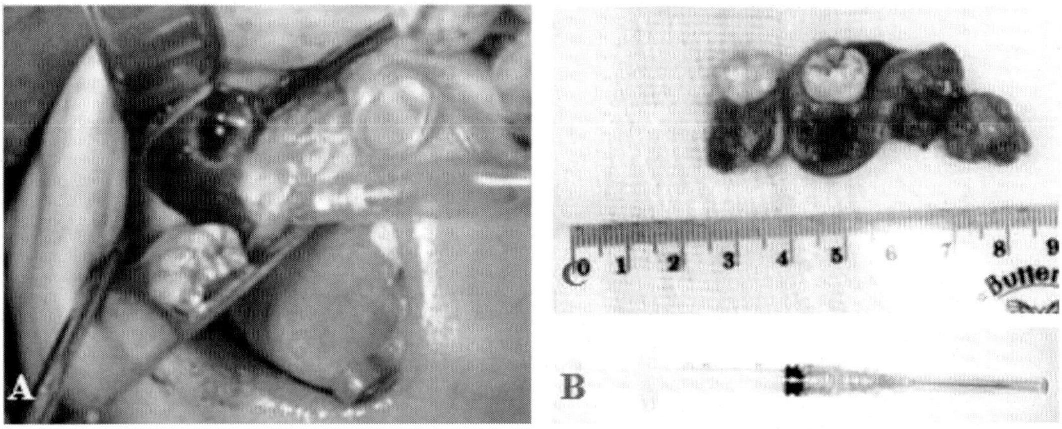

Figure 2. The cavity after mass is removed) A); The mass has been enucleated, the teeth involved have been extracted (B); Yellowish fluid on aspiration ©.

Then, the cavity was irrigated with povidone iodine and NaCl 0.9% (Figure 2A). Continuous, interlocking 3-0 silk sutures were used to close the flap. Histopathological examination of the removed cyst identified the visible mass flexed with cyst wall tissue and was coated with thin squamous epithelium with connective tissue stroma. These results were consistent with a plexiform type of ameloblastoma. Panoramic radiographs were obtained every three months for the first year, every six months for the second and third years, and annually for the following two years. During postoperative follow-up, the patient had no untoward complications.

There was no alteration of facial movements postoperatively, demonstrating preservation of the facial nerve (Figure 3A). Follow-up every three months and to date showed no evidence of recurrence (Figure 3B).

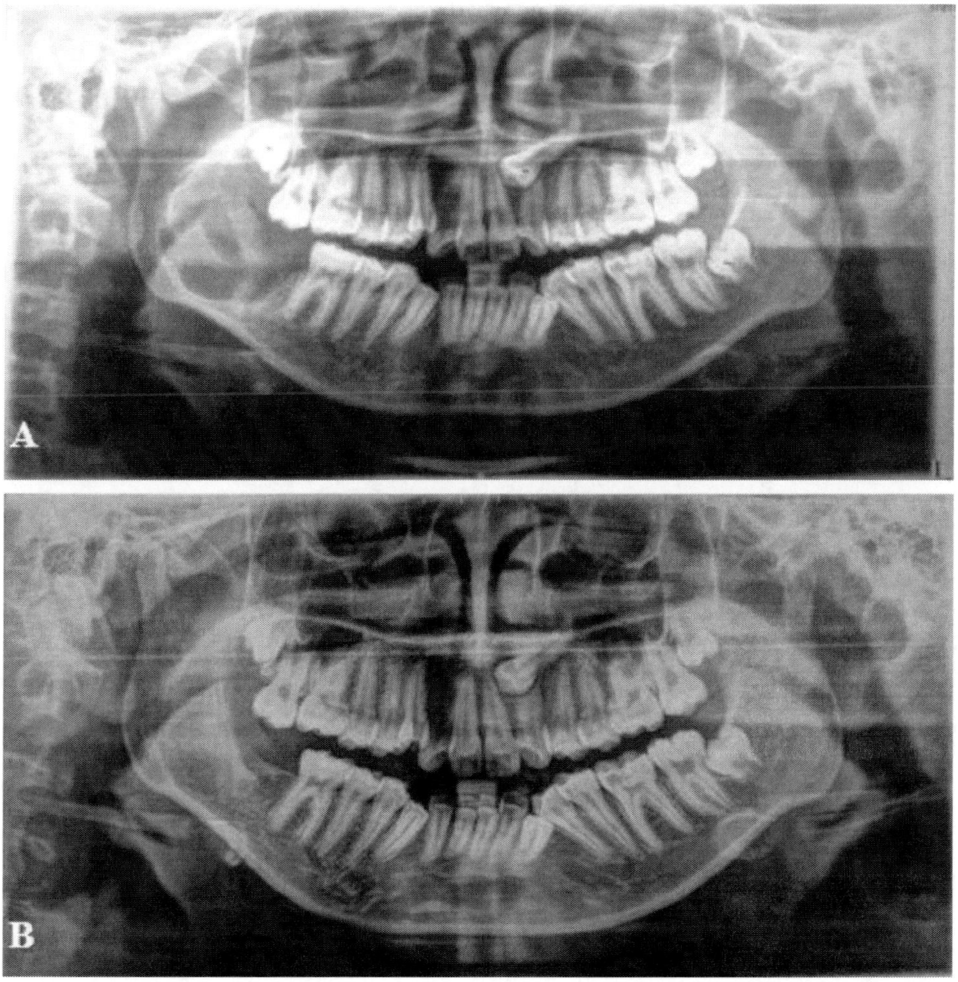

Figure 3. Postoperative orthopantomograph. Taken a month after surgery (A); Orthopantomograph six months postoperatively (B).

3. Discussion

Ameloblastomas account for 1% of all tumors of the jaw that are encountered during the third to fifth decades of life. However, this tumor can also affect children aged 10 – 19 years, although the frequency of occurrence is very rare, at approximately 14.6%. The most common site of tumor occurrence is in the mandible (80% of ameloblastomas), with 70% of tumors located in the area of the molars or in the ascending ramus. In the case of our patient, the tumor occurred in the posterior mandible and displaced the third molar impacted teeth. In our knowledge of the literature, this is the rarest reported case in a young girl [5, 8, 9].

Based on a variety of theories, unicystic ameloblastoma can develop from reduced enamel epithelium, which is associated with teeth or ameloblastoma that develops in dentigerous cysts or in other preexisting odontogenic cysts. This further degenerates into cysts and causes unicystic ameloblastoma. However, no satisfactory evidence exists to prove this particular theory. Some investigators claim that unicystic ameloblastoma begins (de novo) from a cystic neoplasm. Furthermore, the afore-mentioned case is also a demonstration of conservative therapy in a case of ameloblastoma [8, 9].

Histopathological examination demonstrated that the lesion was a plexiform ameloblastoma. This might have been caused by a dentigerous cyst that can develop into ameloblastoma. Based on the study, 15% – 20% of unicystic ameloblastomas form from the dentigerous cyst wall [10]. The literature explains that ameloblastoma as a tumor has a history as a slow-growing mass, with malocclusion and loose teeth or, more rarely, paresthesia and pain; however, many lesions are detected incidentally on radiographic studies done on asymptomatic patients. Slow progress is common, and the tumors are locally invasive and will infiltrate through the medullary spaces and can erode cortical bone [3, 11, 12]. In our case study, the patient reported a slowly progressive swelling and a little discomfort in mastication. There was no history of pain, trauma, or any discharge from the swelling.

Treatment of ameloblastoma is either conservative or radical. Enucleation is a conservative treatment performed by removing the lesion in toto. The enucleation process must be performed carefully to prevent recurrence of the tumor. When removing the lesion, the remaining tissue in the exposed cavity is cleared and no fragments remain [11, 13]. In addition, smoothing the surrounding tissue and irrigation are both important before closure of exposed areas. However, this treatment showed a high recurrence rate of ameloblastoma (60%); therefore, some studies recommend radical treatment in the form of resection.

The number of regions taken varies, depending on the site and extent of the tumor. It is important to understand the tumor growth characteristics, and to remove the whole tumor including the surrounding tissue since remaining tumor cells cause recurrence. The first recommendation is surgery with extensive resection, because it reduces the recurrence rate of solid or multicystic ameloblastomas. A 1.5 – 2cm margin beyond the radiological limit is used to ensure that all microcysts are removed. Recurrence rates are up to 90% – 100% after curettage, and 13% – 15% after resection [10, 13]. Previous studies suggest appropriate treatment is an important prognostic factor, particularly those studies involved in treatment being the cause of recurrence [12, 13].

In the case of our young patient, although the lesion was removed conservatively by enucleation, the lesion cavity showed good bone remodeling at six months after treatment with no signs of recurrence. Routine evaluation is important because most tumors recur within the first five years; however, some tumors have been observed as recurring at >10 years after initial treatment [7].

CONCLUSION

Ameloblastoma is derived from the tooth-forming epithelium of the mandible or maxilla. Potential epithelial sources include epithelial enamel, rest of Malassez, epithelial layer cysts, and especially dentigerous cysts. Based on the results of our case study, we concluded that ameloblastoma requires appropriate radical treatment to limit its recurrence rate. Long-term follow-up is necessary to determine this recurrence rate.

REFERENCES

[1] Cawson, R. A., Odell, E. W. (2002). *Cawson's Essentials of Oral Pathology and Oral Medicine*. 7th ed. Churchill Livingstone.

[2] Gardner, D. G., Heikinheimo, K., Shear, M., Philipsen, H. P., Coleman, H. (2008). *Ameloblastoma.* In: Barnes, L., Eveson, J. W., Reichart, P., Sidransky, D. World Health Organization classification of tumours: pathology and genetics of head and neck tumours. Lyon: IARC Press, 296 - 300. Hupp, J. R., Ellis, E., Tucker, M. R. Contemporary Oral and Maxillofacial Surgery. 5th ed. St. Louis: Mosby Elsevier.

[3] Bhushan, N. V. V., Rao, N. M., Navantha, M., Kumar, B. (2014). Ameloblastoma Arising from A Dentigerous Cyst-A Case Report. *J. Clin. Diagn. Res.,* 8:23 - 25.

[4] Miloro, M., Ghali, G., Larsen, P., Waite, P. (2004). Peterson's Principles of Oral and Maxillofacial Surgery. 2nd ed. Hamilton, Ontario: B C Decker.

[5] Neville, B. W., Damm, D. D., Allen, C. M., Bouquot, J. E. (2009). *Oral and Maxillofacial Pathology*. 3rd ed. Saunders Elsevier.

[6] Regezi, J., Sciubba, J., Jordan, R. (2012). *Oral Pathology*. 6th ed. St. Louis, Mo: Elsevier/Saunders.

[7] Soluk-tekkesin, M., Wright, J. (2017). The World Health Organization Classification of Odontogenic Lesions: A Summary of the Changes of the 2017 (4th) Edition. *Turkish J. Pathol.,* p. 2.

[8] Laxmidevi, B., Mohammed, M., Ashok Kumar, K. (2015). Unicystic Ameloblastoma with Impacted Third Molar Mimicking Dentigerous Cyst. *J. Interdiscipl. Denti.,* 5:37.

[9] Olsen, J., Muhrbeck, T. (2016). *Surgical Removal of Ameloblastoma and Keratocystic Odontogenic Tumors in Maxilla and Mandible*, a Literature Review on Surgical Techniques and Risk of Recurrence. https://pdfs.semanticscholar.org /77e8/fd765bc69075720cb99209fa03ac12915581.pdf.

[10] Tanveer, K., Suresh, P. L., Dinesh, S. K. (2013). Unicystic Ameloblastoma Mimicking a Dentigerous Cyst. *Indian J. Dent. Adv.*, 5:1235 - 1238.

[11] Abdulai, A. E. (2011). Treatment of Ameloblastoma of the Jaws in Children. *Ghana Medical Journal,* 45:35 - 37.

[12] Dandriyal, R., Gupta, A., Pant, S., Baweja, H. H. (2011). Surgical Management of Ameloblastoma: Conservative or Radical Approach. *National Journal of Maxillofacial Surgery,* 2:22 - 27.

[13] Ecande, C., Andre, C., Philippe, M. et al. (2009). A Treatment Algorythmn for Adult Ameloblastomas according to the Pitie´-Salpetriere Hospital Experience. *J. Cranio-Maxillofacial. Surg.,* 37:363e369.

In: Clinical Reports in Dentistry
Editor: Lisa R. Amir

ISBN: 978-1-53617-328-4

Chapter 17

COMPARISON OF IMAGING CHARACTERISTICS AND MARGIN OF AN AMELOBLASTOMA BETWEEN CONE BEAM COMPUTED TOMOGRAPHY AND COMPUTED TOMOGRAPHY: A CASE REPORT

M. Adhitya Latief[1,*], Benny S. Latief[1] and Menik Priaminiarti[2]

[1]Department of Oral and Maxillofacial Surgery, Faculty of Dentistry, Universitas Indonesia, Jakarta, Indonesia

[2]Department of Dentomaxillofacial Radiology, Faculty of Dentistry, Universitas Indonesia, Jakarta, Indonesia

ABSTRACT

Introduction: Ameloblastomas are rare, benign, odontogenic tumors that mainly affect the mandible. They are slow-growing tumors with an affinity for bone, and they have a high recurrence rate if not adequately removed. Tumor removal needs attention with regard to the assessment of the correct free tumor margin. Computed tomography (CT), as the gold standard, allows good assessment and contrast enhancement is helpful. Advancements in imaging technology have resulted in the development of cone beam computed tomography (CBCT) as an alternative imaging approach. We present a patient with an ameloblastoma, who underwent both CT and CBCT. We compared the imaging characteristics and tumor margin between these imaging approaches in this patient.

Case Report: The patient was a 34-year-old woman with swelling in the right lower jaw. She underwent both CT and CBCT. The lesion was identified as an ameloblastoma. We found that both approaches provided good image quality with regard to anatomy; however, there was a slight difference in measurement results.

* Corresponding Author's Email: adhityalatief@yahoo.com.

Conclusion: Our findings suggest that CBCT provides good image quality for surgical guidance with regard to measuring ameloblastomas and determining the free tumor margin and that CBCT results are as good as CT results in the assessment of ameloblastomas.

Keywords: CBCT, MSCT-Scan, ameloblastoma

1. INTRODUCTION

In 2005, the World Health Organization described ameloblastomas as benign, locally invasive, polymorphic neoplasms that include proliferating odontogenic epithelium (usually with a follicular or plexiform pattern) and are present in a fibrous stroma [1]. They are slow-growing tumors with an affinity for bone but not soft tissue, and they can recur (recurrence rate up to 60%-80%) if not adequately removed [2]. They are often asymptomatic and are frequently incidentally detected during routine panoramic radiography. A painless swelling of the jaw is the usual clinical presentation. Ameloblastomas arising within the jaw bones are subclassified as "solid" (formerly "multilocular"), "unicystic" and "desmoplastic" types [1].

It is important to determine whether the lesion is unicystic or solid, as a unicystic ameloblastoma responds well to conservative surgery, enucleation and adjuvant treatment (usually Carnoy's solution), whereas a solid ameloblastoma requires resection to minimize recurrence [3]. Additionally, it is important to understand the tumor margin, which divides the free tumor margin in an ameloblastoma, as this will help obtain better results with minimum risk of recurrence [4]. As ameloblastomas are difficult to recognize in the early stages, they are often relatively large at diagnosis and can fill the ramus or body of the mandible. The radiological appearance of an ameloblastoma can be unilocular, multilobular, or multilocular [5].

Radiological imaging technology has advanced through the use of computed tomography (CT) or helical CT, and this is considered as the gold standard radiological examination especially for the oral and maxillofacial regions [4]. Advancements in radiology have resulted in the development of cone beam computed tomography (CBCT), which allows exposure to be specifically limited to only the oral and maxillofacial regions, and the wide use of CBCT in dentistry has improved imaging when compared with conventional radiography [6]. CBCT can provide submillimeter spatial resolution for images of the craniofacial complex with scanning times comparable with those of panoramic radiography, and the radiation dose is generally lower with CBCT than with fan-beam or helical CT [7]. CBCT is becoming an increasingly frequent imaging option for oral and maxillofacial regions, and it needs to be compared with CT, as it does not involve the use of contrast and has limited Field of View scan for assessing lesions in the maxillofacial region [8]. Here, we present a case of a patient with an ameloblastoma, who underwent both CT and CBCT. We compared the imaging characteristics and tumor margin between these two imaging approaches in this patient.

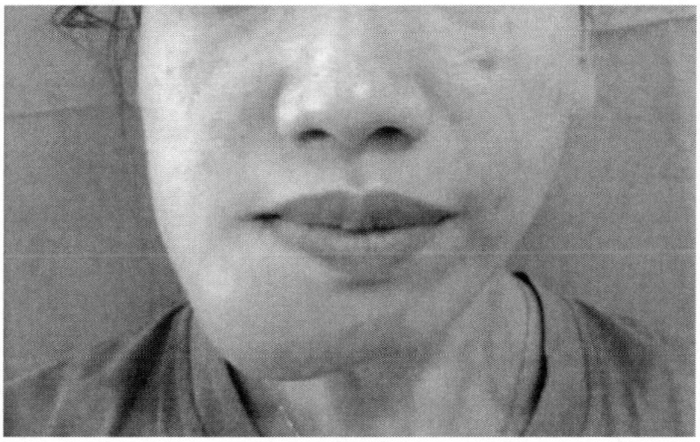

Figure 1. Patient profile.

2. CASE REPORT

A 34-year-old female patient with swelling in the right lower jaw was referred to the Oral and Maxillofacial Surgery Division at Cipto Mangunkusumo Hospital in January 2018 (Figure 1). She had swelling in the right lower jaw 3 years previously, and there was no pain, trismus, or dysphagia. Examination revealed a diffuse and bulging intra-oral mucosa that was prominent in the buccal region, and the swelling was intra-oral and extra-oral. There was no purulence or fluid discharge, and aspiration with a syringe revealed a reddish dark fluid.

About 1 year previously, she underwent biopsy at Fatmawati Hospital, and histopathological findings revealed an ameloblastoma. Initially, surgery was postponed as she had early signs of lung tuberculosis (TB). She then decided to seek further treatment for the ameloblastoma at Cipto Mangunkusumo Hospital, and she was treated with TB medication 3 months prior to surgery. Patient is planned to have surgical resection with reconstruction using Titanium Plate 2.4, based on oralpanthomography, a segmental resection is prepared to out take tumor which involve half of anterior symphysis up to angular mandibula since inferior border of mandible is very thin and fragile for pathologic fracture. Surgical planning is needed to decide tumor margin and free tumor margin.

To have surgical free tumor margin, patient is usually measured 1 cm from outline of tumor margin, this measurement is based on CT Scan or CBCT data. However, measuring tumor volume cannot be accurately done since data slice is on 2D imaging. To have good outcomes, surgical simulation is done by producing 3D Model from CT Scan or CBCT data. An imaging examination is prepared.

She underwent CT with contrast enhancement for better imaging as orthopantomography could not appropriately differentiate the tumor margin (Figure 2). A 128-slice CT scan using contrast (iopamidol) was performed 5 days prior to surgery. However, she lost her original CD of the CT scan data and decided to undergo CBCT without contrast. Both data sets were assessed using InVesalius ver. 3.1 (CTI, Campinas, São Paulo, Brazil), and multi-slice data were measured using the measurement function caliper in mm. The point of measurement was confirmed with a 3D feature that enables ballpoint markers that are equivalent to point marks in multi-slice data (axial/coronal/sagittal view). Point markers are measured with the same points in the same positions between CT and CBCT data (Figure 3).

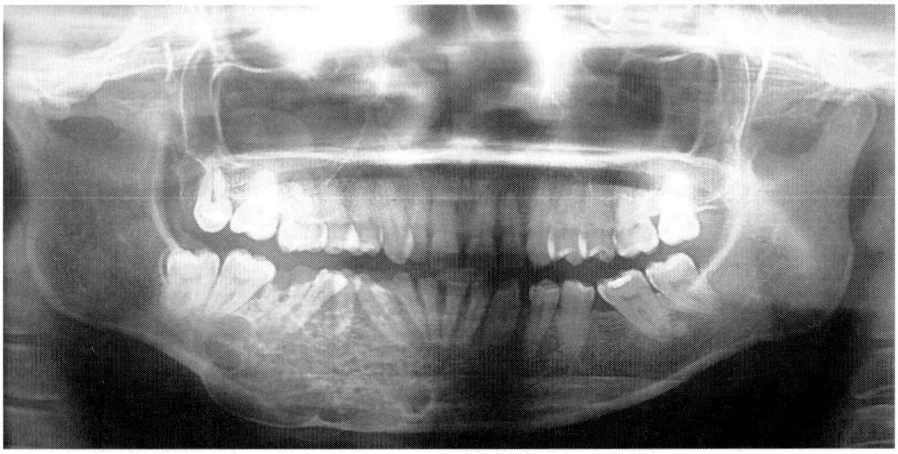

Figure 2. Lesion on orthopantomograph (OPG). The lesion is expanding from region 41 to 48, the "bubble soap" appearance is identified from cervical of alveolar bone to inferior border of ramus mandibula. Foramen mentalis cannot be identified on this OPG.

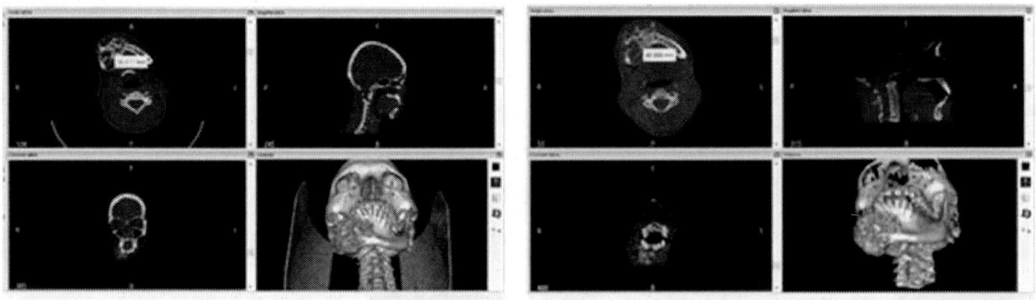

Figure 3. Comparison of measurements between computed tomography (left side) and cone beam computed tomography (right side) data using InVesalius.

Table 1. Comparison of measurements between computed tomography and cone beam computed tomography data

Variables	CT	CBCT	Differences
Tumor length (mm)	50.58	49.90	0.68
Tumor height (mm)	31.74	31.25	0.49
Tumor thickness (mm)	37.40	37.30	0.10
Symphysis height (mm)	30.12	30.03	0.09
Symphysis thickness (mm)	10.42	10.12	0.30
Angular angulation (degree)	115.67	114.53	1.14
Mentalis nerve preservation	None	None	None

Based on the measurement results, all CBCT values were lower than the corresponding CT values (Table 1). In the tumor region and normal bone region, there were value discrepancies. In the tumor region, the highest discrepancy was for the tumor length (difference of 0.68 mm), and the lowest discrepancy was for the tumor thickness (difference of 0.10 mm). On the other hand, in the normal bone region, the thickness of the mandible had a difference of 0.30 mm between CBCT and CT. Additionally, angulation was lower with CBCT than with CT, and the difference was 1.14°.

However, the same result was obtained for the involvement of the mentalis nerve between CBCT and CT. The mentalis nerve was evaluated to assess whether the result differs between soft tissue measurement and bone measurement, which in CT Scan will produce high contrast of radiopaque appearance for bone.

In regard to size dimension, there were differences in tumor length, height, thickness, volume, and angulation between CT and CBCT, although those were very small. The dimension differences are associated with different fields of view between the radiographic approaches. CBCT can only assess the oral and maxillofacial regions from condyle to condyle and from menton to supraorbital bone. On the other hand, CT can assess almost the entire body and can focus on a specific area.

3. Discussion

An ameloblastoma is relatively common among young patients, and it is frequently located in the mandible [1]. In regard to preservation of the mandible, the tumor is usually associated with important anatomical structures, such as inferior alveolar nerve, foramen mentalis, and teeth; thus, care should be taken during surgical removal [2]. The present case was atypical primary tumor because the tumor size was large, which made difficulties to manage such tumor as well as poor outcome.

During the management of an ameloblastoma, it is extremely important for the surgeons to select the most appropriate approach and to decide the extent of resection with a radical approach or assess the consequences of a conservative approach that may be associated with frequent relapses. Preoperative examination involving radiographic assessments will determine the tumor size and help decide whether to select a radical or conservative approach, and if a radical approach, such as resection, is needed, the radiographic findings will help determine the free tumor margin, with consideration of important structures in cases involving the mandible [9].

Considering the CBCT and CT data in our ameloblastoma case, it was found that the data differed and that CBCT results were lower than CT results by about 0.30-1.34%. These findings are consistent with the findings in the study by Lechuga et al., which concluded that CBCT results differ from CT results and that image quality affects the assessment of scanning findings, with better image quality for CT than for CBCT [10]. The difference in image quality might be associated with a larger field of view and higher radiation dose in CT than in CBCT, as CT requires more time and radiation exposure for scanning of the maxillofacial region [10, 11]. Another study has reported different measurement results between CBCT and CT; however, both results were highly accurate for the identification of bone lesions [12].

In the present case, the different findings on CBCT and CT with regard to the ameloblastoma size might not affect the treatment outcome as the free tumor margin has been decided as 1 cm from the outer tumor margin. However, for assessments that need highly accurate measurements in mm, such as implant planning, a measurement difference in mm will affect the treatment plan.

CONCLUSION

Our findings suggest that although CBCT or CT Scan shown slight differences in their results, however, both methods provide good image quality for surgical guidance in regard to measure ameloblastomas and determine the free tumor margin. We demonstrated that a sound judgment is required to select the surgical technique for the treatment of ameloblastomas.

The course of action should be appropriate for each case, especially when a radical treatment is selected. The use of appropriate radiographic examinations, such as CT and CBCT, will help in comparing the consequences of a radical intervention with those approaches that are more conservative, according to the unique features of ameloblastomas on clinical assessment and imaging.

Conflict of Interest

All authors disclose any financial interest and personal relationship to organisations and companies that are mentioned in the article. The patient has given their consent to use photograph for publication.

References

[1] Barnes L, Eveson JW, Reichart P, Sidransky D. World Health Organization Classification of Tumors. *Pathology & Genetics Head and Neck Tumors IARC WHO Classification Head and Neck Tumors.*

[2] Pogrel MA, Dds DMM. (2009). Is there a role for enucleation in the management of ameloblastoma?. *Int. J. Oral Maxillofac. Surg.*, 38:807-812. doi:10.1016/j.ijom. 2009.02.018.

[3] Gosau M, Draenert FG, Müller S, Frerich B, Bürgers R, Reichert TE, et al. (2010). Two modifications in the treatment of keratocystic odontogenic tumors (KCOT) and the use of Carnoy's solution (CS) - a retrospective study lasting between 2 and 10 years. *Clin. Oral Investig.*, 14:27-34. doi:10.1007/s00784-009-0264-6.

[4] Handschel J, Naujoks C, Depprich RA, Kübler NR, Kröpil P, Kuhlemann J, et al. (2012). CT-scan is a valuable tool to detect mandibular involvement in oral cancer patients. *Oral Oncol.* 2012;48:361-366. doi:10.1016/j.oraloncology.2011.11.009.

[5] Chapelle KA, Stoelinga PJ, de Wilde PC, Brouns JJ, Voorsmit RA. (2004). Rational approach to diagnosis and treatment of ameloblastomas and odontogenic keratocysts. *Br. J. Oral Maxillofac. Surg.,* 42:381-390. doi:10.1016/j.bjoms. 2004.04.005.

[6] Güngör E, Doğan MS. (2017). Reliability and accuracy of cone-beam computed tomography voxel density and linear distance measurement at different voxel sizes: A study on sheep head cadaver. *J. Dent. Scim.* 12:145-150. doi:10.1016/j.jds. 2016.11.004.

[7] Brown AA, Scarfe WC, Scheetz JP, Silveira AM, Farman AG. (2009). Linear accuracy of cone beam CT derived 3D images. *Angle Orthod.*, 79:150-157. doi:10.2319/122407-599.1.

[8] Carter JB, Stone JD, Clark RS, Mercer JE. (2016). Applications of Cone-Beam Computed Tomography in Oral and Maxillofacial Surgery: An Overview of Published Indications and Clinical Usage in United States Academic Centers and Oral and Maxillofacial Surgery Practices. *J. Oral Maxillofac. Surg.*, 74:668-679. doi:10.1016/ j.joms.2015.10.018.

[9] Wolff C, Mücke T, Wagenpfeil S, Kanatas A, Bissinger O, Deppe H. (2016). Do CBCT scans alter surgical treatment plans? Comparison of preoperative surgical

diagnosis using panoramic versus cone-beam CT images. *J. Cranio-Maxillofacial Surg.*, 44:1700-1705. doi:10.1016/j. jcms.2016.07.025.

[10] Lechuga L, Weidlich GA. (2016). Cone Beam CT vs Fan Beam CT: A Comparison of Image Quality and Dose Delivered between Two Differing CT Imaging Modalities Methods and materials. *Cureus*, 8. doi:10.7759/cureus.778.

[11] Stratis A, Zhang G, Lopez-rendon X, et al. (2017). Physica Medica Two examples of indication specific radiation dose calculations in dental CBCT and Multidetector CT scanners. *Phys. Medica*, 41:71-77. doi:10.1016/j.ejmp.2017.03.027.

[12] Gaia BF, Sales MA, Perrella A, Fenyo-Pereira M, Cavalcanti MG. (2011). Comparison between cone-beam and multislice computed tomography for identification of simulated bone lesions. *Braz. Oral Res.*, 25:362-368.

In: Clinical Reports in Dentistry
Editor: Lisa R. Amir
ISBN: 978-1-53617-328-4

Chapter 18

FACIAL LIPOMA: A CASE REPORT

Hardi S. Riyadi[1], Abdul Latif[2,*] and Eky Nasuri[3]

[1]Oral and Maxillofacial Surgery Residency Program, Faculty of Dentistry,
Universitas Indonesia, Jakarta, Indonesia
[2]Department of Oral and Maxillofacial Surgery, Faculty of Dentistry,
Universitas Indonesia, Jakarta, Indonesia
[3]Department of Oral and Maxillofacial Surgery,
Cipto Mangunkusumo Hospital, Jakarta, Indonesia

ABSTRACT

Introduction: Lipomas are common, benign, soft-tissue tumors containing mature adipose tissues that rarely develop in the head and neck region; however, these should be considered as one of the potential diagnoses of a neck mass. Most lipomas develop in subcutaneous tissues, but deeper tissues may also be involved. Between 15% and 20% of lipomas involve head and neck masses and between 1% and 5% involve benign oral cavity neoplasms. We reported the case of a patient with lipoma on the left sub-mandibular region of the face.

Case report: A 54-year-old man was admitted to Cipto Mangunkusumo hospital with an initial complaint of swelling on the left mandible with a painless, mobile, and smooth surface that had been present for 1 year prior to admission. Computed tomography revealed a radiolucent image of the left mandible. The diagnosis was a lipoma on the left mandible. Complete surgical excision should be performed on lipomas because of the potential for recurrence after inadequate surgery.

Conclusion: A submandibular incision can provide good visualization of the tumor and also lead to a better esthetic end result for the patient.

Keywords: maxillary tuberosity, maxillary sinus, impacted upper third molar, odontectomy

* Corresponding Author's Email: hartantodentz@yahoo.com

1. Introduction

Lipomas are benign tumors containing mature adipose cells without atypical cells that can occur at all body sites consisting of fatty tissues. Lipomas in the facial region are rare, with 15%-20% of lipoma cases found in the head and neck region and 1%-5% in the oral cavity [1-3].

Lipomas can be divided into three types: superficial lipomas, deep lipomas, and periosteal lipomas [4]. Some studies have correlated the etiology and pathogenesis of lipomas with inflammatory, endocrine, and mechanical processes, however, these correlations remain to be clearly defined [1].

The age of onset for lipomas is usually in the 5th or 6th decade of life, while the occurrence in children is very uncommon. A few studies have indicated that lipomas occur in approximately 5% of patients, with no gender predilection. Lipomas may occur at various sites in the oral cavity, including the vestibular region, major salivary glands, buccal mucosa, the roof of the mouth, lips, and tongue; these lipomas account for 1%-4.4% of all benign oral lesions [1,2]. Some studies have reported that the cheeks are the most common site of lipoma development [5]. The characteristics of this tumor are soft, painless, nodular masses with a smooth, mobile surface. Sometimes this tumor interfere speech and mastication. We report the case of a patient with lipoma in the oral and maxillofacial region. The treatment for lipomas is surgical excision, and the incidence of recurrence is rare.

2. Case Report

A 54-year-old man visited Cipto Mangunkusumo Hospital with an initial complaint of a lump in his left mandible that had been existed for 1 year prior to admission. Clinical examination revealed a soft, painless lump (90×60×90 mm) on the left mandible, with a smooth, mobile surface, well-defined borders, no tenderness, and the color was similar to its surroundings, with no visible fluid discharge and no signs of inflammation that would cause difficulty in swallowing (Figure 1). Computed tomography (CT) showed an encapsulated mass growth in the buccal soft tissue (with a maximum diameter of around 7×5 cm), with dense adipose tissue on the left side of the face extending adjacent to the body of the left mandible (Figure 2).

The patient underwent surgery under general anesthesia. A transcutaneous approach via a submandibular incision was chosen for this procedure to gain a clearer visualization of the tumor. Furthermore, a blunt layered dissection was performed to release the mass from the surrounding tissue (Figure 3).

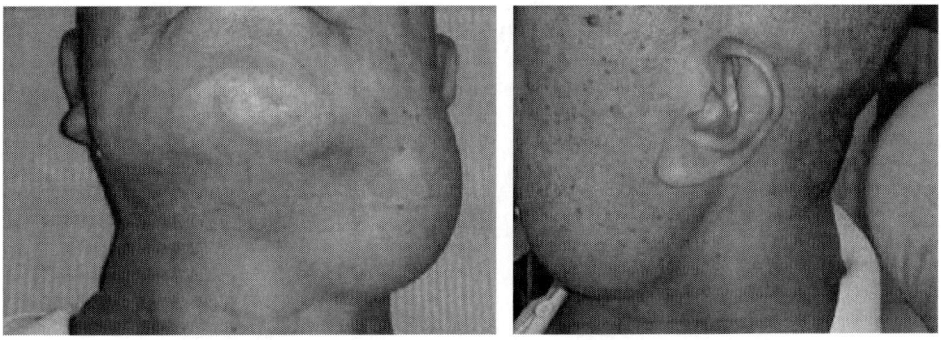

Figure 1. Clinical appearance of the tumor on the left side of the face.

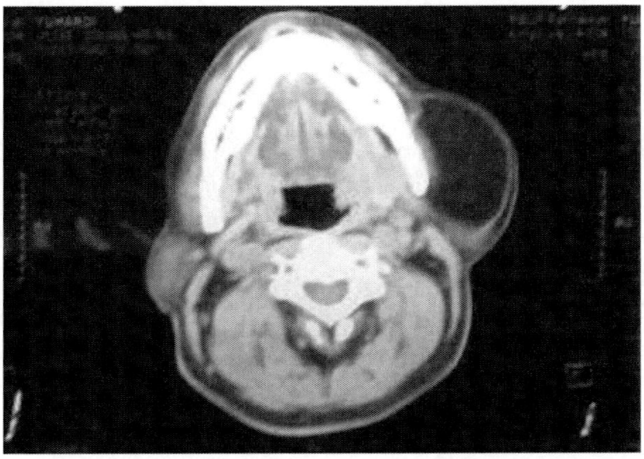

Figure 2. Axial CT section showing a tumor-like mass located in the left mandible (masseteric).

Surgical cavity irrigation was then performed with Povidone iodine, and the muscle layers were sutured using Vicryl suture 3.0 for muscle tissue and Promilene suture 4.0 for skin. The 70 × 50 × 20-mm tumor was yellowish and was found to be well encapsulated (Figure 3).

3. Discussion

Lipomas are benign, subcutaneous, and submucosal tumors that usually grow without any symptoms and cause cosmetic problems [3,6]. These tumors rarely occur and can be characterized by their mostly well-circumscribed, encapsulated, smooth, or lobulated appearance [1,2,6]. Usually, lipomas can be classified depending on the clinical and microscopic features of the tumor. Lipomas may invade muscle tissue or grow between the muscles, resulting in the formation of infiltrating or intramuscular lipomas [6]. Intermuscular lipomas can occur between skeletal muscles. While the etiology for these tumors remains to be verified.

Lipomas are normally triggered by local irritation, caused by activities such as smoking and alcohol. The most common location of lipomas in the oral and maxillofacial region is in cheek mucosa, followed by the tongue, lips, oral cavity, palate, and retromolar space. According to a study by Furlong et al. 125 cases of lipomas in the oral and maxillofacial region have been reported, showing that the parotid region has the highest prevalence of lipomas, followed by oral mucosa, with most tumors having diameters of 0.5-2 cm; a maximum size of 5.5 cm in diameter has been reported, but it is not common [1,4,6].

Imaging of tumors is necessary for diagnosis, and many techniques such as CT, magnetic resonance imaging (MRI), and ultrasonography are present. On CT, the soft-tissue mass appears as a homogenous hypo-attenuated mass with a number from -60 to 120 HU and does not typically show contrast enhancement [6]. In MRI, fatty tissue has typical intensity, and MRI provides better information because it has superior soft-tissue contrast resolution and presents clearly defined locations [6].

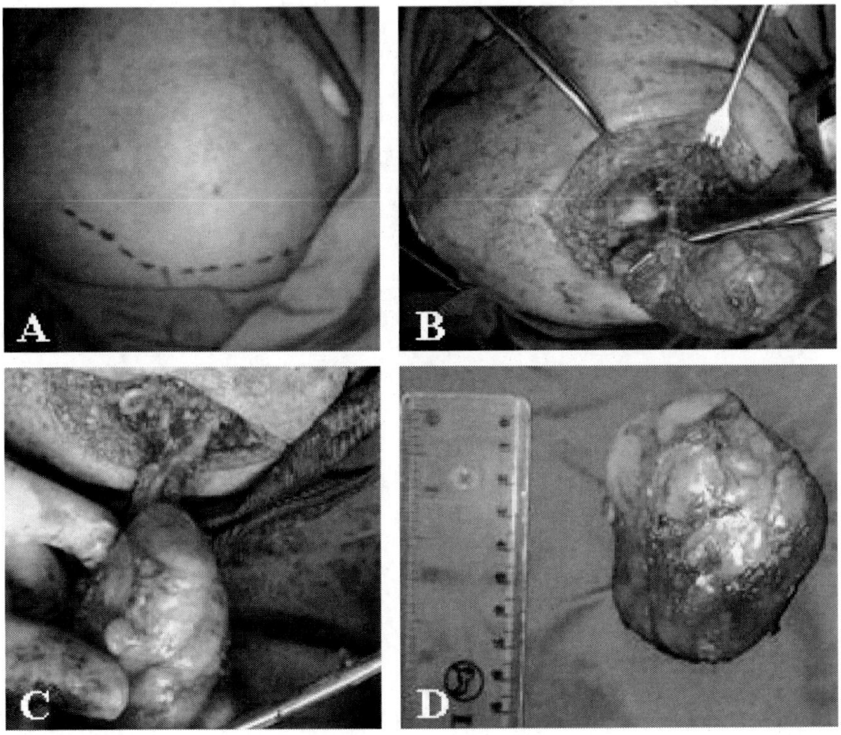

Figure 3. Marking of the intended incision site (sub-mandibula incision) (A); the dissection process (B); The release of the mass from the surrounding area (C), and the mass (D)

The clinical differential diagnoses for this type of lesion include dermoid cysts, pleomorphic adenomas and mucoepidermoid carcinomas, angiolipomas, fibrolipomas, and malignancy [4]. The treatment for lipomas is a conventional surgical excision, and the access to the tumor depends on its location [1]. An intra-oral incision can be performed if tumors extend into the buccal region. In this case report, the tumor presented on the face with no buccal extension. Based on these observations, the extra-oral access considered as a good option to obtain complete tumor excision. However, as a complication, the instrument may damage the facial nerves and blood vessels during dissection procedure, which may lead to the compromised function and aesthetics of the stomatognathic system of the patient [1,4]. To avoid aesthetic problems, thus, a submandibular incision was performed. Histopathological findings confirmed that the lump was a simple lipoma. The well-encapsulated mass contained the proliferation of fat tissue without the presence of any atypical cells and no sign of malignancy was found.

The prognosis for lipomas is always good. Their recurrence after complete surgical excision in adult patients is rare, although a long-term monitoring is recommended to ensure the success of the procedure [1,5].

Conclusion

Complete surgical excision should be undertaken for lipomas because of their infiltrating nature and potential for recurrence after inadequate surgery. A submandibular incision can provide good visualization of the tumor and lead to a better aesthetic result. Imaging, using techniques such as CT and MRI, is very important for determining the nature of anatomical extensions. After surgery, it is very important to monitor the patient to avoid the recurrence of tumors.

References

[1] Oliveira R., Tavares S. S., Peixoto T. S., Arag S., Godoy G. P., (2014). Unusual facial lipoma. *RGO-Revista Gaúcha de Odontologia* [*RGO-Gaúcha Journal of Dentistry*], 62:425-430.

[2] Kawasaki G., Yanamto S., Hirata K., Mizuno A., Fujita S., Ikeda T., (2006). Spindle cell lipoma of the cheek: A case report and review of literature. *Oral. Oncol. Extra,* 42:301-304.

[3] Chia C. Y., Rovaris D. A., Fontana R. (2016). Giant lipoma of the buccal fat pad: case report and literature review. *Rev. Bras. Cir. Plástica-Brazilian. J. Plast. Surg.,* 31: 112-117.

[4] Sathiaki D. C., Swarup J. *The case report lipoma of the submandibular space*, 2: 4329-4331.

[5] Saluja H., Mahindra U., Kasat V., Dehane V., Chaudhari R. K. (2013). Excision of a large soft tissue lipoma of the cheek through an intra-oral approach. *J. Cranio. Max. Dis.,* 2:201-204.

[6] Salvatore C., Antonio B., Del Vecchio W., Lanza A., Tartaro G. P., Giuseppe C. (2003). Giant infiltrating lipoma of the face: CT and MR imaging findings. *Am. J. Neuroradiol.*, 24:283-286.

In: Clinical Reports in Dentistry
Editor: Lisa R. Amir
ISBN: 978-1-53617-328-4

Chapter 19

MANAGEMENT OF MAXILLARY DENTIGEROUS CYST IN A 14-YEAR-OLD FEMALE: A CASE REPORT

Ahdadiansyah[1,*], Evy Eida Vitria[2] and Eky Nasuri[3]

[1]Oral and Maxillofacial Surgery Residency Program, Faculty of Dentistry, Universitas Indonesia, Jakarta, Indonesia
[2]Department of Oral and Maxillofacial Surgery, Faculty of Dentistry, Universitas Indonesia, Jakarta, Indonesia
[3]Division of Oral and Maxillofacial Surgery, Cipto Mangunkusumo National Hospital, Jakarta, Indonesia

ABSTRACT

Introduction: Dentigerous cyst is the most common odontogenic cyst in the jaw after radicular cyst and more frequently occurs in males at the 20s – 30s years. This cyst is commonly associated with impacted or embedded teeth, such as the third mandibular molar. Dentigerous cyst is frequently discovered accidentally when radiographs are used to investigate a failed tooth eruption or missing tooth, and it can could grow to be an ameblastoma. This case report described the diagnosis and management of a right maxillary dentigerous cyst.

Case Report: A 14-year-old female visited the Oral and Maxillofacial Surgery Clinic of Cipto Mangunkusumo Hospital because she has had a swelling in her right maxilla from 3 months ago. Enucleation of the cyst along with odontectomy of the unerupted tooth were performed under general anesthesia. The diagnosis was a maxillary dentigerous cyst due to an impacted maxillary canine.

Conclusion: An adequate and appropriate treatment to prevent further maxillary damage and recurrence is necessary in the rare case of maxillary dentigerous cyst.

Keywords: dentigerous cyst, impacted canine, enucleation

* Corresponding Author's Email: ahdad99@gmail.com.

1. Introduction

The dentigerous cyst is usually formed by fluid accumulation between the reduced enamel epithelium and results from the proliferation of this epithelium after the enamel formation of an impacted tooth [1]. This cyst is a benign odontogenic lesion that occurs in the permanent dentition. Usually, no pain or discomfort is associated with the cyst unless it becomes larger or there is pain from secondary infection [2]. A dentigerous cyst can cause local destruction, bony expansion, root resorption, or teeth displacement, which more commonly occurs with long-standing lesions [3].

Radiographically, dentigerous cyst typically appears as a well-defined unilocular radiolucency with a radiopaque border and surrounds the crown of an impacted or unerupted tooth. Microscopic features of dentigerous cyst must be evaluated because it can potentially develop into an aggressive ameloblastoma or squamous cell carcinoma [4]. The early detection and removal of the cyst is required to prevent the foreboding associated with the lesion because the prognosis is very good and recurrence is rare if completely removed. The treatment protocol for a dentigerous cyst involves the surgical enucleation and extraction of the impacted or unerupted tooth associated with the cyst [5].

2. Case Report

A 14-year-old female was referred to the Oral and Maxillofacial Surgery Clinic of Cipto Mangunkusumo Hospital with the chief complaint of right cheek swelling from 3 months ago. The swelling was initially small and slowly became larger.

There was no history of pain or discharge related to the swelling. On a general examination, she was healthy and denied any allergy, heart disease, hypertension, and diabetes mellitus. There was no history of past illness or hospitalization or trauma to the jaw.

On an extra-oral examination, facial asymmetry with a single mild, approximately 4×3×1cm swelling was found overlying the right maxillary sinus region (Figure 1). The swelling consistency was cystic with an ill-defined border. The mucosa over the swelling was normal, and the color and temperature were the same as those of the surrounding tissue with no active discharge of pus. On intra-oral examination, oral hygiene was moderate. There was swelling on the right maxillary vestibule area approximately 3×2×2cm, extending from regions 11 to 16. The mucosa over the swelling appeared normal, the color was the same as the surrounding tissue, and there was no evidence of discharge from the swelling region (Figure 2A). On palpation, the swelling was immobile and had a smooth surface, no tenderness, and a cystic consistency. All permanent teeth were present except for the maxillary right canine. The deciduous right maxillary canine was present in the first quadrant with grade II mobility. No other caries lesion or periodontal condition was present.

Orthopantomography revealed a well-defined radiolucent lesion extending from the distal aspect of the lateral right maxillary incisor to the distal aspect of the second permanent right maxillary molar with lesion margins attached to the neck of the unerupted permanent canine, which was located near the orbital floor.

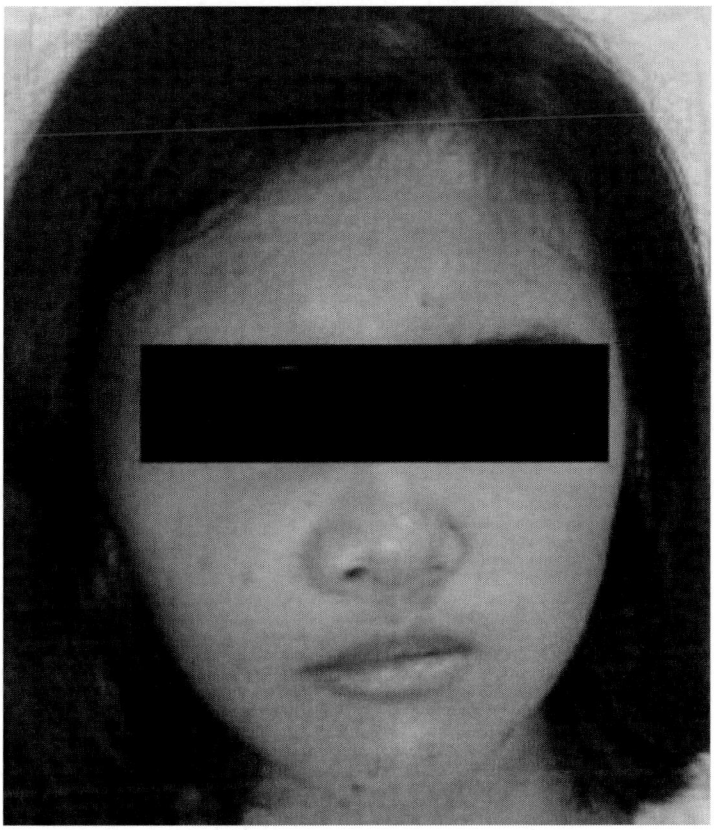

Figure 1. Facial asymmetry with a single mild swelling.

Radiographs demonstrated a deciduous canine with complete and partial root resorption of the first and second premolars (Figure 2B). Aspiration of the swelling yielded a straw-colored fluid. Laboratory examination were within the normal limits. The presumptive diagnosis was a cyst [6].

Surgical enucleation of the lesion and removal of impacted teeth were performed with the patient under general anesthesia. The patient was intubated in a supine position, and povidone iodine was used for asepsis and antisepsis of the operative site. The lesion was identified, and local anesthetic with vasoconstrictor was injected around it. A full-thickness mucoperiosteal flap was elevated to expose the lesion using a No. 15 blade from the distal tooth 21 to the distal tooth 16. A soft-consistency lesion fenestrating the alveolar ridge was observed.

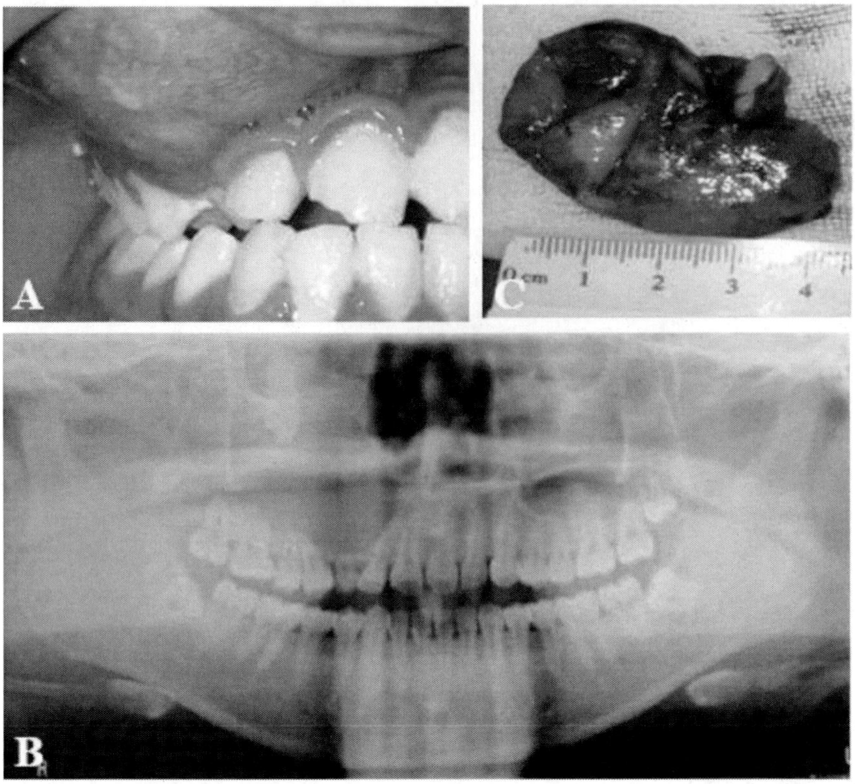

Figure 2. Cyst after enucleation.

The buccal mucosa was dissected to reach the lesion, cyst was enucleated, and impacted maxillary canine tooth was removed, followed by extraction of teeth 53, 14, 15, and 16. The incision was closed using 3 - 0 silk sutures, and the specimen was sent for histopathological investigation (Figure 2C).

On histopathological examination, the cyst wall comprised connective tissue lined by squamous and cuboidal, one layer to stratified epithelium. The subepithelial layer showed an infiltration of acute and chronic inflammatory cells and focus tissue granulation. There were groups of odontogenic epitheliums. On one side of the cyst wall, there was hyperplastic epithelium, which formed a plexiform layer. Histological analysis results were in accordance with a dentigerous cyst with a hyperplastic epithelium focus.

3. Discussion

Dentigerous cyst is the second most common odontogenic cyst in the jaws after radicular cyst. It develops from fluid accumulation between the enamel epithelium and crown of the permanent tooth germ and usually covers the crown of an unerupted tooth, attaches to the cement–enamel junction of the tooth, and expands the follicle [7]. The mandibular and maxillary third molars are the most common unerupted teeth affected followed by the maxillary permanent canines. Generally, a dentigerous cyst occurs in males between ages 20s and 30s. Usually, it is asymptomatic, unless it becomes secondarily infected or becomes large and produces bone deformation or adjacent tooth retention or displacement [8]. Clinical and radiographic examinations are needed for the diagnosis of this cyst. Radiographically, other lesions may share the same radiologic features as dentigerous cysts, such as periapical cysts, residual cysts, odontogenic keratocysts or unicystic ameloblastomas [9]. The involvement of the tooth, cortical expansion, and radicular resorption are characteristics that are more relevant to dentigerous cyst. It presents as a well-defined unilocular radiolucency, often with a sclerotic border, and this radiolucency surrounds the crown of an impacted tooth [10]. Treatment options for dentigerous cyst include marsupialization or enucleation, depending on the size and location of the cyst, patients 'age, and the proximity of the cyst to vital structures. The cyst should be treated to avoid bone destruction, resorption of teeth roots, displacement, and obliteration of the maxillary antrum and nasal cavities [11]. In our case, total enucleation and curettage of the cyst with the removal of the impacted tooth were chosen.

Conclusion

This report described a rare presentation of inflammatory dentigerous cyst occurring at a young age and being discovered after the patient complained of swelling on her face. The lesion could have destroyed more anatomical areas if she did not have a complaint. All specialists, including general dental practitioners, must evaluate missing teeth so that an accurate diagnosis and adequate treatment can be planned for the best management of these patients.

References

[1] Devi, P., Thimmarasa, V. B., Mehrotra, V., Agarwal, M. (2015). Multiple Dentigerous Cysts: A Case Report and Review. *J. Maxillofac. Oral Surg.*, 14:47 - 5. DOI 10.1007/s12663-011-0280-3.

[2] Kaushik, A., Chaudhry, A., Saluja, P., Kumar, M., Varshney, M. (2015). Non-syndromic Bilateral Dentigerous Cysts of Maxillary and Mandibular Canines: A Case Series and Review of Literature. *J. Oral Maxillofac. Surg. Med. Pathol.,* 27(4):562 - 566.

[3] Gendviliene, I., Legrand, P., Nicolielo, L. F. P., Sinha, D., Spaey, Y., Politis, C. et al. (2017). Conservative Management of Large Mandibular Dentigerous Cysts with

A Novel Approach for Follow Up : Two Case Reports. *Stomatologija, Baltic Dent. Maxillofac. J.,* 19:24 - 32.

[4] Natarajan, S., Inbarajan, A., Seenivasan, M., Banu, F. R., Saravanan, T. T., Saran, P. (2018). Prosthetic Management of Dentigerous Cyst Associated with Impacted Mandibular Molar. *Dent. Med. Res.*, 6:15 - 18.

[5] Chhimwal, P., Shrivastava, H., Shah, N., Bhavasar, R. (2016). Dentigerous Cyst Associated with Impacted Permanent Maxillary Canine: A Case Report. *Inter. J. Recent Sci. Res.,* 7(4):10496 - 10498.

[6] Mert, T., Cem, Ö., Burak, Ç. A., Sami, Y., Levent, B. (2016). Conservative Approach to A Large Dentigerous Cyst in An 11-Year-Old Patient. *J. Istanbul Univ. Fac. Dent.,* 50(3):51 - 56.

[7] Xu, G. Z.,Yang, C., Fan, X. D., Hu, Y. K., Yu, C. Q. (2015). Functional Surgery for the Treatment of Dentigerous Cyst in the Maxillary Sinus. *J. Craniofac. Surg.,* 26(2):e84 - 86.

[8] Contar, C. M. M., Thome, C. A., Pompermayer, A., Sarot, J. R., Vinagre, R. O., Machado, M. A. N. (2015). Marsupialization of Dentigerous Cyst: Report of a Case. *J. Maxillofac. Oral Surg.,* 14(Suppl. 1):S4–S6. DOI 10.1007/s12663-011-0172-6.

[9] Thambi, N., Anjana, G., Sunil, E. A., Manjooran, T., Nair, A., Jaleel, D. (2016). Inflamed Dentigerous Cyst: A Case Report and Review. *Oral Maxillofac. Pathol. J.,* 7(2):744 - 747.

[10] Jain, N., Gaur, G., Chaturvedy, V., Verma, A. (2018). Dentigerous Cyst associated with Impacted Maxillary Premolar: A Rare Site Occurrence and a Rare Coincidence. *Inter. J. Cli. Pediatr. Dent.,* 11(1):50 - 52.

[11] Gendviliene, I., Legrand, P., Nicolielo, L. F. P., Sinha, D., Spaey, Y., Politis, C. et al. (2017). Conservative Management of Large Mandibular Dentigerous Cysts with A Novel Approach for Follow Up: Two Case Reports. *Stomatologija, Baltic Dent. Maxillofac. J.,* 19:24 - 32.

In: Clinical Reports in Dentistry
Editor: Lisa R. Amir

ISBN: 978-1-53617-328-4

Chapter 20

SURGICAL MANAGEMENT OF LARGE FIBRO-EPITHELIAL HYPERPLASIA: A CASE REPORT

Yayan Andrian[1], Iwan Tofani[2,*] and Etty Soenartini[3]
[1]Oral and Maxillofacial Surgery Residency Program,
Faculty of Dentistry, Universitas Indonesia, Jakarta, Indonesia
[2]Department of Oral and Maxillofacial Surgery, Faculty of Dentistry,
Universitas Indonesia, Jakarta, Indonesia
[3]Department of Oral and Maxillofacial Surgery, Persahabatan Hospital,
Rawamangun, Indonesia

ABSTRACT

Introduction: Fibro-epithelial hyperplasia is a localized or generalized proliferative fibrous lesion of oral mucosa resulting from local irritation and response to injury. This pathological lesion can impair the gingival functions of mastication and their aesthetic appearance. This case study is a diagnostic and management report of a patient with 10-year-long slowly progressive gingival enlargement with several systemic complications. This patient has been managed by excisional surgery.

Case report: A 69-year-old female patient came to the oral and maxillofacial clinical department in Persahabatan Hospital with a chief complaint of gum enlargement starting 10 years ago, accompanied by systemic complications. Panoramic radiographic showed no bone destruction. The fibrous inflammatory gingival tissue was surgically excised under general anesthesia. Post-surgery, the enlarged gingival tissue was significantly reduced and no post-operative complications were noted.

Conclusion: Cognizant and careful treatments are needed in patients with large fibro-epithelial hyperplasia accompanied by systemic complications.

Keywords: fibro-epithelial hyperplasia, gingiva, local irritation, surgical management

* Corresponding Author's Email: iwan.tofani@yahoo.com.

1. Introduction

Gingival tumors are challenging because many differential diagnoses can be inferred from a single complaint. Gingival tumors can be categorized by their location, etiopathogenesis, size and various other factors [1]. Patients with gingival tumors should be managed cautiously, as prevention and curative action require a flawless diagnostic approach [2]. Moreover, as gingival enlargement is a symptom of several systemic diseases, the correct diagnosis can potentially save a patient's life and improve their quality of life when treatment is started promptly [3].

Etiopathogenesis inducers of gingival enlargement include inflammation, associated systemic diseases, side effects of drug administration and neoplasia. Enlargements can even be false [1]. On the basis of the visual appearance of their distribution, gingival tumors can be isolated, discrete, or regional [4]. Isolated gingival growth is clearly limited to one or two teeth adjacent to the gingival location. Discrete lesions are described as tumor-like enlargements with isolated sessile or pedunculated characteristics; they can also be observed as a fibroma or pyogenic granuloma. Regional enlargements, which involve three or more teeth, may occur in single or multiple areas within the oral cavity. Generalized enlargements involve almost all parts of the gingiva adjacent to the presented teeth [1].

Fibroepithelial hyperplasia can manifest as a non-inflammatory an isolated-to-regionally distributed gingival enlargement [4]. The condition sometimes presents in hypertensive patients treated with calcium channel blockers [5,6]. Although gingival hyperplasia is a common side effect of nifedipine, several case reports have also mentioned amlodipine as an inducer of fibroepithelial hyperplasia [6,7]. The surgical approach should be selected in a cautious manner. Patients with gingival enlargement can be treated through conventional periodontal management, such as scaling or root planning. However, patients with a significant fibrotic component within the enlarged gingiva, including those with fibroepithelial hyperplasia, may not respond to these modalities. As the patient in our case study has had enlarged gingiva for 10 years, and a history of routine amlodipine consumption, excisional surgery is the preferred treatment and diagnostic tool.

2. Case Report

A 69-year-old female patient came to the oral and maxillofacial clinical department in Persahabatan Hospital with a chief complaint of gum enlargement starting 10 years ago, accompanied by systemic complications. The patient's chief complaint was a progressively enlarging bump on the left upper jaw. Initially the approximate size of a soybean, the bump had slowly enlarged over the past 10 years. No history of pain accompanied the growth. As the bump enlarged, the surrounding teeth became unsteady. Until examination, the bump has been filling the oral cavity and the intrusion was felt by the patient (Figure 1). The bump was felt to move when the patient swallowed. A previous history of shortness of breath or drastic weight loss was denied. The patient has a history of hypertension and is currently treated with amlodipine.

Physical examination revealed a normal extra-oral region with no lymph node enlargement. In the intra-oral region, a bump of size (10 x 8 x 5) cm^3 was identified near #27 tooth, growing from a stalk and expanding into the palate and oropharynx area. The growth was of solid consistency, similar color to the surrounding tissue, not easily bled, non-tender, and painless on palpation. The diagnosis was a tumor of gingival origin that was planned to be removed by excisional surgery. No visible bone destruction was detected in panoramic radiograph (Figure 2).

The patient was managed by excisional biopsy under general anesthesia. Prior to surgery, the patient was given cefazoline (2 g) as a prophylactic antibiotic. A triangular flap incision was made in the distal part of teeth 23-28 (Figure 3A). The flap was opened with a raspatory until the mass became identifiable (Figure 3B). The peduncle of the mass was fixed with an Ellis clamp and moved with the raspatory (Figure 3C). The mass was faultlessly removed, followed by the extraction of 24, 27 and 28 teeth. The buccal mucosa tissue was dissected to achieve primary wound closure (Figure 3D). The removed mass (Figure 3E) was stored in 10% formalin liquid and transferred to the Pathological Anatomy Department of Persahabatan Hospital for histopathological examination. The remaining sharp bone was mashed with a Fraser bur until a good arch maxilla was obtained. The wound was irrigated with 0.9% NaCl, and the flap was repositioned and sutured with silk 3.0. 16, 17, 18, 34, 36, 44, and 48 Teeth were also extracted as indicated. The wound was then irrigated with povidone iodine and 0.9% NaCl 0.9% and sutured using silk 3.0.

Histopathological examination revealed a polypoid mass covered by hyperplastic and erosive stratified squamous epithelial tissue, as well as granulation tissue with comminuting acute and chronic inflammatory cells accompanied by myxoid degeneration.

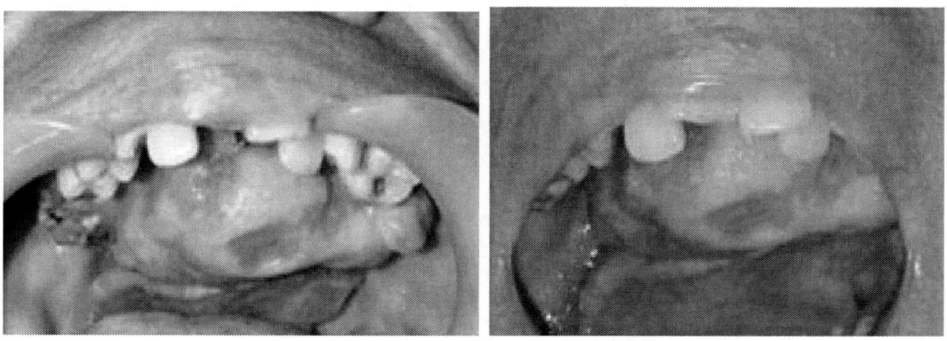

Figure 1. Pre-operative assessment of the patient in the case study.

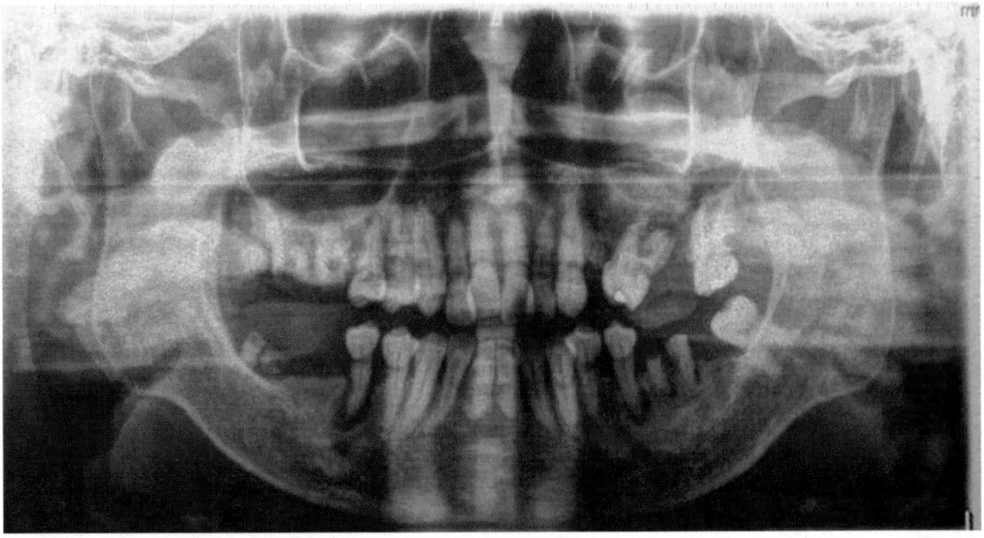

Figure 2. Panoramic radiograph showing no visible bone destruction.

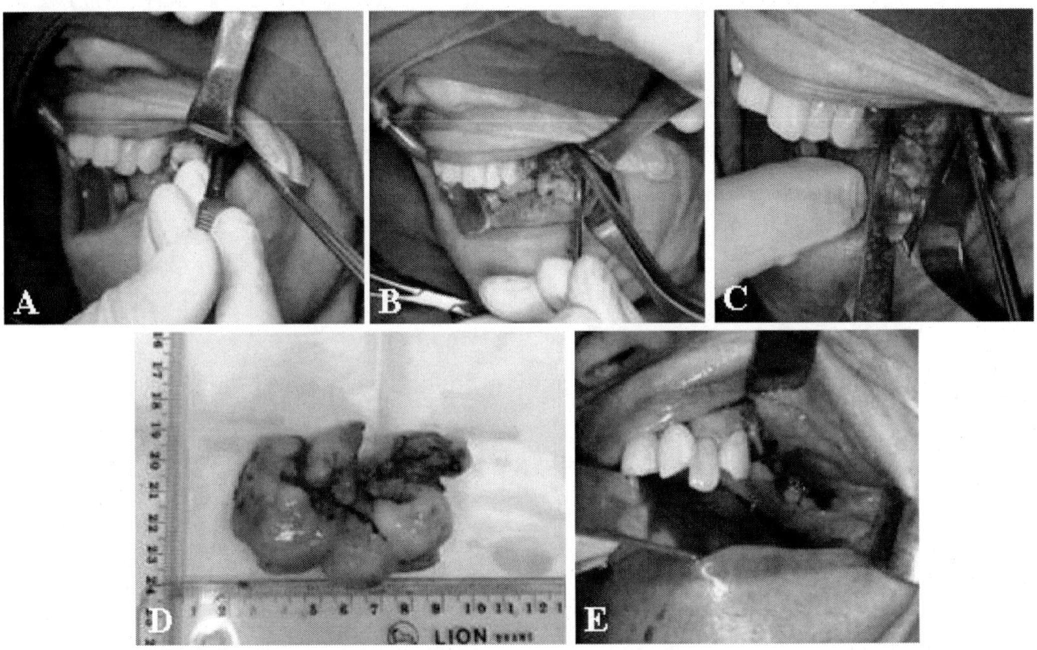

Figure 3. The excision procedure. Making the flap incision with blade no. 15 (A); Separating the mass using the rasparatorium (B); Extracting the mass using an Ellis clamp (C); Suturing the wound with silk 3-0 (D); Solid mass after removal, size $(8 \times 5 \times 3)\ cm^3$ (E).

The mass was diagnosed as a secondarily infected fibro-epithelial hyperplasia with pyogenic granuloma. The patient control plan was observation and suture removal within 1 week and observation at 1-month post-surgery (Figure 4A, B).

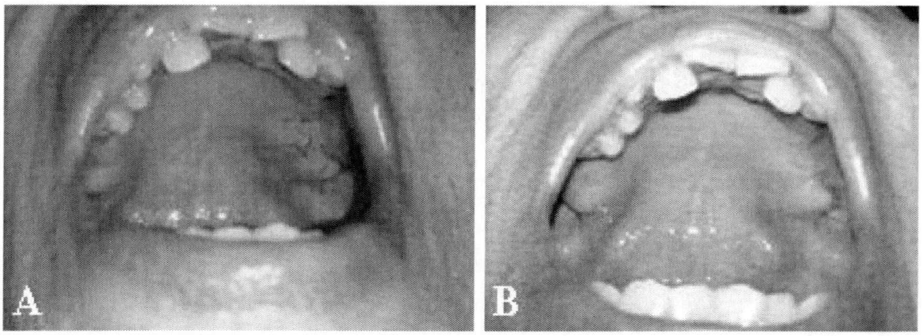

Figure 4. Post-surgery appearances. 1 week after of post-surgical control, the patient presented without further complaint (A); After 1 month of post-operative control, the patient again reported no complaint (B).

3. Discussion

Either reactive or neoplastic conditions can induce fibrous growth within the oral cavity. Most fibroepithelial hyperplasias arise through repetitive mechanical stress or injury. Mechanical stress may be caused by particulate matter such as calculi and foreign bodies or by physical processes such as teeth biting [8]. Clinically, they appear as sessile or elevated pedunculated growths with a smooth surface and normal color. The case-study patient did not complain of jaw misalignment or ill-fitting restorations but presented with a history of hypertension and amlodipine consumption. Therefore, amlodipine was considered as the main culprit in this case [7, 9].

Drug-induced gingival overgrowth has also occurred in several patients who systemically use anticonvulsants and immunosuppresants [6]. An association between erythromycin and trimethropim-sulphamethoxazole consumption with gingival enlargement has also been reported, albeit to a lesser degree. Gingival hyperplasia is less commonly seen in patients consuming vigabatrin, sodium valproate, primidone, and phenobarbital drugs than in patients consuming phenytoin. Among the calcium channel blocker class, nifedipine is the most widely prescribed drug, followed by amlodipine, verapamil, nicardipine, oxodipine, nitrendipine, felodipine, and lastly diltiazem [5, 6]. Our patient denied the consumption of any calcium channel blocker except amlodipine.

Amlodipine is a member of the dihydropiridine sub-class of calcium channel blockers. The drug lowers the blood pressure but may induce gingival hypertrophy. The prevalence of gingival enlargement among amlodipine consumers is fairly low (1.7-3.3% of all cases) [9]. Nifedipine-induced gingival hypertrophy is much more common, presenting in 20% of nifedipine consumers. In total, calcium channel blockers are believed to contribute up to 38% of gum hypertrophy cases. Prevalence-wise, men appear to be more commonly affected than women [9].

Gum enlargement in drug-induced gingival overgrowth begins with a firm, modular enlargement of the interdental papilla, usually within 3 months of starting the suspected medication. Initially limited to the keratinized portions of the gingiva, the slowly growing bump eventually involves other part of the gum. The connective tissue component is thought to increase through activation of the gingival fibroblasts. The growth may be accompanied by gingival inflammation, mostly due to mechanical injury causing secondary infection. All of these observations suggest that such lesions emerge through interactions among the gingival fibroblasts, drug metabolites, and cellular and biochemical mediators [6].

Although the causative link between bacterial plaque and gingival overgrowth remains ill-defined, poor oral hygiene is a risk factor of any form of gingival enlargement. Despite lack of a concrete explanation, several development pathways have been proposed for gingival enlargement. Gingival enlargement can be dichotomized into inflammatory and non-inflammatory types. The suggested non-inflammatory mechanism includes changes in collagenase activity following a prior history of decreased folic acid intake, aldosterone synthesis blockage, adrenocorticotropic changes in hormone levels and upregulation of keratinocyte growth factor. On the other hand, inflammatory gingival enlargements are considered as a direct toxic effect of a concentrated drug and its metabolites, which may or may not be accompanied by bacterial plaques. In turn, this inflammation may upregulate several cytokine factors, including transforming growth factor beta [6]. In managing patients with gingival overgrowth, the surgical approach is preferred over other conventional modal treatments. Patients presenting with large bumps that aesthetically and functionally impair the oral cavity are encouraged to undergo surgical management [10].

Conclusion

Large fibroepithelial hyperplasia can impair the gingival functions of mastication and their aesthetic appearance. Cognizant and careful treatments are needed in patients with large fibroepithelial hyperplasia accompanied by systemic complications.

References

[1] Agrawal, A. A. (2015). Gingival enlargements: Differential diagnosis and review of literature. *World Journal of Clinical Cases*, 3:779.

[2] Sabharwal, S., Shukla, P., Dahiya, V. & Kataria P. (2014). Inflammatory hyperplasia: From diagnosis to treatment. *Journal of Indian Society of Periodontology*, 18:92.

[3] Shivakumar, M. A., Mathew, M., Govindaraju, P. & Suvarchala, D. P. (2016). Gingival hyperplasia and quality of life. *Journal of Research in Medical and Dental Science*, 4:75.

[4] Varghese, J., Raizada, S., Bhat, K. & Gupta, K. (2016). Isolated gingival overgrowths: A review of case series. *Contemporary Clinical Dentistry*, 7:265.

[5] Carty, O., Walsh, E., Abdelsalem, A. & MaCarthy, D. (2015). Case report: Drug-induced gingival overgrowth associated with the use of a calcium channel blocker (amlodipine). *Journal of the Irish Dental Association*, 61:248-251.

[6] Madi, M., Shetty, S., Babu, S. & Achalli, S. (2015). Amlodipine induced gingival hyperplasia a case report and review. *West Indian Medical Journal*, 64:279-282.

[7] Koratala, A., Jamalpur, I. & Mogili, H. R. (2017). Amlodipine-induced gingival enlargement. *Clinical Case Reports*, 5:1714-1715.

[8] Jain, M., Singh, A. V., Leekha, S. & Prashar, S. (2017). Firboepithelial hyperplasia: A case report. *International Healthcare Research Journal*, 1:16-19.

[9] Sharma, S. & Sharma, A. (2012). Amlodipine-induced gingival enlargement - a clinical report. *Compendium of continuing education in dentistry (Jamesburg, NJ: 1995)*, 33:78-82.

[10] Srivastava, A., Kundu, D., Bandyopadhyay, P. & Pal, A. (2010). Management of amlodipine-induced gingival enlargement: Series of three cases. *Journal of Indian Society of Periodontology*, 14:279.

In: Clinical Reports in Dentistry
Editor: Lisa R. Amir
ISBN: 978-1-53617-328-4

Chapter 21

SURGICAL APPROACH TO RADICULAR CYST WITH REPOSITIONING OF THE INFERIOR ALVEOLAR NERVE: A CASE REPORT

Riadin J. Patomo[1], Adhitya Latief[2,*] and Benny S. Latief[2]

[1]Oral and Maxillofacial Surgery Residency Program,
Faculty of Dentistry, Universitas Indonesia, Jakarta, Indonesia
[2]Department of Oral and Maxillofacial Surgery,
Faculty of Dentistry, Universitas Indonesia, Jakarta, Indonesia

ABSTRACT

Introduction: Radicular cysts are the most common cystic lesions in the jaw, with a prevalence of approximately 52% to 68% cysts affecting the jaw. These cysts are associated with non-vital teeth. Nonsurgical treatment includes root canal therapy, where the lesion is localized, or surgical treatment such as enucleation of a large lesion. In this case report, we described the surgical approach of a right mandibular radicular cyst with relocation of the inferior alveolar nerve due to surgical enucleation.

Case Report: A 61-year-old female patient attended the division of oral and maxillofacial surgery at Jakarta Hospital with the chief complaint of pain, swelling and paresthesia of the right posterior jaw. Intra-oral clinical examination revealed swelling at the buccal mucosal region #44–46. Unilocular periapical radiolucency associated with teeth #44–46 was revealed on a panoramic radiograph. The patient was treated by surgical enucleation under general anesthesia.

Conclusion: Enucleation with relocation of the inferior alveolar nerve was performed to remove the radicular cyst. Depending on the size and extent of the lesion, surgical enucleation of a radicular cyst is necessary for optimal treatment and prevention of recurrence.

* Corresponding Author's Email: adhityalatief@yahoo.com.

Keywords: radicular cyst, mandible, enucleation, inferior alveolar nerve

1. Introduction

Cysts are pathologic epithelial cavities containing fluid or semifluid material. Odontogenic cysts are derived from the epithelium due to dental growth. Some types of cysts are classified according to the stages of odontogenesis. Odontogenic cysts can be formed due to dental tooth infection, epithelial cell rests of Malassez, epithelium derived from dental crowns, dental lamina remnants, or possibly the basal layer of the oral epithelium. Cysts are often found in the mouth and maxillofacial areas, and those developing in the jaw bone region are fluid-filled cavities or semifluid materials surrounded by epithelium. Cystic fluid has a higher osmotic pressure compared to its surroundings, resulting in fluid entering the tissue in the cystic cavity, causing cyst enlargement and damage to the surrounding hard tissue [1, 2].

The most common cyst in the jaw is the radicular cyst. This cyst is caused by dental caries with untreated necrotic pulp and periapical infection with a prevalence of 52% – 68%. They are formed by chronic inflammatory processes and grow over long periods of time. Radicular cysts are also known as apical periodontal cysts and root canal cysts. Radicular cysts become very large due to their ability to expand and extend to adjacent tissues accompanied by rapid growth and high recurrence rates [2, 3].

These cysts are generally not accompanied by symptoms, and some cases are diagnosed as radicular cysts following radiological examination. Therapy for radicular cysts includes nonsurgical treatment, such as root canal treatment, or surgical treatments such as enucleation, marsupialization, or decompression. Surgical treatment becomes more difficult when the larger cysts, especially if it is positioned near the structure of the inferior alveolar nerve [4, 5].

Here, we described a case of radicular cysts of the right lower jaw surrounding the first molars and first and second premolars of the right mandible. Treatment includes surgical enucleation, tooth extraction and relocation of the inferior alveolar nerve.

2. Case Report

A 61-year-old woman presented to the Oral and Maxillofacial Surgery Division of Jakarta Hospital with the chief complaint of pain and swelling in the right lower jaw (Figure 1). She had been suffering from paresthesia in the right lower jaw for several months, but her facial expression muscles were fully functional. There was no previous history of systemic or allergic disease, and she denied trauma to the right lower jaw. A panoramic radiographic examination was performed, which detected swelling around the right mandibular first molar and right mandibular first and second premolars.

Based on panoramic radiographs in the right mandibular region, a periapical unilocular radiolucency was suspected as a radicular cyst surrounding the distal roots of the first molar teeth and the right mandibular first and second premolars. The floor of the cyst wall was very close to the lower jaw, compressing the nerve so that the image of the inferior alveolar nerve bundle disappears, changing the position of the mental foramen (Figure 2).

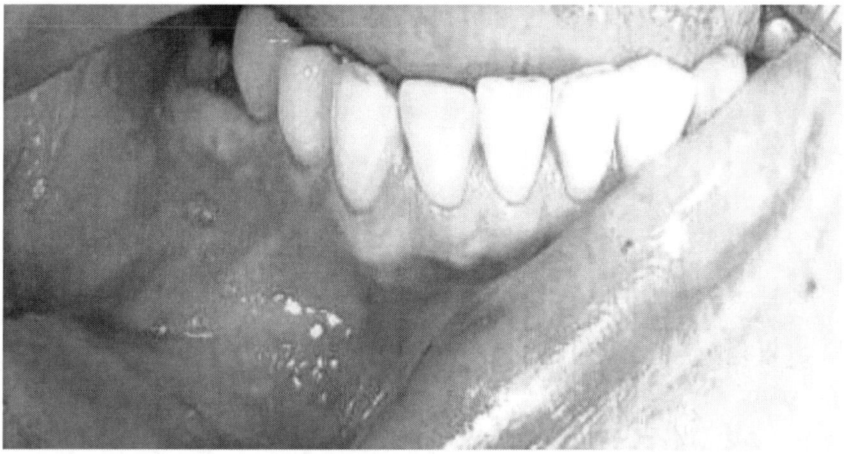

Figure 1. Intra-oral appearance and swelling on the right mandible.

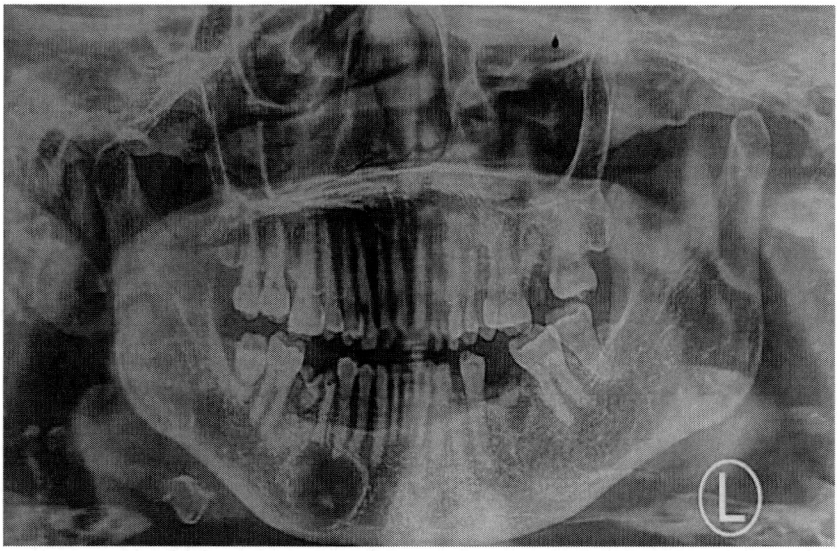

Figure 2. Radiographic appearance of 3 teeth surrounded by a large radicular cyst.

Our treatment of this case was based on clinical and radiological examination and was performed surgically under general anesthesia with the aim of removing the entire cyst using enucleation technique and simultaneously removing the infected teeth causing the formation of the cyst. This operation was based on minimally invasive techniques to protect the inferior alveolar nerve, with relocation of the nerve. The patient was placed in the supine position, and asepsis and antisepsis were performed in the operating room under general anesthesia, with the area of operation covered by a sterile drape. A lidocaine HCl with epinephrine 1:80000 injection was performed as a vasoconstrictor in the mucobuccal fold of the mandibular canine region, followed by a vertical incision of mesial region 43 – 47 and opening the mucoperiosteal flap with a raspatory.

The inferior alveolar nerve exiting the mental foramen was separated from the cyst wall by osteotomy. In conventional techniques, a window is made in the buccal portion of the lower jaw by removing the cortico-cancellous bone (Figure 3). In this surgery, repositioning the inferior alveolar nerve is determined by the surgeon's experience and skills. The surgeon should attempt to perform osteotomy while keeping the inferior alveolar nerve away from the surgical site [6].

The mandibular bone was opened with a round bur to identify the cyst wall area, and the cysts were removed with enucleation and extraction of the involved teeth.

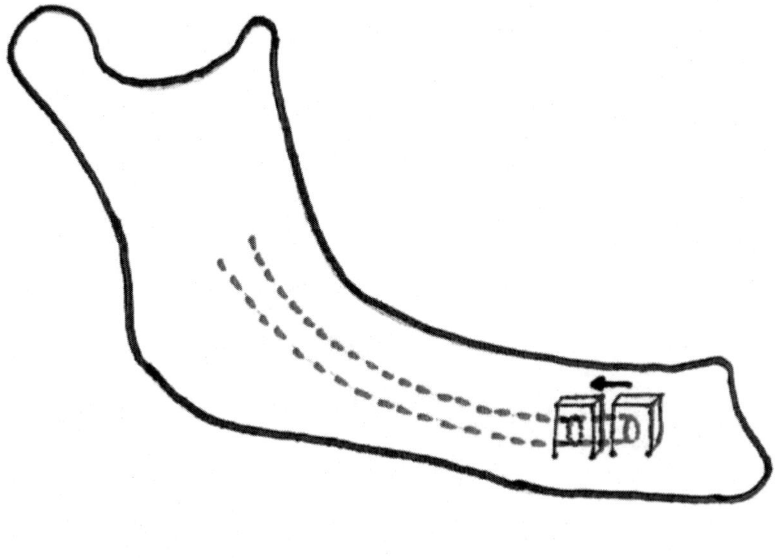

Figure 3. Illustrating the osteotomy technique with inferior alveolar nerve repositioning.

Special care is taken when relocating the inferior alveolar nerve in order to maintain nerve integrity. After the cyst was enucleated, we separated the compressed nerve from the cyst, which was clearly visible at the bottom of the bone cavity. Carnoy solution was applied and rinsed with 0.9% NaCl solution, and Suprasorb was applied in the cyst cavity in addition to primary approximation of the mucoperiosteal flaps using Vicryl 3-0. The specimens were sent to pathology for examination with a diagnosis of suspected radicular cysts (Figure 4). Postoperative intra-oral appearance was shown in Figure 5.

3. Discussion

Radicular cyst is one of the most common cystic lesions in the jaw, with a prevalence of 52% to 68%, and typically occurs in the anterior maxillary region. The cyst is most commonly found in men in the third to fifth decade, with a ratio of 3:2. According to Shear et al., these cysts are not usually asymptomatic, grow slowly, and are not accompanied by extraoral swelling [3, 7, 8, 9]. Intra-oral swelling begins with the formation of the radicular cyst, which is usually bony hard, but because the cyst becomes larger, the bone covering the cyst can become very thin.

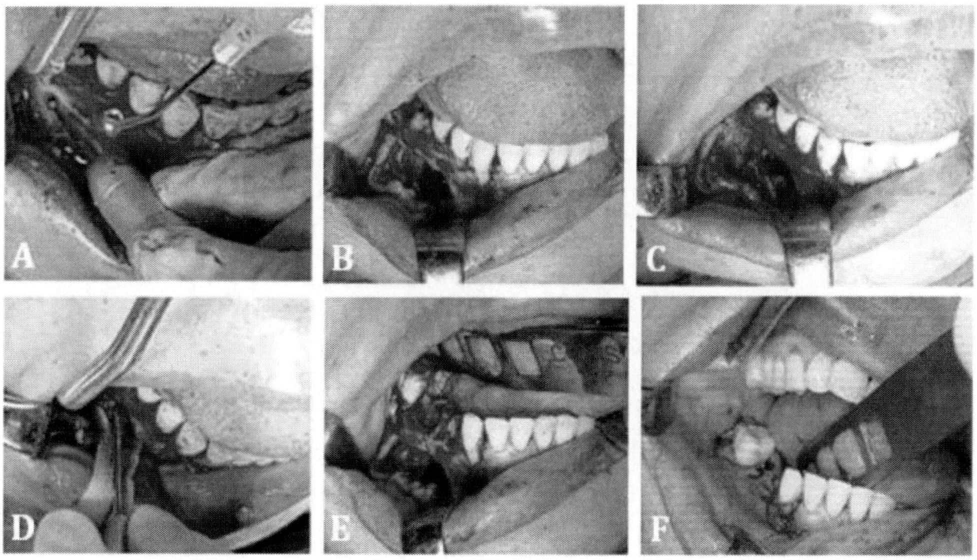

Figure 4. The surgical approach.

The involved teeth are always non-vital and indicate discoloration.

Although the teeth do not usually show root resorption, they may have smooth tooth root resorption [2]. Radicular cysts are also referred to as periapical cysts, periodontal cysts, root cysts, or dental cysts, originating from Malassez epithelial cells in the periodontal ligament as an inflammatory process due to pulpal or traumatic necrosis. Moreover, it is the most common inflammatory odontogenic cystic lesion primarily formed in the periapical region of the involved teeth [3, 7, 8, 9]. Cyst pathogenesis occurs in 3 phases. The first phase involves inflammatory effects leading to the development of Malassez epithelial cells, which is also due to the influence of bacterial antigens, development of epidermal cell agents, and metabolites detached by several cells within periapical lesions. In the second phase, an epithelium-lined cavity is seen. The third phase is cyst growth, and is generally attributed to osmosis, but the mechanism remains unknown [3].

In this article, we reported a case of radicular cysts sized approximately 4 cm in diameter, and enucleation of the involved teeth was performed with extraction of cystic discharge. The floor of the cyst wall was very close to the lower jaw, and compression of the inferior alveolar nerve bundle disappeared and changed the position of the anterior mental foramen. Proper planning was essential to avoid radical surgery in this case and ensure adequate access for cyst enucleation and relocation of the inferior alveolar nerve. The inferior alveolar nerve exiting the mental foramen was separated from the cyst wall by osteotomy. The goal was to relocate the inferior alveolar nerve with osteotomy to return the mental foramen to the normal position and ensure the cystic epithelial lesions were free from the surrounding tissue.

This is a complicated surgical procedure involving large cystic lesions and multiple teeth in the right mandible in addition to suppressing and covering the inferior alveolar nerve. Therefore, special planning is required, incisions are longer, and the flaps become wider, to facilitate relocation of the inferior alveolar nerve and enucleation of the cyst [10, 11]. The flaps were helpful in performing the operation due to the presence of large radicular cysts in the region compressing the mandibular nerve.

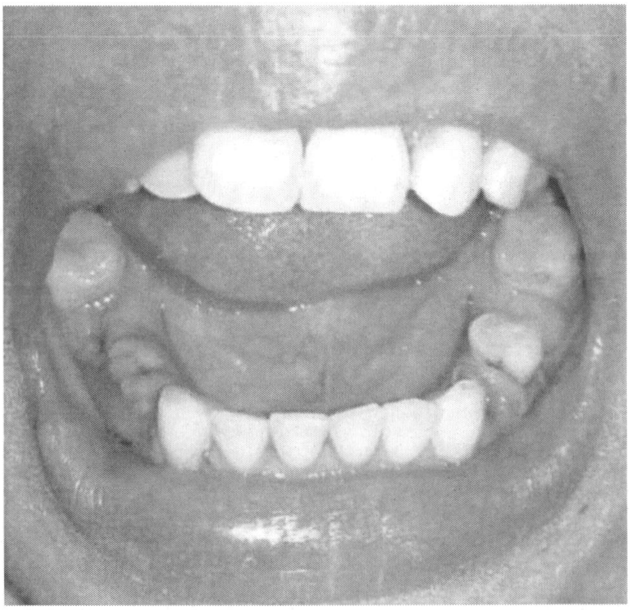

Figure 5. Postoperative view at 2 weeks.

Special care was taken when relocating the inferior alveolar nerve and maintaining integrity of the nerve, then the cystic membrane wall was released, and the entire cyst enucleated. Immediately after cyst removal, the inferior mandibular nerve was released and replaced to its normal position. At 2-week follow-up, the patient did not complain of symptoms of paresthesia of the right mandible (Figure 5).

Conclusion

The surgical approach to the radicular cyst in this patient was enucleation, with relocation of the inferior alveolar nerve. Depending on size and extent of the lesion, surgical enucleation is necessary for achieving optimal treatment, preventing recurrence, and maintaining integrity of the nerve.

References

[1] Harshita, K. R. (2015). Radicular Cyst: A Case Report. *Int. J. Dent. Sc.,* 1(4): 20 - 22.

[2] Brave, D., Madhusudan, A. S., Ramesh, G., Brave, V. R. (2011). Radicular cyst of anterior maxilla. *Int. J. Dent. Sc.*, 3(2):16 - 17.

[3] Parmar. (2018). The diagnostic dilemma of an infected radicular cyst: a case report. *International Journal of Applied Dental Sciences,* 4(2): 168 - 170.

[4] Mantu, V. K., Mitra, R. (2015). Radicular cyst: a case report and its histopathological analysis. *Int. J. Adv. Health Sci.*, 2:9 - 12.

[5] Han, Y. S., Lee, H., Seo, B. M. (2018). Fate of mandibular canals displaced by enlarged cystic lesions: does the inferior alveolar neurovascular bundle relocate to its original position? *Br. J. Oral Maxillofac. Surg.,* 56:292 - 298.

[6] Mahmood-Hashemi, H. (2006). A modified technique of inferior alveolar nerve repositioning: results in 11 patients. *J. Oral Maxillofac. Surg.,* 44:273 - 276.

[7] Kadam, N. S., De Ataide, I. D., Raghava, P., Fernandes, M., Hede, R. (2014). Management of large radicular cyst by conservative surgical approach: a case report. *J. Clin. Diagn. Res.,* 8:239.

[8] Shivhare, P., Singh, A., Haidry, N., Yadav, M., Shankarnarayan, L. (2016). Multilocular radicular cyst – a common pathology with uncommon radiological appearance. *J. Clin. Diagn. Res.,* 10:ZD13.

[9] Chander, V. V., Koduri, S., Basoya, S., Arya, L. (2014). Radicular cyst of maxillary primary tooth: report of two cases. *J. Oral Res. Rev.,* 6:61.

[10] Aziz, S. R., Pulse, C., Dourmas, M. A., Roser, S. M. (2002). Inferior alveolar nerve paresthesia associated with a mandibula dentigerous cyst. *J. Oral Maxillofac. Surg.,* 60:457 - 459.

[11] Sumer, M., Bas, B., Yildiz, L. (2007). *Inferior alveolar nerve parestesia caused by a dentigerous cyst associated with three teeth*, 12:388 - 390.

In: Clinical Reports in Dentistry
Editor: Lisa R. Amir

ISBN: 978-1-53617-328-4

Chapter 22

ORBITAL DEFECT REHABILITATION IN AN ADOLESCENT: A CASE REPORT

Yayuk S. Rahayu[1], Inge Paramitha[1] and Nina Ariani[2*]

[1]Prosthodontics Residency Program, Faculty of Dentistry,
Universitas Indonesia, Jakarta, Indonesia

[2]Department of Prosthodontics, Faculty of Dentistry,
Universitas Indonesia, Jakarta, Indonesia

ABSTRACT

Introduction: Disfigurement associated with the loss of an eye causes significant physical and emotional complications. Prosthetic rehabilitation of such patients leads to improvement in their appearance as well as psychological status. Growth of adolescent patients and disease recurrence are important considerations when managing such cases. The present report described the ocular and orbital prostheses fabricated for an adolescent over the course of several years.

Case Report: A 13-year-old female was referred to the Department of Prosthodontics, Faculty of Dentistry, Universitas Indonesia in 2015 for ocular prosthesis fabrication for the rehabilitation of orbital meningioma. Her medical history revealed tumor recurrence requiring several surgeries. Enucleation of the left eye had been performed in 2009, followed by a second surgery in 2010. Tumor debulking and radiation therapy had been performed in 2014 due to recurrence. In early 2015, the defect area did not provide sufficient space for inserting an ideal ocular prosthesis, but for psychological reasons, the first ocular prosthesis was fabricated at this time. In mid-2015, a second ocular prosthesis was fabricated. In 2017, the patient visited the department with a loose-fitting ocular prosthesis. By this time, the defect area was large enough to accommodate an orbital prosthesis. Lastly, an adhesive-retained silicone orbital prosthesis utilizing the anatomical undercut was fabricated.

Conclusion: Selection of a maxillofacial prosthesis should follow the patient's condition to achieve optimal results. Several factors should be taken into consideration,

*Corresponding Author's Email: nina.ariani02@ui.ac.id.

such as the patient's tissue condition, defect size, disease behavior, age and economic status. Over several years, different types of prostheses may be indicated.

Keywords: orbital, ocular, maxillofacial prosthesis, adolescent

1. INTRODUCTION

The eyes are vital organs that provide vision and are an important component of facial expression. The loss of an eye could result from congenital disease, trauma, or neoplasm and will likely have a negative effect on the patient's psychology, leading to the requirement for rehabilitation [1]. Neoplasms often require partial or complete eye removal. Surgical procedures for eye removal are classified into the following three general categories: enucleation (removal of the globe and parts of the optic nerve), evisceration (removal of intra-ocular content of the globe), and exenteration (removal of the entire orbital contents) [2]. Exenteration is the most radical of these three procedures, often resulting in deep deformity; hence, surgical reconstruction is not the best option for rehabilitation. Orbital prosthesis presents an attractive and viable alternative when local surgical reconstruction is deemed too difficult to achieve esthetic and functional demands [3].

Prosthetic rehabilitation options for the anophthalmic socket can be either ocular or orbital prostheses, depending on the defect area. An ocular prosthesis is a maxillofacial prosthesis that artificially replaces a missing eye, while an orbital prosthesis is a maxillofacial prosthesis that artificially restores the eye, eyelids, and adjacent hard and soft tissues [4]. An orbital prosthesis is also indicated for severely contracted sockets to which an ocular prosthesis cannot be fitted [5]. This prosthesis is generally fabricated following complete healing (usually 2-4 months) [6]. Several factors should be considered in the selection of a prosthesis to achieve optimal results, such as the patient's tissue condition, defect size, disease behavior, age, and economic status [7]. The present case report describes both ocular and orbital prostheses sequentially fabricated for an adolescent patient during the course of several years. The unideal contracted socket and shallow periorbital defect were the complicating factors in performing treatment. Growth in adolescent patients and disease recurrence are important considerations when managing this kind of case.

2. CASE REPORT

A 13-year-old female was referred from Department of Ophtalmology, Cipto Mangunkusumo National Hospital, Jakarta, Indonesia to the Department of

Prosthodontics, Faculty of Dentistry, Universitas Indonesia, Jakarta, Indonesia in January 2015, with the chief complaint of a missing left eye. Patient's legal guardian consented for patient's case to be published. Her medical history revealed orbital meningioma of the left eye with tumor recurrence requiring several surgeries. Enucleation surgery had been performed in 2009, followed by a second surgery in 2010.

Tumor debulking, bone shaving, exenteration and radiation therapy had been performed in October 2014 due to disease recurrence. Extra-oral examination in January 2015 showed a contracted eye socket with a shallow peri-orbital defect area. In 2017, the patient returned because of an ill-fitting prosthesis. Her left eye socket had become smaller and the peri-orbital defect area deeper (Figure 1A). Inflammation was not present in the defect area and there was continuous discharge from the lacrimal duct. The patient had been advised by her ophthalmologist to undergo graft surgery to line the socket, but she had declined due to socioeconomic reasons and the additional time required. There was no pain or discomfort in the defect area.

2.1. Case Management

In early 2015, the defect area did not provide sufficient space for an ideal ocular prosthesis. The socket was already contracted when the patient was first referred; however, for psychological reasons, the first ocular prosthesis was fabricated. In mid-2015, the first ocular prosthesis became loose and a new one was fabricated (Figure 1C). In 2017, the patient returned with an ill-fitting ocular prosthesis. By this time, the defect area was sufficiently large and deep to accommodate an orbital prosthesis (Figure 1B). The anophthalmic socket and defect area were examined; an undercut was available on the superior and lateral borders of the socket. Following a discussion with her parents regarding the treatment options, which were an ocular or an adhesive-retained silicone orbital prosthesis, the latter option was chosen despite the inadequate defect size and shape. The anatomical undercut available was used as an aid for prosthesis retention and to overcome the inadequate depth of the defect.

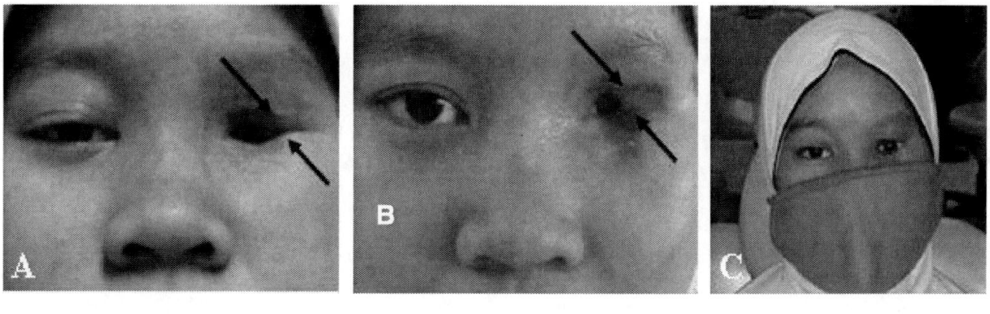

Figure 1. Eye sockets and periorbital defect area in 2015 (A); in 2017 (B); The patient with a new ocular prosthesis fabricated in mid-2015 (C).

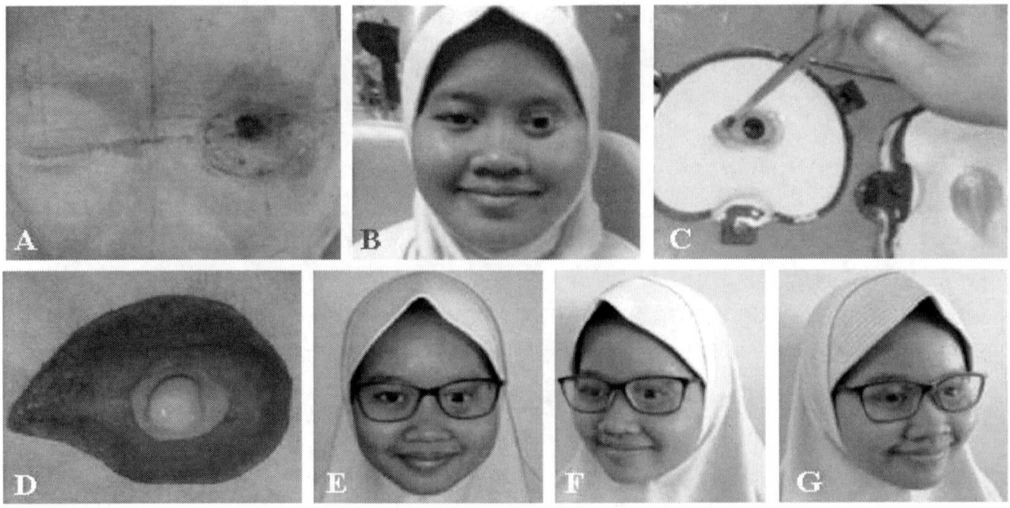

Figure 2. Procedure to fabricate an adhesive-retained silicone orbital prosthesis: Cast showing orientation lines (A); Wax try-in to check the symmetry and shape of the orbital prosthesis (B); The intaglio side of the prosthesis (C); The ocular part extends into the undercut to aid retention; Final prosthesis (D-F).

First, an impression of the defect was obtained. Orientation marks denoting facial midline, center of iris, and inner and outer canthi were indicated for symmetry of the orbital prosthesis. These lines were transferred to the cast and provided orientation for the wax-up. Impression was obtained using a combination of light body polyvinyl siloxane (EXAFLEX, GC America) for the eye socket and irreversible hydrocolloid (Aroma Fine Plus Normal Set, GC Europe) for the orbital area. The cast was poured with a type IV dental stone (Figure 2A).

The wax carving for the orbital prosthesis was performed, and the existing ocular prosthesis was used for the ocular part of the new prosthesis. A wax try-in was performed to check the orientation of the pupil, eye opening, and the volume of sclera available compared with the contralateral eye. The orbital wax-up was checked and adjusted in accordance with the contralateral eye in all directions (Figure 2B). The wax prosthesis was then made into master mold in a metal flask. A room-temperature-vulcanizing medical-grade silicone VST-50HD (Factor II, Lakeside, AZ, USA) base was mixed with four silicone-based pigments (red, yellow, blue, and white pigments; Factor II, Lakeside, AZ, USA) for obtaining the skin shade of the patient. Nylon flocks (Thackray Ltd., England) were added to achieve high similarity to the skin color.

The catalyst was subsequently added according to the manufacturer's instructions and the silicone was carefully poured into the mold, avoiding entrapment of air bubbles. The mold was approximated, secured, and kept in a bench press for 24 hours. Following polymerization, the prosthesis was deflasked. Extrinsic pigments and ready-made eyelashes were used. Retention was achieved through the undercut (Figure 2C) and adhesive. The eyeglass frame was selected and tried on the patient (Figure 2D-F).

Instructions for adhesive application and home care were provided. The patient was satisfied with the prosthesis, since it made her socially presentable again.

3. Discussion

In early 2015, the patient presented with a contracted eye socket and shallow peri-orbital defect that did not provide a sufficient space for inserting an ideal ocular prosthesis. Socket contracture can be the result of irradiation of the socket following enucleation, severe socket infection, not wearing an artificial eye, keloid-like mass formation in the socket, tissue loss due to injury, or scarring of the conjunctiva due to various factors [8]. In this case, several surgeries and radiation therapy may have contributed to socket contraction. Moreover, no conformer or prosthesis was used for approximately five years following the first enucleation surgery. Conformer placement minimizes changes in socket size and prevents scar tissue contracture during tissue healing [9]. In the present case, a prosthodontist/anaplastologist was not involved in treatment planning prior to surgery. A multidisciplinary management approach is essential in providing optimal and efficient rehabilitation for patients.

Two years later, growth of this adolescent patient had promoted tissue changes, and the peri-orbital defect had become larger and deeper, which then required an orbital prosthesis although the defect was not sufficiently deep for optimal ocular and silicone thickness. An orbital prosthesis sometimes calls for additional retention such as remaining anatomical structures besides adhesive [10]. Careful examination of the remaining undercut was performed for identifying possible areas that could increase the retention of the prosthesis. The advantage of using an undercut is that the prosthesis tends to move less during functional movement; thus, there is less open margin and the need for an additional osseointegration implant procedure is reduced [10]. If a prosthesis is properly designed and patient is motivated to care for the underlying and supporting tissue, then an anatomical undercut can be successfully used to retain an orbital prosthesis [11]. For achieving optimal results regarding anatomical undercut retention of the prosthesis, light body polyvinyl siloxane is used at the impression stage to obtain maximum adaptation of the underlying tissue and available undercut inside the socket [11].

Although implants enhance the retention of facial prostheses, implant success with an orbital defect (35%) is lower than that with nasal (71%) or auricular (100%) defects. Orbital sites are the most difficult for patients to clean and have the highest rate of peri-implant tissue reaction. The questionable survival of implants placed in irradiated bone, the need for additional invasive procedures, and financial constraints are other considerations for implant-retained prostheses [12]. Therefore, during the growth period of adolescent patients, the selection of a reasonable maxillofacial prosthesis should be the goal for the rehabilitation of defects resulting from diseases with recurrence.

CONCLUSION

The selection of a maxillofacial prosthesis should follow the patient's condition to achieve optimal results. In the adolescent patient in this case, the defect area had become sufficiently large and deep to accommodate an orbital prosthesis two years after her first ocular prosthesis. The defect size may change over time and different types of prostheses may be indicated. In the present case report, defect changes were advantageous for orbital prosthesis fabrication.

REFERENCES

[1] Pai UY, Ansari NA, Gandage DS. (2011). A Technique to Achieve Predictable Iris Positioning and Symmetry in Ocular and Orbital Prostheses. *J. Prosthodont.*, 20:244-246.

[2] Peyman G, Sanders D, Goldberg M. (1987). *Principles and Practice of Ophtalmology*. 3rd ed.

[3] Pruthi G, Jain V. (2013). Light Weight Prosthesis for a Patient with Bilateral Orbital Exenteration - a Clinical Report. *J. Prosthodont. Res.*, 57(2):135-139.

[4] Driscoll CF, Freilich MA, Guckes AD, et al. (2017). The Glossary of Prosthodontic Terms. *J. Prosthet. Dent.*, 17(5):e1-e105.

[5] Gupta S, Gupta S. (2016). Orbital Prosthesis Fabrication. *Delhi J. Ophthalmol.*, 27:136-138.

[6] Soni BW, Soni N, Bansal M, Dabreo EL. (2014). Orbital Prosthesis: a Novel Reconstructive Approach. *J. Oral Health Dent. Manag.*, 13:690-692.

[7] Pruthi G, Jain V, Rajendiran S, Jha R. (2014). Prosthetic Rehabilitation after Orbital Exenteration: a Case Series. *Indian J. Ophthalmol.*, 62:12-15.

[8] Kronish J, Russell G, Dortzbach R, et al. (1990). The Pathophysiology of the Anophthalmic Socket Part I. Analysis of Orbital Blood Flow. *Ophtalmic Plast. Reconstr. Surg.*, 6(2):77-87.

[9] Hafezeqoran A, Koodaryan R. (2010). A Technique for Fabrication of an Orbital Prosthesis: A Case Report. *J. Dent. Res. Dent. Clin. Dent. Prospect.*, 4(2):69-73.

[10] Chang T, Garrett N, Roumanas E, Beumer J. (2005). Treatment Satisfaction with Facial Prosthesis. *J. Prosthet. Dent.*, 94:275-280.

[11] Wadud A, Jamayet N Bin, Srithavaj T, Alam MK. (2015). Use of Anatomical Undercut in Adhesive Retained Orbital Prosthesis: An Alternative to

Osseointegration to Improve Retention and Reduce Margin Gap. *Br. J. Med. Med. Res.*, 6(8):841-847.

[12] Jain S, Jain P. (2016). Rehabilitation of Orbital Cavity after Orbital Exenteration Using Polymethyl Methacrylate Orbital Prosthesis. *J. Indian Prosthodont. Soc.*, 16(1):100-104.

In: Clinical Reports in Dentistry
Editor: Lisa R. Amir
ISBN: 978-1-53617-328-4

Chapter 23

ORBITAL CAVITY RECONSTRUCTION USING ORBITAL AND TITANIUM MESH PLATES AFTER ENUCLEATION OF RUPTURED EYEBALL DUE TO TRAUMA

Nissia Ananda[1], Amru Sungkar[2] and Dwi Ariawan[3,*]
[1]Oral and Maxillofacial Surgery Recidency Program,
Faculty of Dentistry, Universitas Indonesia, Jakarta, Indonesia
[2]Department of Plastic Surgery, Faculty of Medicine,
Universitas Sebelas Maret – RSUD Dr. Moewardi, Surakarta, Indonesia
[3] Department of Oral and Maxillofacial Surgery, Faculty of Dentistry,
Universitas Indonesia, Jakarta, Indonesia

ABSTRACT

Introduction: Orbital trauma often occur in patients with multiple facial traumas. On the other side, injury of the soft tissue in the facial region must consider ocular trauma as one of the most significant factors contributing to visual impairment. Accurate diagnosis of eye injury requires expertise in ophthalmology, which makes it possible to identify mild ocular injury in maxillofacial trauma patients. Computed Tomography is the main modality used for orbital trauma because of its sensitivity to detect fracture and soft tissue injury accurately.

Case Report: We reported a case of ocular trauma with eyeball rupture and medial orbital wall fracture. This case was treated by eyeball enucleation and orbital wall reconstruction. Material used for orbital wall reconstruction was titanium mesh because it was superior to autogenous bone graft and porous polyethylene sheets (PPE). Surgery was performed carefully by opportune manipulating of bone, reconstruction material, and soft tissue.

* Corresponding Author's Email: dwiariawan75@gmail.com.

Conclusion: Proper healing at the surgical approach site was observed, patient had no complaint and no post-surgery complication was noted. Eyeball prosthesis will be cast to reach an optimum aesthetic result.

Keywords: orbital fracture, orbital wall reconstruction, titanium mesh, eyeball rupture, eyeball enucleation

1. Introduction

Maxillofacial trauma is physical trauma which can affect soft tissue, hard tissue, or both on the maxillofacial region [1]. Fracture is a traumatic injury which caused bone discontinuity. The orbital position in the facial landmark tends to be prominent, and this is considered a predisposing factor for the orbital trauma [2]. Orbital trauma often occurs in patients with multiple facial trauma. The injury can only affect the orbital region or also involve other extensive craniofacial bone fractures.

According to Kramp et al. the incidence rate of isolated orbital wall fracture is 4% - 16% of all facial fracture cases, while the incidence rate of orbital wall fracture combined with middle face fracture is at 30% - 55%. The most common orbital fracture involved the orbital base which is around 69% of all orbital fractures then followed by fractures of the medial orbital wall (19%) [3].

On the soft tissues, ocular trauma is one of the most significant factors contributing to visual impairment [4]. Ocular trauma on the soft tissues can be manifested in various degrees of injuries such as eyelid laceration, corneal abrasion, inflammation of the iris, scleral hemorrhage, lens injury, detached of retinal layer, traumatic optic neuropathy, retrobulbar hematoma, orbital fracture, and eyeball rupture. Notably, eyeball rupture can lead to permanent loss of vision [4-6].

It is best to save the eyeball by doing immediate treatment. However, there are some considerations and evaluations to be made in order to determine whether eyeball enucleation is needed [7]. Furthermore, careful planning of the definitive treatment is prompt specifically by selecting the optimum reconstruction material. Herein, we reported a case of ocular trauma with eyeball rupture and medial orbital wall fracture. This case was treated by eyeball enucleation and orbital wall reconstruction using titanium mesh.

2. Case Report

The case involved a 42-years-old woman with a history of right orbital trauma after MVA (Motor Vehicle Accident). She was admitted to Moewardi Hospital with a chief complaint of injury and protrusion of the right eyeball.

The patient was not able to see with her right eye and there was no light perception. Physical examination revealed an open wound at the superior palpebra extending to the nasofrontal junction with a size of 4x1x1 cm and at the inferior palpebra with a size of 3x2x1 cm. There was proptosis of the right eyeball, and visual acuity of the right eye was 0 (Figure 1).

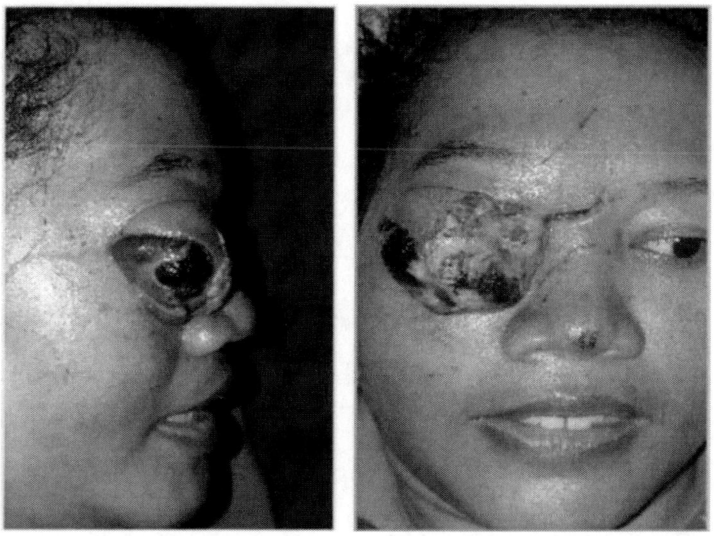

Figure 1. Properative clinical picture

MSCT (Multi Slice Computed Tomography) Scan without contrast revealed some injuries. Rupture of the right eyeball which caused proptosis and rupture of the rectus, superior, lateral, and right medial oblique muscles were identified as the soft tissue injuries (Figure 2A).

Three-dimensional imaging revealed some fractures, namely, fracture of the right orbital bone, lateral wall of the right frontal sinus, lateral wall of the right ethmoid sinus, anterior wall of the right sphenoid sinus, and superior wall of the right maxillary sinus (Figure 2B).

Nine days after the accident, the patient underwent surgery. The ophthalmologist did enucleation of the right eyeball and a plastic surgeon examined the orbital wall fracture and revealed a medial orbital rim wall fracture that extended to the medial wall of the orbit.

Orbital plate and titanium mesh were used to reconstruct the orbital cavity, followed by repair of the orbital soft tissues (Figure 3A,B). An orbital prosthesis was fabricated after the surgical wound healed. At the follow-up period, the patient had no complaint and there was an epithelized orbital socket and the postoperative wound had healed. (Figure 4A, B).

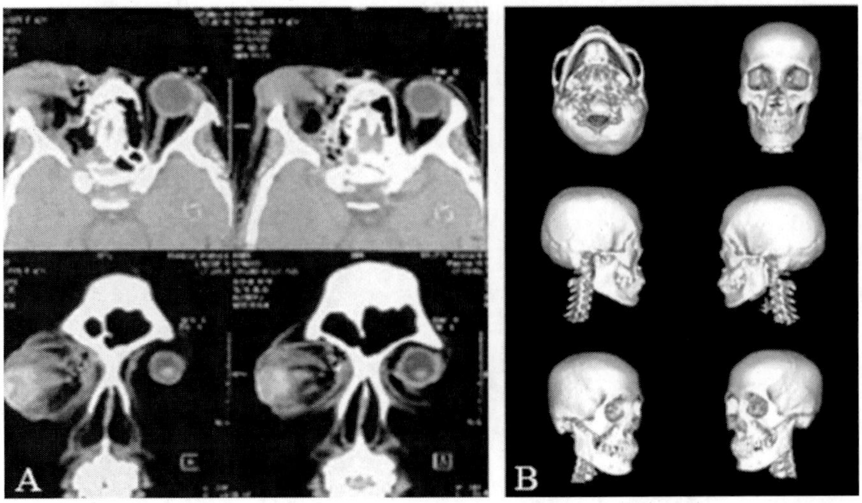

Figure 2. MSCT Scan of the head without contrast (A); Three-dimensional imaging from the MSCT Scan of the patient (B).

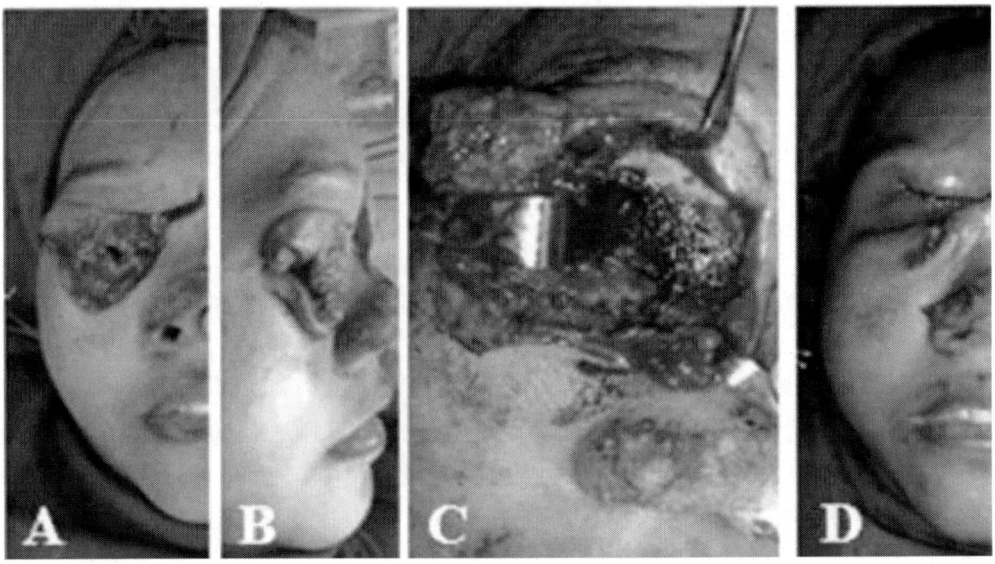

Figure 3. Clinical picture post eyeball enucleation (A,B), orbital reconstruction (C), Clinical picture post soft tissue repair (D).

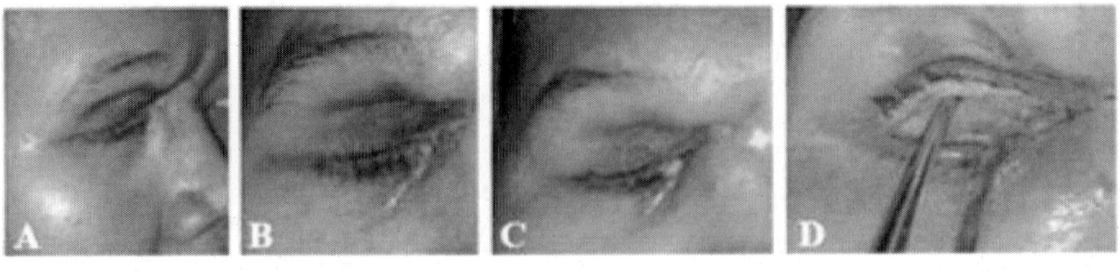

Figure 4. Clinical photo at one-month follow-up of patient's condition (A-C), at 1,5-month follow-up (D).

The patient was ready to use an orbital prosthesis. (Figure 4C,D). The patient was informed that her case report would be submitted for publication and she agreed to give authorization by signing an informed consent.

3. Discussion

Maxillofacial fractures, especially fractures that occur in the upper face and frontal areas, are significantly associated with ocular trauma where orbital wall involvement occurs approximately 85% of all cases of mid-facial fracture [8]. Guly et al., stated that the risk of ocular trauma is higher in patients with facial fractures than those without facial fractures [9]. Mid-facial fractures are often complicated by eye trauma and the severity of the fractures is varied, so are the complications [10]. In the presented case, the ocular injury was manifested as a right eyeball rupture accompanied by a fracture in the medial wall of the orbit.

In the presented case, the cause of ocular trauma was vehicle accident. This was confirmed by Chen H. et al. who stated that the main cause of injury or trauma in the orbital region is vehicle accident [11]. Several previous studies also reported the same cause of maxillofacial and ocular trauma [5, 9]. Brookes reported maxillofacial trauma with an ocular injury due to vehicle accidents is generally caused by the release of high kinetic energy and vehicular condition affected by acceleration and abrupt decelerations [9].

In this case, the patient complained of prominent right eyeball after the accident; conclusively, the patient had an avulsion of the right eyeball. Avulsion of the eyeball caused by trauma is rare and it is usually accompanied by the trauma of other maxillofacial structures [7]. Avulsion of the eyeball due to trauma is associated with the presence of sharp objects or fractured bone fragments that injured the optic nerve and extra-ocular muscles [12]. Decreased orbital volume resulting from inwardly shifted frontal bone and laterally shifted medial bone of the orbit can also lead to protruding eyeball [13]. Detail anamnesis regarding the history of iatrogenic eyeball penetration such as cataract surgery is also essential for this condition significantly, as this is related to a higher rate of post-traumatic eyeball rupture, which was not found in this patient [1].

It is suggested that early repositioning of the eyeball may increase the chance to save the eyeball even though the visual prognosis is poor. Early diagnosis and prompt treatment should be done within 24 hours prior to the accident to handle eyeball rupture [6]. If ultimately the visual function cannot be restored, enucleation of the eyeball could be done after several period of evaluation [7,14]. In this case, enucleation of the right eyeball and orbital bone reconstruction were performed in nine days after the accident. If the golden period to treat eyeball rupture had passed, then it is preferable to have definitive treatment within 1 - 2 weeks post-accident to wait until inflammation process have finished [15,16]. Orbital reconstruction should avoid soft tissue entrapment, and it is important when the tissue swelling caused by the inflammation process had subsided. Soft tissue entrapment during can lead to ischemia of the muscle, fat tissue, or connective tissue which increases risk of fibrosis, necrosis, strabismus, and even permanent motility of the extra-ocular muscles [16].

Accurate diagnosis of eye injury requires expertise in ophthalmology, which makes it possible to identify mild injury in maxillofacial trauma patients. This will surely affect the incidence rate of ocular injury in the study, and the rate will be higher if the case was assessed by ophthalmologist compared to non-ophthalmologist. It is noticeably in study by al-Qurainy et al. result of his study revealed that more than 90% of mid-facial fracture patients have ocular injury (which assessed by an ophthalmologist) [9].

Treatment modalities to examine orbital and eye region include radiography, ultrasonography, MRI (Magnetic Resonance Imaging) and CT (Computed Tomography). Generally, radiographic imaging is relatively sensitive to detect bone fracture, but it is not sensitive to detect soft tissue injury. For early evaluation of the eyeball, the use of ultrasonography is good enough; however, in certain cases, such as suspicion of eyeball rupture, it is not recommended. MRI has an advantage in differentiating soft tissue, but is not recommended for initial evaluation of trauma, and it is contraindicated in cases where there is suspicion of a foreign object in the eye. CT is the main modality used for orbital trauma because of its sensitivity to detect fracture and its ability to reform three-dimensional imaging which is useful to plan surgery. Moreover, CT is capable of detecting soft tissue injury accurately [17]. In this case, MSCT Scan without contrast revealed rupture of the right eyeball and fracture in the right orbital bone.

Orbital bone reconstruction is important because the structure must be able to isolate orbital content from the nasal cavity and paranasal sinuses, which also provide adequate support to prevent enophthalmus and diplopia. The selection of the ideal material for reconstruction of the orbital floor and walls remains highly controversial. The ultimate goals of orbital reconstruction are to restore anatomy, volume, function, and aesthetics of the bony orbital defect [18].

Titanium mesh is considered highly appropriate as orbital wall reconstruction material, as it can provide precise anatomical reconstruction. The biocompatibility aspect of titanium mesh is good enough, and also the material can be easily manipulated to follow the desired shape. Application of titanium mesh gives space for connective tissue to grow through and around the implant, preventing the migration of the mesh [17]. However, it should be noted that titanium mesh is not appropriate for patients who are still in a growth period [19].

There are three types of titanium mesh, the first type is patient-specific molding, then freehand bending, and last preformed titanium mesh. Patient-specific molding type is contoured using trimmed and molded traditional titanium mesh sheet onto the preinjury STL (stereolithiography) models. Freehand bending type is bent and trimmed traditional titanium mesh sheet by the surgeon intraoperatively without using a template. Preformed mesh type is industrially machined preformed titanium mesh sheets [20]. The patient in this case was treated with surgical enucleation of the right eyeball and reconstruction of the fractured orbital medial and inferior wall using freehand bending titanium mesh nine days after the accident.

Other alternative materials for reconstruction is autogenous bone graft, such as calvarium and iliac crest. Bone graft was once the main standard for orbital wall reconstruction due to strength aspect, biocompatibility and osteogenic - osteoconductive - osteoinductive potential but it was slowly began to be abandoned because of morbidity from donor sites, varying resorption rates, prolonged surgery, postoperative postoperative pain, limited quantity, and the difficulty of manipulating the material to achieve the desired shape [17]. In addition, temporalis fascia patch graft combined with porous polyethylene can also be used as another option of the autogenous graft [21].

PPE (porous polyethylene sheets) is also one of the orbital reconstruction materials with advantageas of easy contouring and smooth edges, but they are not radiopaque and lack of rigidity in heavily displaced fractures with massive tissue herniation into the maxillary sinus. Nevertheless, infection is the most trappy complication when PPE was used in orbital wall reconstruction [21].

Moreover, there is also a composite of porous polyethylene and titanium which used to prevent postoperative enophthalmus, but there are several reports of late complication such as infection, diplopia, and implant migration associated with this material [21]. Therefore it can be said that titanium mesh is the current gold standard for orbital wall reconstruction materials.

To obtain appropriate post-enucleation eyeball socket, good surgical techniques along with detail analysis of the size defect using CT Scan are required. Careful sub-periosteal dissection is done to prevent injury to the muscle and to assure complete release of the soft tissue from the bone segment during reconstruction. It is advisable to pay attention in inspecting soft tissue entrapment, especially when using metallic mesh material. Soft tissue entrapment can be prevented by eliminating sharp edges of the mesh and not letting intra-orbital tissue passed through or trapped on mesh edges [22].

In this case, the patient showed no infection on the surgical site and no other complications associated with alloplastic materials such as implant migration, extrusion of implant or hypersensitivity. Epiphora was noted in this patient which resolved considerably within 6 weeks. The patient was planned to have prosthesis in the orbital region during the rehabilitation phase.

Ocular prosthesis is an artificial substitute for enucleated eyeball with the aim to restore the volume of the orbit, to facilitate motility, and to improve the appearance of the socket which also helps to improve the psychological state of the patient, increases patient's level of confidence and raise the esthetic value [23, 24]. Intimate contact between the ocular prosthesis and the tissue bed is needed to distribute even pressure.

Stable orbital socket post enucleation (fully resolved chemosis and orbital inflammation) which is formed by epithelized tissue and the well-fit orbital prosthesis is required to achieve ideal rehabilitation.

CONCLUSION

This paper reported a case of 42 year old woman with right ocular trauma manifested as right eyeball rupture and medial orbital wall fracture caused by a vehicle accident. This case was treated by teamwork of ophthalmologist and plastic surgeon. Enucleation of the right eyeball was performed by the ophthalmologist, and bone reconstruction and vulnus repair were performed by plastic surgeon. During the post-surgical period, proper healing at the surgical approach site was observed and no post-surgery complication was noted. Eyeball prosthesis will be cast to reach optimum aesthetic result.

REFERENCES

[1] Hollier, L. J. and Kelley, P. (2007). Soft tissue and skeletal injuries of the face. In: C. H. Thorne, R. W. Beasley, S. J. Aston, S. P. Bartlett, G. C. Gurtner, S. L. Spear (Eds.), *Grabb And Smith's Plastic Surgery* (6th edition, pp. 315 - 332). Philadelphia: Lippincott Williams & Wilkins.

[2] Chen, C.-T., Chen, R.-F. and Wei, F.-C. (2006). Craniofacial trauma and reconstruction. In: J. Lumley (Ed.). *Plast. Reconstr. Surg.,* (pp. 275 - 296). London: Springer.

[3] Hardt, N. and Kuttenberger, J. (2010) *Craniofacial trauma.* Berlin: Springer.

[4] Press, D. (2013). Traumatic ruptured globe eye injuries in a large urban center. *Clin. Opthalmol.,* 7:485 - 488.

[5] Zimmerer, R. M., Gellrich, N., von Bülow, S. et al. (2018). Is there more to the clinical outcome in posttraumatic reconstruction of the inferior and medial orbital walls than accuracy of implant placement and implant surface contouring? A prospective multicenter study to identify predictors of clinical outcome. *J. Cranio-Maxillo-Facial Surg.*, 1-10.

[6] Burstein, E. S. and Lazzaro, D. R. (2013). Traumatic ruptured globe eye injuries in a large urban center. *Clin. Ophthalmol.,* 7:485 - 488.

[7] Narayani, R., YB, R., R. A. (2013). Traumatic avulsion and bilateral eye loss: report of two cases. *Nepal J. Ophthalmol.,* 5(10):272 - 274.

[8] Mast, G., Ehrenfeld, M., Litschel, R., Tasman, A. and Cornelius, C. (2015). Maxillofacial fractures: midface and internal orbit — part I: classification and assessment. *Facial Plast. Surg.,* 31:351 - 356.

[9] Zhou, H., Liu, Q. and Yang, R. (2014). Ocular trauma in patients with maxillofacial fractures. *J. Craniofac. Surg.,* 25:519 - 523.

[10] Politis, C., Kluyskens, A. and Dormaar, T. (2017). Association of midfacial fractures with ophthalmic injury. *Craniomaxillofac Trauma Reconstr.,* 10(2): 99 - 105.

[11] Chen, H., Pan, C., Leow, A., Tsay, P. and Chen, C. (2016). Evolving concepts in the management of orbital fractures with enophthalmos: A retrospective comparative analysis. *Formos. J. Surg.,* 49:1 - 8.

[12] Gupta, H., Natarajan, S., Vaidya, S. et al. (2017). Traumatic eye ball luxation: A stepwise approach to globe salvage. *Saudi J. Ophthalmol.*, 31:260 - 265.

[13] Khadamy, J., Khademi, P. and Kashkouli, M. (2017). Missing globe: a case of severe head trauma, eyelid laceration, and traumatic enucleation missing globe: a case of severe head trauma, eyelid laceration, and traumatic enucleation. *Cureus,* 9(12): e1988.

[14] Warrak, E. L. and Sammouh, F. K. (2015). Complete visual rehabilitation in a patient with no light perception after surgical management of a penetrating open-globe injury : a case report. *Case Rep. Ophthalmol.,* 6:204 - 209.

[15] El-ghafar, A. A. (2015). Influence of time on the management of complications of orbital floor fracture. *J. Egypt Ophthalmol. Soc.,* 108:47-51.

[16] Harris, G. J., (2015). Avoiding complications in the repair of orbital floor fractures. *JAMA Facial Plast. Surg.,* 16:290 - 295.

[17] Lima, L. B., Barjona, R., Miranda, M. De et al. (2015). Reconstruction of orbital floor for treatment of a pure blowout fracture. *Rev. Port. Estomatol. Med. Dentária e Cir. Maxilofac.,* 56:122-126.

[18] Singh, M., Mamatha, N. S., Kedarnath, N. S., Kumar, R. S., Vijayanand, S. and Haidry, N. (2014). Reconstruction of the orbital floor using titanium mesh: a study of three cases. *International Journal of Medical and Dental Case Reports,* ID:201114.

[19] Arslan, E., Arslan, S., Kalkisim, S., Arslan, A. and Kuzeyli, K. (2016). Long-term results of orbital roof repair with titanium mesh in a case of traumatic intraorbital encephalocele: a case report and review of literature. *Craniomaxillofac. Trauma Reconstr.,* 9:255-259.

[20] Strong, E. B., Fuller, S. C., Wiley, D. F., Zumbansen, J., Wilson, M. D. and Metzger, M. C. (2013). Preformed vs intraoperative bending of titanium mesh for orbital reconstruction. *Facial Plast. Reconstr. Surg.*, 149:60-66.

[21] Banica, B., Ene, P., Vranceanu, D. and Ene, R. (2013). Titanium preformed implants in orbital floor reconstruction – case presentation, review of literature. *A J. Clin. Med.,* 8:34-39.

[22] Collin, R. and Rose, G. (2001). *Fundamentals of clinical ophthalmology: Ophthalmology plastic and orbital surgery* (1st edition). London: BMJ Books.

[23] Sethi, T., Kheur, M., Haylock, C. and Harianawala, H. (2014). Fabrication of a custom ocular prosthesis. *Middle East Afr. J. Ophthalmol.,* 21:271-275.

[24] Wladis, E. J., Aakalu, V. K., Sobel, R. K., Yen, M. T., Bilyk, J. R. and Mawn, L. A. (2017). Orbital implants in enucleation surgery a report by the American Academy of Ophthalmology. *Ophthalmology,* 125:311-317.

In: Clinical Reports in Dentistry
Editor: Lisa R. Amir

ISBN: 978-1-53617-328-4

Chapter 24

CLOSED MOUTH IMPRESSION TECHNIQUE IN RESORBED MANDIBULAR RIDGE: A CASE REPORT

***Sharren Teguh*[1] *and Lindawati S. Kusdhany*[2,*]**
[1]Prosthodontics Residency Program, Faculty of Dentistry,
Universitas Indonesia, Jakarta, Indonesia
[2]Department of Prosthodontics, Faculty of Dentistry,
Universitas Indonesia, Jakarta, Indonesia

ABSTRACT

Introduction: A highly resorbed mandibular ridge poses an inevitable challenge for prosthodontists. Denture base is required to be extended adequately. A good and retentive set of dentures is a desirable outcome besides good aesthetic and functional values.

Case report: A female aged 72 years visited our Hospital and reported about losing her old dentures. She required a new set of dentures. Her examination revealed highly resorbed mandibular ridge or an order V pattern of alveolar ridge resorption, as described by *Atwood*. Closed mouth technique was used to develop border molding, where the patient's muscle and muscular activity provided maximum support to the denture-bearing area. This technique aimed to obtain an accurate impression of undisturbed and uncompressed tissues. Impression using a soft liner has also shown a wider denture support area. A new set of dentures was confirmed showing good retention and stability despite the resorbed ridge, by functional and speaking examination.

Discussion: Various methods have been used to achieve retention, stability, and support. The closed mouth technique was chosen owing to the stability of the material when stored.

Conclusion: The proposed method is an excellent option to overcome highly resorbed mandibular ridge in a fully edentulous patient.

*Corresponding Author's Email: lindaskusdhany@gmail.com.

Keywords: closed mouth technique, resorbed mandibular ridge

1. Introduction

Tooth loss has a multifactorial pathology, and it progresses with age. The alveolar ridge changes its form after tooth extraction. The anatomy, resorption pattern, and denture-bearing area are the main features that make resorption in the mandibular region more challenging than that in the maxillary region [1, 2]. Reduction in ridge height affects denture stability [1]. This condition poses several challenges in complete denture fabrication [2]. A completely edentulous patient requires dentures to improve not only masticatory function due to tooth loss but also facial appearance to increase self-confidence.

Categories of bone resorption need to be created for edentulous patients for a better denture treatment outcome and to develop an efficient guide for dental educators, general dentists, and even prosthodontists [3, 4]. A simple classification of mandibular resorption was described by *Atwood* using bone specimens under microradiographs: Order I (before extraction), Order II (after extraction), Order III (high well-rounded), Order IV (knife-edge), Order V (low well-rounded), and Order VI (depressed). This order ranges from uncomplicated to an increasingly complex situation [4] and is applicable even today [3]. Decreasing bone volume affects the denture-bearing area, remaining tissue for reconstruction, facial muscle support/attachment, total facial height, and ridge morphology. Patients with a more advanced level of resorption should be referred to the graduate program of prosthodontics or to practicing prosthodontics in order to decrease the incidence of retreatment [3]. An accurate impression will provide sufficient retention, stability, and support [2]. An impression technique is an essential step in defining the support of the prosthesis [5]. The technique will then improve the material through further studies and with new materials born. The use of new materials in the dental industry results in improved impression technique [6].

According to *Rao* and *Zinner*, the closed mouth technique was introduced between 1900 and 1929 using a free-flowing material, as described for border molding with sucking and swallowing action and peripheral musculature movement in the direction of the attachment [6, 7]. The closed mouth technique is a functional impression technique to record the functional form of the edentulous ridge. This method involves creating a dynamic impression using a tissue conditioner. This material is used for conditioning abused soft tissue under the denture surface from the post-extraction period, or ill-fitting denture, thus permitting the tissue to return to its normal form. The effect of this material has been well established. Using tissue conditioner as an impression materials, this method will record tissue, as in complete denture need a static tissue on ridge and functional of the muscle. This method captures the tissue in a static condition and functional state [8]. Various modifications of this method using tissue conditioner have been reported to date [9-12].

2. Case Report

A 72-year-old female visited the Prosthodontics Department of Universitas Indonesia to request for a new set of dentures because she lost her older lower dentures. She had been using a full denture set for the upper and lower jaw for more than 10 years. The patient was unable to determine how long she had been in an edentulous state. Her intra-oral examination revealed a normal maxilla but a resorbed mandibular ridge (Atwood Order V) (Figure 1). The preliminary impression was made using a perforated stock tray and a reversible hydrocolloid material (GC Aroma Fine Plus Alginate Normal Set); this was then poured into the cast with type-III dental stone and a base. From this first impression, a cold-curing acrylic resin base and occlusal rim were prepared in the cast for later using dynamic impression on the resin base inside the patient's mouth.

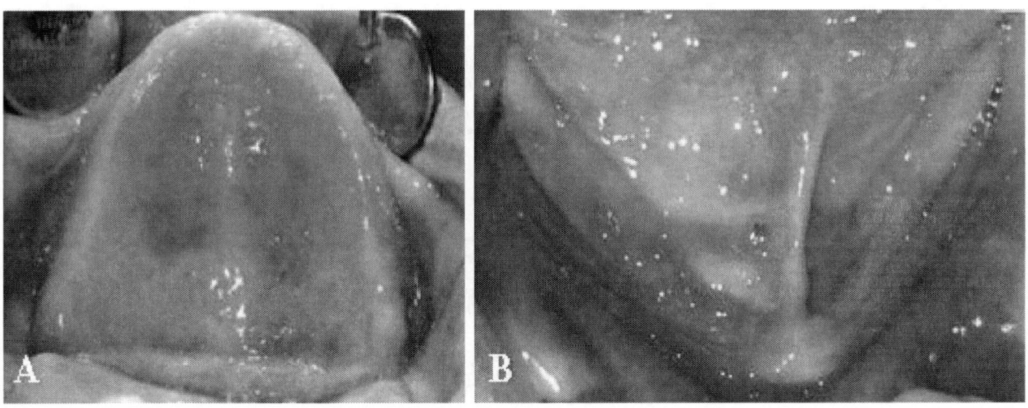

Figure 1. Intra-oral view of patient normal maxilla (A); and resorbed mandibular ridge (B).

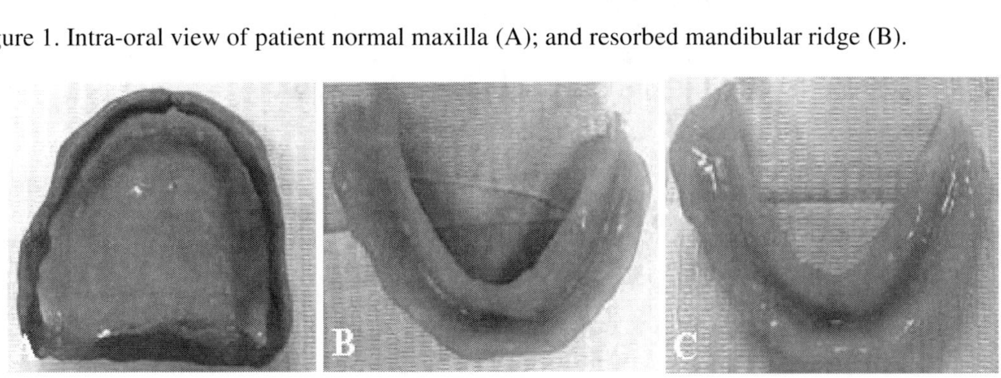

Figure 2. Border molding in the maxilla (A); First application of a soft relining material (B); Final result after application of soft relining material and green stick compound (C).

Occlusal vertical dimension and centric relation were determined at this stage with a 4-mm chosen freeway space from the rest position in order to reduce pressure on this resorbed mandibular ridge. Border molding on the maxilla was performed using a green stick compound (GC Peri Compound) (Figure 2A) and a tissue conditioner (GC Soft Liner). The tissue conditioner was applied three times on the tissue surface of the mandibular base (Figure 2B and 2C); both the processes were performed with functional movements of blowing, puffing, whistling, and smiling [10].

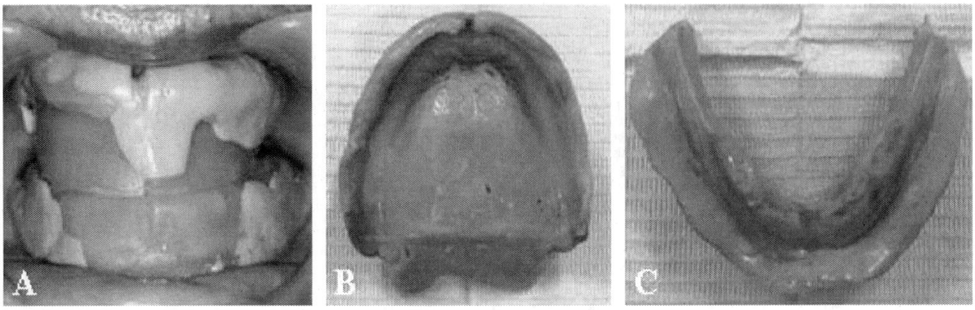

Figure 3. Repeating functional movement of wash impression with a light-body material; (A) final wash impressions (B,C).

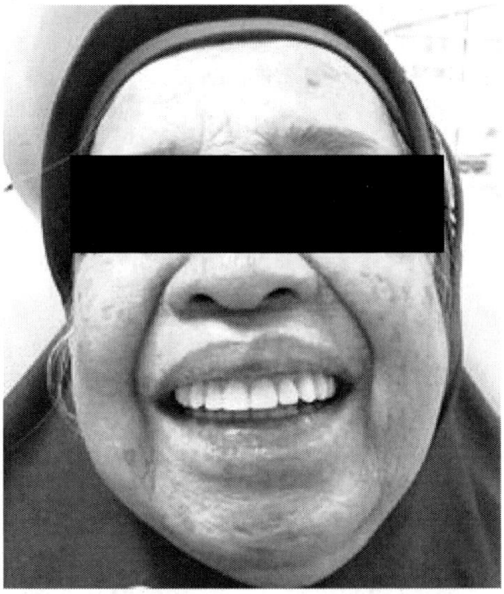

Figure 4. Denture insertion into the patient's mouth.

This tissue conditioner comprises three different viscosities, from thick to watery, which can be regulated by maintaining the powder and liquid ratio. Each application is made in 8-10 min, depending on the material setting time, which is different for each manufacturer. The final impression repeating the functional movement was made with a light-body material and poured into type-III dental stone for preparing the final working model (Figure 3). The face-bow transfer was performed with different upper occlusal rims and mounted in a semi-adjustable articulator. Tooth arrangement was set and tested in the patient's mouth. A final check for aesthetic, vertical dimension, and speaking in the final stage was essential before processing the denture in the dental laboratory. The denture base processing from flasking, packing, and polishing was performed using a conventional method. The denture was then inserted into the patient and checked for stability, occlusion and speaking function (Figure 4).

The compatibility of a new set of dentures was examined in the patient's mouth to show good retention of the lower jaw despite the resorbed mandibular ridge. Lateral and protrusive movement was evaluated using an articulating paper; the impression surface was evaluated for the mucose contact between tissue and denture using pressure indicator paste. This technique provided a thicker buccal border than the conventional technique (open mouth technique). Pronunciation assessment was performed to test the freeway space and word pronunciation efficiency. Patient has given consent to use the clinical photograph for publication.

3. Discussion

The method of recording denture-bearing tissue for complete dentures is crucial to achieve good, functional dentures. The success of every complete denture can be scored by three fundamental properties of retention, stability, and support. A mandibular denture usually presents with difficulties caused by its anatomy and other factors, such as cohesion, adhesion, fluid viscosity, atmospheric pressure, musculature and occlusion.

Various impression techniques were employed to achieve good retention, stability and support. Admixed, all green, closed mouth, cocktail and elastomer impression techniques using various materials to provide better retention and support of the denture. The admixed technique by *McCord* and *Tyson* was developed using a kneaded mix of impression compound and green tracing compound in a 3:7 ratio on a secondary tray after placement in a 60°C water bath [10, 13]. In this method, a custom tray was fabricated with 4-mm wax spacer and removed before loading with a kneaded mix material [13]. The all green technique involves a secondary impression using heated low-fusing compound with functional movement and a final wash impression with light-viscosity polyvinyl siloxane [2] or zinc oxide eugenol [10]. The cocktail technique is a combination of different impression techniques used to obtain a definitive impression. Admixed impression material and closed mouth technique using a custom tray were combined, with elevated cylindrical rest on the posterior region [10, 14]. The elastomer impression technique involves a secondary impression that uses a silicone putty with extended working time on the border of a secondary tray with adhesive and a light-body addition material loaded [10]. Severe bone resorption and musculature insertion near the ridge crest will cause greater muscle-induced denture displacement. A functional technique such as the closed mouth technique is highly recommended in this case, which shows a more significant score in retention [10]. GC Soft Liner is one of the chosen materials for this technique because of the stability in dimension and the low percent of water absorption when stored for 7 days. Other brand materials can also be used such as Visco Gel (Dentsply), Hydro-Cast (Kay-See Dental Mfg.) or FITT (Sybron/Kerr) [15]. This functional method is referred to by various different names by several authors, such as closed mouth technique, introduced by *Lieberthal* in 1919, or dynamic impression method, introduced by *Tryde* in 1965 [6]. Until this year, although a soft liner is still not available, to achieve this impression method, *Lieberthal* used a modeling compound and *Tryde* used an irreversible hydrocolloid [6]. Using this method, authors have claimed that the denture base is extended more buccally and lingually [16].

CONCLUSION

Dynamic impression by the closed mouth technique and functional movements of blowing, puffing, whistling and smiling using a soft liner are excellent methods to achieve maximum support in a highly resorbed mandibular ridge in a fully edentulous patient.

REFERENCES

[1] Zarb GA, Jacob R. (2012). Eckert S: *Prosthodontic Treatment for Edentulous Patients*, 13/E. Elsevier India, Mosby.

[2] Tunkiwala A, Ram S. (2013). Management of mandibular poor foundation: conventional complete dentures. *Dent. Pract.,* 1:34-37.

[3] Mcgarry TJ, Skiba DDSJF, Ahlstrom RH, Smith CR, Koumjian JH. (1999). Classification system for complete edentulism. *J. Prosthet. Dent.,* 8:27-39.

[4] Atwood DA. (1963). Postextraction changes in the adult mandible as illustrated by microradiographs of midsagittal sections and serial cephalometric roentgenograms. *J. Prosthet. Dent.,* 13:810-824.

[5] Gandage Dhananjay S, Kini Ashwini Y, Gangadhar SA, Lagdive SB, Pai UY. (2012). Two-step impression for atrophic mandibular ridge. *Gerodontol.,* 29:e1195-1197.

[6] Rao S, Chowdhary R, Mahoorkar S. (2010). A systematic review of impression technique for conventional complete denture. *J. Indian Prosthodont. Soc.,* 10:105-111.

[7] Zinner ID, Sherman H. (1981). An analysis of the development impression techniques of complete denture. *J. Prosthet. Dent.,* 46:242-249.

[8] Lee BK, Park SH, Lee CH, Cho JH. (2014). Implant overdenture impressions using a dynamic impression concept. *J. Adv. Prosthodont.,* 6(1):66-69.

[9] Singh N, Singh A, Singh S. (2014). CASE REPORT Impression of Severely Atropied Ridge Using Soft Liner : A Case Report. *Int. J. Dent. Med. Res.*, 1(4):61-63.

[10] Yadav B, Jayna M, Yadav H, Suri S, Phogat S, Madan R. (2014). Comparison of different final impression techniques for management of resorbed mandibular ridge: a case report. *Case Rep. Dent.,* 2014:1-6.

[11] Chugh D, Phull S, Rana A, Saini Y. (2015). Modified functional impression technique for resorbed mandibular ridge: Two case studies. *Inter. J. Med. Dent.,* 5:148.

[12] Kresnoadi U, Rostiny R. (2007). Closed mouth method with dynamic and muco compressive impression on upper and lower jaw flat ridges for aid full denture retention. *Dent. J. (Majalah Kedokt Gigi),* 40:193.

[13] Manoj SS, Chitre V, Aras M. (2011). Management of compromised ridges: A case report. *J. Indian Prosthodon.t. Soc.,* 11:125-129.

[14] Praveen G, Gupta S, Agarwal S, Agarwal SK. (2011). Cocktail impression technique: A new approach to atwood's order vi mandibular ridge deformity. *J. Indian Prosthodont. Soc.,* 11:32-35.

[15] Murata H, Kawamura M, Hamada T, Saleh S, Kresnoadi U, Toki K. (2001). Dimensional stability and weight changes of tissue conditioners. *J. Oral Rehabil.,* 28: 918-923.

[16] Tryde G, Olsson K, Jensen SA, Cantor R, Tarsetano JJ, Brill N. (1965). Dynamic impression methods. *J. Prosthet. Dent.,* 15:1023-1034.

SECTION 3: CONSERVATIVE DENTISTRY AND PERIODONTOLOGY

In: Clinical Reports in Dentistry
Editor: Lisa R. Amir
ISBN: 978-1-53617-328-4

Chapter 25

SINGLE VISIT ROOT CANAL TREATMENT IN BILATERAL MAXILLARY FIRST MOLARS WITH MULTIPLE PULP STONES: A CASE REPORT

***Muchlis Fauzi*[1] *and Endang Suprastiwi*[2,*]**
[1]Conservative Dentistry Residency Program, Faculty of Dentistry,
Universitas Indonesia, Jakarta, Indonesia
[2]Department of Conservative Dentistry, Faculty of Dentistry,
Universitas Indonesia, Jakarta, Indonesia

ABSTRACT

Introduction: The pulp stones are calcified mass in the pulp chamber and often present in teeth that have experienced trauma or injury. The pulp stones can cover part or all of the pulp chamber so that it can close access to the root canal.

Case report: A 27-year-old man came to the Conservative Dentistry Clinic, Faculty of Dentistry, Universitas Indonesia with a chief complain of severe pain in the upper left and right back teeth since last week. The patient experienced intermittent pain even though he has been taking pain killer medication. The radiographic examination showed the presence of stone-like formation in the pulp chamber that covers some areas of root canals in bilateral maxillary first molar. The precise combination of magnification and minimal invasive instrument will remove the multiple pulp stones entirely till the root canal treatment in this patient has done very well in single visit on each tooth. During 1-year follow-up, there was no more pain and cone beam computed tomography (CBCT) evaluation demonstrated good tissue healing.

Conclusion: The successful treatment in a difficult endodontic case can be obtained through proper magnification and minimally invasive instruments.

Keywords: pulp stones, ultrasonic instrument, single visit root canal treatment

* Corresponding Author's Email: endang.suprastiwi@ui.ac.id.

1. INTRODUCTION

The success of endodontic treatment depends on triad of endodontics: access opening, root canal preparation and hermetic obturation of root canal. All procedures must be done sequentially and correctly, because the previous procedure will affect the results of next procedure. One of the complications in endodontic treatment is that the presence of pulp stones in the pulp chamber can cover the orifices during root canal preparation [1, 2]. The pulp stones are calcified mass in the pulp chamber and often present in teeth that have experienced trauma or injury. Pulp stones commonly occur in post-traumatic tooth if there are irritants on the teeth chronically altering the pulp chamber to undergo calcification changes and lead to pulp necrosis. The pulp stone may be free in pulp tissue, attached to the wall of the pulp chamber, or embedded within the dentine. The pulp stones can generally be seen through radiographic examination as radiopaque mass seen in the pulp chamber with varying sizes [1, 2].

The obstruction caused by pulp stones often complicates the endodontic treatment. The pulp stones can cover part or all of the pulp chamber so that it can close access to the root canal. Therefore, combination of magnification and ultrasonic instrument is needed to get good visibility in pulp chamber area and surroundings so that the root canal treatment can be well done [2, 3]. In this case report, we will discuss about the removal of the embedded pulp stones on bilateral maxillary first molar teeth with an ultrasonic device.

2. CASE REPORT

A 27-year-old man came to the Conservative Dentistry Clinic, Faculty of Dentistry, Universitas Indonesia with a chief complaint of severe pain in the upper left and right back teeth since last week. The patient experienced intermittent pain even though he has been taking pain killer medication. Clinically there is a filling material in 16 tooth and no cavities in the 26 tooth (Figure 1A-B). There was no swelling of the gingiva and pocket depth of about 3 mm. Vitality test had showed a response. There was a tenderness on percussion test in both teeth. The periapical and panoramic radiographic examinations showed the presence of a stone-like formation in the pulp chamber that covers some areas of root canals in both teeth (Figure 2A-B). The diagnosis of these teeth was symptomatic irreversible pulpitis: symptomatic apical periodontitis with multiple pulp stones.

Treatment plan for both 16 and 26 teeth were endodontic treatments, however the final restorations were different. First, the rubber dam for the isolation was placed (Figure 3A-B). Open access started from the occlusal area on both teeth, removing the old filling in 16 tooth with open access bur (Dentsply). The pulp stones were clinically visible as an irregular translucence attached to the walls and the floor of the pulp chamber in mesial and distal area (Figure 3C-D). An ultrasonic tapered and active tip Start-XTM #3 (Dentsply® Maillefer) was introduced to remove the embedded pulp stones. It is able to smoothly plane embedded pulp stones away when used with a brush-like motion without gouging the floor. Finally, a Start-X tip no. 5 was used to smooth the pulp floor and walls of the access cavity (Figure 3C-D). All canals were negotiated to working length, using a combination of C+ #8 and K-Files #10 (Dentsply/Maillefer). After that, a SX rotary was used to preflaring the 2/3 of root canal (Dentsply® Maillefer).

Initially it was seen that there were four root canals in both teeth and negotiated using K-file #10 on the mesial and distal and K-file #25 on the palatal root canal. From radiograph view, it was showed that there were two mesio buccal canals (mb 1 & mb 2). The working length in both teeth was determined by Pixie apex locator for the four root canals and confirmed by a radiograph. After that, the glide path was enlarged with pathfiles rotary in the mesial and distal of root canals and subsequently followed by root canals preparation with protaper next. Root canals preparation in both teeth was done with ProTaper Next X1 and X2 for the mb 1, mb 2 and distal root canal, whereas in large palatal root canals the preparation is done until the protaper next X4. All of the four root canals in both teeth were thoroughly irrigated with a 5.25% NaOCl and Glyde (Dentsply/Maillefer). Both solutions were activated with the EndoActivator (Dentsply/Maillefer).

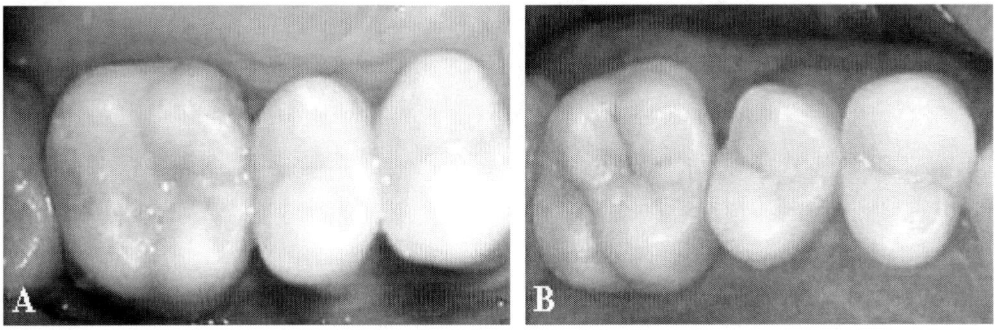

Figure 1. Composite filling was present in #16 tooth (A); No cavity was observed in #26 tooth (B).

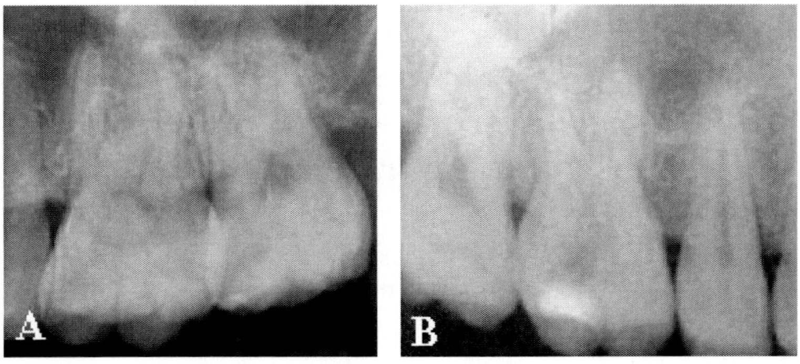

Figure 2. Pre-operative periapical radiograph showed the presence stone-like in the pulp chamber in #16 (A) and #26 (B).

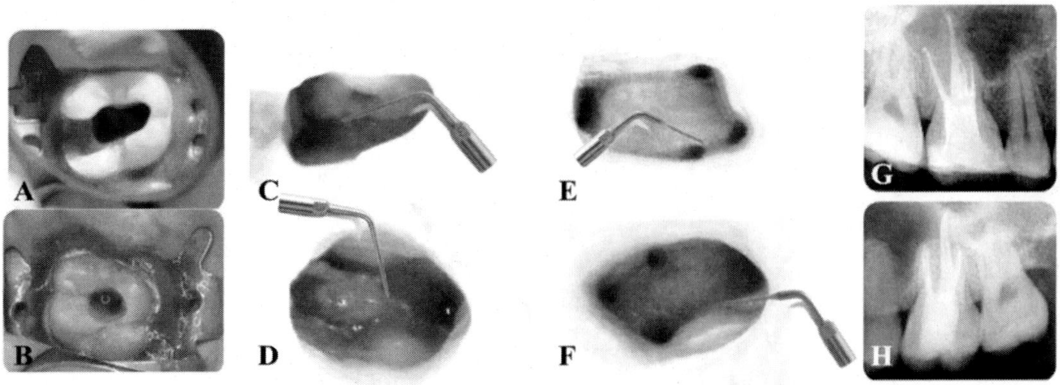

Figure 3. 16 and 26 teeth were isolated with rubber dam prior access opening and preparation (A-B); An ultrasonic tapered and active tip were used to remove (C-D) and smoothen the pulp floor and walls of the access cavity (E-F) Radiographic images of the obturated root canals of 16 and 26 teeth (G-H).

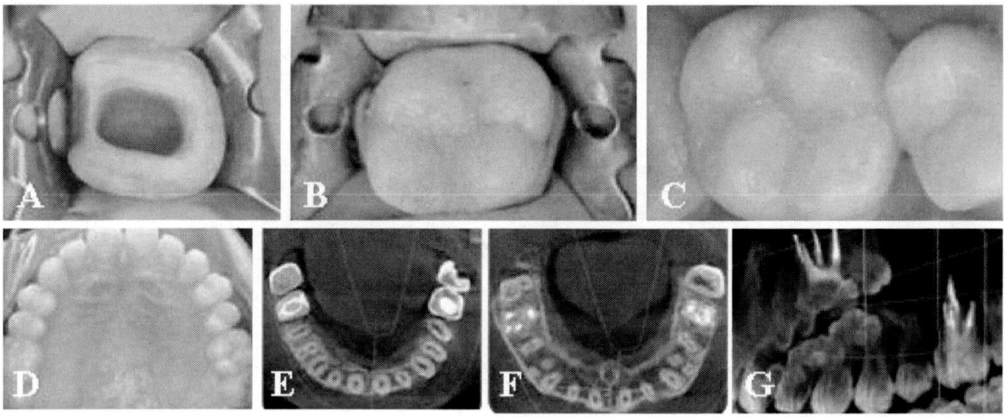

Figure 4. Restoration with Ceram-X Universal SphereTech composite resin (A-C); evaluation the obturation and restoration of 16 and 26 teeth clinically and cone beam computed tomography evaluation (CBCT) (D-G).

Rinsing was done using distilled water solution each turn of irrigation solution. X2 and X4 GuttaCore verifiers (Dentsply/Maillefer) were fitted in the prepared root canals and checked radiographically by Gutta percha protaper next. The both canals were obturated with AH Plus Cement and X2 and X4 GuttaCore obturators (Dentsply/Maillefer) heated in the ThermaPrep 2 oven (Dentsply/Maillefer)(Figure 3G-H).

Coronal seals were done by using bulkfill SDR Dentsply. The access cavity of 16 tooth was restored with composite overlay and 26 tooth was restored with Ceram-X Universal SphereTech composite resin with enhance and pogo as finishing and polishing materials (Figure 4A-C). Evaluation has been done in 6 months clinically and radiography with CBCT (Figure 4D-G).

3. Discussion

Pulp stone is a calcified mass that can be located in the pulp chamber or root canal [7]. In this case, the embedded pulp stones in the pulp chamber can block access to the root canal and inhibit the process of cleaning and shaping the root canal, which influences the success of root canal treatment. Radiographic examination before treatment are very important in detecting the presence of pulp stones both in size and location [3, 7]. If root canal treatment is performed on teeth with multiple pulp stones, elimination of pathogenic bacteria in the root canal will be inhibited. Therefore, the multiple pulp stones in the pulp chamber or root canal should be removed as much as possible [3, 4, 7]. In general, the prevalence of pulp stones is quite high. In this case, pulp stones occur in restored and intact teeth. The presence of pulp stones can be detected by radiographic or histological examination. The radiographic examination is a non-invasive examination. So that the presence of pulp stones before opening access can be more predictable [3, 5].

From the literatures, the methods of pulp stones removal can be done by using a bur or ultrasonic tips. Ultrasonic tips removal can be considered the best choice because it is relatively easier to do and it can be used up into narrow root canals [5]. In addition, according to Plottino et al., the use of ultrasonic tips is very useful to get ideal access to the root canals, making identification of mesio buccal (mb) 2 root canal in maxillary first molars, calcified canals, and removal of multiple pulp stones easier [13,14]. The pulp stones removal in this case were done using an ultrasonic device start X no.3. This instrument has an 8 mm long micro-blade with a maximum diameter of 0.9 mm, tapering down to 0.64 mm, ending with a fine instrument tip which is ideal for the pulp stones removal [4, 5]. After pulp stones removal, the residual of the attachment between the pulp stones and the pulp floor were then smoothed with start X no.5 so that orifice access can be seen. The start X no.5 has a concave end which has almost the same convexity as the pulp floor of the molar teeth which facilitates the removal of calcification without changing the original anatomy and helps localize the presence of the orifice. The advantage of using ultrasonic tips is the incontinuous rotary like using a bur but still have high the cutting efficiency. These instruments are created at an angle of 110° so as to optimize the visibility during clinical use either with a microscope or with dental loupe [4, 5].

To optimize the root canal preparation procedure, the combination of 5.25% Sodium hypochlorite (NaOCl) as an organic solvent and 17% Ethylenediaminetetraacetic acid (EDTA) also carried out as an inorganic solvent are needed. EDTA also has the ability to dissolve inorganic material so that it can eliminate the attachment of pulp stones to the pulp chamber. In this case, an optimal mechanical cleansing effect can occur because the pulp stones in the pulp chamber has been removed completely and the root canal can obturated well in single visit [7, 11].

During one year evaluation with CBCT, there was no more complaint from the patient on his teeth. For this case, the evaluation from CBCT can give us information about the healing process in periapical area and success rate of 3D obturation in root canal treatment, it can be seen from the aspects of endodontic and restoration. The literatures have indication high success rate (90%), if good endodontic treatment with the 3D obturation and restoration was achieved [1, 6, 8].

Conclusion

Successful root canal treatments in this patient was achieved, partly due to the multiple pulp stones that blocked access to canal orifices and alter the internal anatomy of the pulp can be removed entirely. For this case, the combination of using proper magnification and minimally invasive instruments such as endodontic ultrasonic devices, may lead a better visibility and overcome success in such difficult cases of endodontic treatment. Thus, the cleaning and shaping process that aims to eliminate bacteria in the root canal with the chemo-mechanical procedure can be achieved.

References

[1] Luukko K, et al. (2011). Structure and Functions of the Dentin-Pulp Complex. In: Hargreaves KM, Cohen S, editors. *Cohen's Pahway of the Pulp*. 10th ed. Missouri: Mosby Elsevier, p. 494-497.

[2] Berés F, et al. (2016). Comparative Physicochemical Analysis of Pulp Stone and Dentin. *J. Endod.*, 42(3):432-438.

[3] Nanjannawar GS, et al. (2012). Pulp Stone-An Endodontic Challenge: Successful Retrieval of Exceptionally Long Pulp Stones measuring 14 and 9.5 mm from the Palatal Roots of Maxillary Molars. *J. Contemp. Dent. Pract.,* 13(5):719-722.

[4] Cantatore G, et al. (2011). Refining Access Cavities with the Start X Ultrasonic Tips. *Endodontics* Vol. 1. Ed. Il Tridente.

[5] Park E. (2013). Ultrasonics in endodontics. *Endodont Topics*, 29:125-159.

[6] Al Qassab E, et al. (2014). Evaluation of Three Different Obturation Techniques Using Three-Dimensional Cone Beam Computed Tomography: *In Vitro* Study. *Int. Endod. J.*, 43: 64-68.

[7] Torneck CD, Torabinejad M. (2002). Biology of the Dental Pulp and Periradicular Tissues. In: Walton RE, Torabinejad M, editors. *Principles and Practice of Endodontics*. 3rd ed. Pennsylvania: *WB Saunders*, p. 14-15.

[8] Polesel A. (2014). Restoration of the endodontically treated posterior tooth. *Giornale Italiano di Endodonzia*, 28(1):2-16.

[9] Cantatore G, et al. (2010). The Pathfiles: a new series of rotary Nickel Titanium instruments for mechanical pre-flaring and creating the Glide Path. Retrieved from https://www.oralhealthgroup.com/ features/the-pathfiles-a-new-series-of-rotary-nickel-titanium-instruments-for-mechanical-pre-flaring-and-crea/.

[10] Cassim I, van der Vyver PJ. (2013). The importance of glide path preparation in endodontics: a consideration of instruments and literature. *SADJ: journal of the South African Dental* Association, 68(7):322, 324-327.

[11] Ruddle CJ, et al. (2013). The Shaping Movement: Fifth-Generation Technology. *J. Endod.*, 32(4):94, 96-99.

[12] Lii G-hay et al. (2014). Quality of Obturation Achieved by an Endodontic Core-carrier System with Crosslinked Gutta-percha Carrier in Single-rooted Canals. *J. Dent.*, Sep; 42(9):1124-1134.

[13] Goga R, Chandler N, Ogginni A. (2008). Pulp stones: a review. *Inter. Endod. J.*, 41:457-468.

[14] Plottino, Gianluca, et al. (2007). Ultrasonics in Endodontics: A Review of the Literature. *J. Endod.*, 33(2):81-93.

In: Clinical Reports in Dentistry
Editor: Lisa R. Amir

ISBN: 978-1-53617-328-4

Chapter 26

RETREATMENT OF A FAILED ENDODONTIC THERAPY OF MAXILLARY INCISIVUS: A CASE REPORT

Stiza T. Wiranatakusumah[1] and Dewa A. Artiningsih[2,*]
[1]Conservative Dentistry Residency Program, Faculty of Dentistry, Universitas Indonesia, Jakarta, Indonesia
[2]Department of Conservative Dentistry, Faculty of Dentistry, Universitas Indonesia, Jakarta, Indonesia

ABSTRACT

Introduction: Retreatment of root canals due to a previously failed endodontic treatment on chronic apical periodontitis e.c. pulp necrosis was reported. The aim of this case report was to present the technique that used for retreatment of a failure endodontic therapy of maxillary incisive.

Case report: Patient male, 32-year-old came with the broken post on his maxillary anterior incisor. The failure was due to inadequate restoration made the reinfection of bacteria in the root canal apex. Retreatment procedures for the case of a failure endodontics was performed. Success criteria on retreatment was accomplished one-month post retreatment combined with a appropriate restoration.

Conclusion: The success on retreatment depends on technique used to remove old post, restoration and obturation materials, leaving much of the residual tooth structure intact. If done properly, this increases prognosis of the case.

Keywords: retreatment, chronic apical periodontitis, metal post, restoration, endodontic failure

---

* Corresponding Author's Email: dewaayunpa@yahoo.co.id.

1. Introduction

Root canal treatment without surgery has become a primary procedure in modern dentistry. The technical and scientific advances in endodontic science have successfully maintained the millions of teeth that should have been lost. Unfortunately, not all treatments results in optimal long-term cure. Of the large number of root canal treatments performed, some cases have failed results and a large number of patients require further treatment. The dentists should be able to diagnose persistent endodontic disease and precisely choose a treatment plan [1]. The etiology of treatment failure can be divided into preoperative, operative and postoperative. The pre-operative etiology includes improper diagnosis, endo-perio lesion, calcified root canal, trauma, internal resorption and systemic disease. The operative etiology is varied, ranging from anatomical variation, technical difficulties, infections, poor debridement, broken instruments, flare ups, mechanical and chemical irritants, poor access preparation, bleeding, overfilling, underfilling, silver point corrosion, un-hermetic obturation, post corrosion and iatrogenic errors. Post-operative etiology related to the failure of retreatment, surgical failure, and restoration failure [2]. Coronal seal is the important thing in successful in endodontic treated the tooth. Coronal seal can prevent for the bacteria enter to the root canal. The good endodontic treatment and restoration show the predictable result [1, 3]. Success criteria of endodontic retreatment are normal response to percussion & palpation, normal mobility & function, no sinus tract or periodontal defects, no signs of inflammation and no pain & patient discomfort [1, 2].

2. Case Report

Patient, male, 32-year-old, came to department of conservative dentistry of Universitas Indonesia Dental Hospital with broken composite filling since 4 months ago (Figure 1A). The patient felt pain when biting since last 1 month. Patient had root canal treatment done one year before. No signs of systemic disease were present. Radiographic examination showed broken restoration, metal post and widening of periodontal ligament space (Figure 1B). Clinical examination showed broken composite restoration and presence of metal post on tooth #11, negative vitality and sensitive to percussion (Figure 1C). Diagnosis of tooth #11 was chronic apical periodontitis *e causa* pulp necrosis. We planned non vital retreatment of the root canal and placement of fiber post and tooth-colored crown.

On first visit, we removed the restoration and metal post using transmetal bur until the upper part of metal post was uncovered with the aid of dental loupe 3.5x (Figure 1D). We cleared the rest of composite around the metal post using scaler. By using forceps, we held the post then slowly turn it until it was removed completely. Removal of gutta percha with solvent eucalyptol oil and retreatment file (*(Dentsply, Mailefer, Switzerland).* Working length was determined by using the apex locator *(Denjoy)* and confirmed with radiograph (Figure 2A). The working length and initial file was #25/20 mm. The root canal was then prepared with rotary instrument Protaper Wave One Gold (Dentsply, Mailefer, Switzerland) until F2/20mm (Figure 2B). During preparation, irrigation was done using *Chlorhexidine* 2% and *Ethylenediaminetetraacetic acid* (EDTA) 17%. The root canal was dried by paper point and intracanal medicament was applied using calcium hydroxide (Calcipex®, Shimonoseki, Nippon Sika-Yakuhin, Japan).

The cavity was then restored with temporary material (Caviton, GC Corporation, Japan).

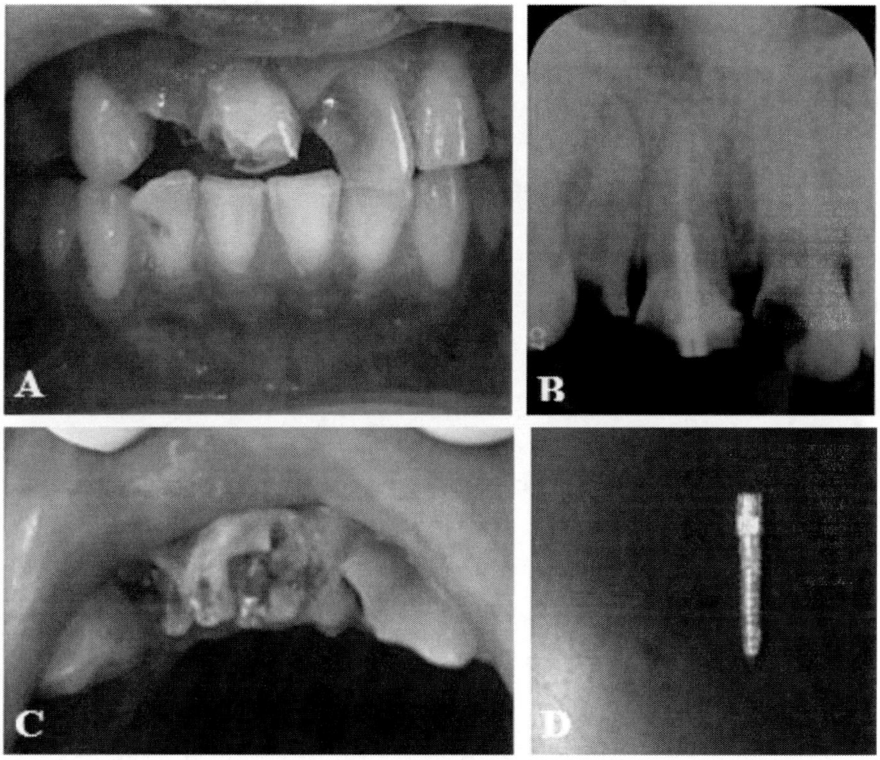

Figure 1. Clinical preoperative of tooth 11. There is remain of resin composite restoration and metal post (A); Preoperative radiograph (B); Clinical condition of metal post after the removal of existing composite restoration (C); Following removal of metal post (D).

On second visit, a week after first visit the patient felt no symptom. Clinical examination showed no gingival swelling, no sinus tract, insensitive to percussion and no pocket deepening. The root canal was irrigated using *Chlorhexidine* 2% and *Ethylenediaminetetraacetic acid* (EDTA) 17%. Sealer AHPlus (Denstply, Maillefer, Switzerland) was used for obturation. Obturation was evaluated radiographically (Figure 2C-E).

Third visit, 1 week after the second visit the patient felt no symptom. Clinically, we found no gingival swelling, no sinus tract and insensitive both to percussion & palpation. We found no deepening of pocket around tooth 11. Radiographically, we found no new lesion on periapical and furcation areas.

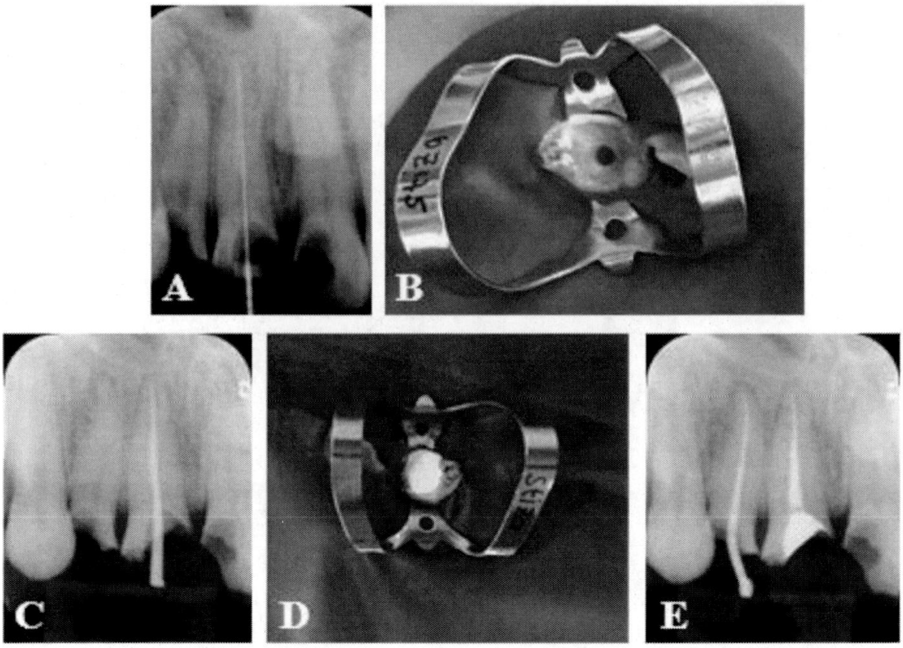

Figure 2. Working length confirmation (A); Access preparation (B); Master apical cone radiograph (C); Cavity restored using temporary material (D) Radiograph of Obturation of the root canal of tooth # 11 (E).

The tooth then was prepared for placement of fiber post. We removed gutta-percha using *gates*-glidden drill bur and drill for fiber post (Kerr Inc, Japan). After that, a 1.25mm fiber post was tried and evaluated radiographically. Then the post was cemented using composite resin cement (Breeze*)* and core buildup was done using dual core resin. We then placed a temporary crown (*easy crown*).

Fourth visit, 1 week after the third visit, the temporary crown was removed using crown retractor. The tooth was prepared for emax crown *post endo*. Impression was made, bite registration was made, color of the crown was chosen. Temporary crown was placed on the tooth.

On fifth visit, one week after the fourth visit, the emax crown was tried and placed. Emax crown was cemented using composite resin cement (*Breeze).* We checked proximal areas of the tooth using dental floss and the occlusion was also checked using articulating paper and evaluation radiograph was made (Figure 3A-C).

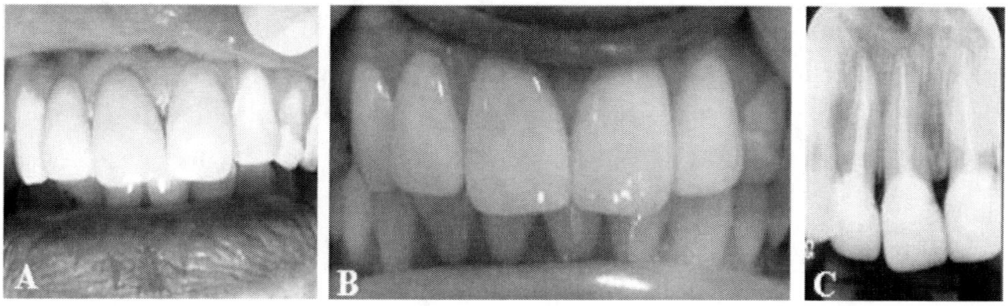

Figure 3. Clinical photograph after sementation (A); on control examination (B); Radiographic condition on control examination (C)

One month after crown placement, our examination showed no clinical symptoms. The tooth was insensitive to percussion. No abnormality on soft tissues and no tooth mobility. The emax crown was clinically satisfactory.

3. Discussion

Before performing root canal treatment, the clinician should be able to detect any problems that occurred during the previous treatment. Difficulties that might occurs during root canal treatment includes un-accessed root canals, additional or undetected root canals, blockades, ledges, perforations, fractured instruments, canal curvature, internal resorption, external resorption, root canal filling materials, posts and core materials [4, 7]. The failure of endodontict treatment is because a wrong diagnosis, inappropriate case selection and treatment procedures [1]. The etiology of treatment failure in this case is due to the loss of post-endodontic restoration of the tooth with poor quality of the post and core materials. If obturation material fails to provide a good seal, then the bacteria will get the nutrient intake from tissue fluid that enters the root canal. Nutrient intakes help the bacteria continue to grow and are able to reach periradicular areas that lead to persistent periradicular infections. The remaining microorganisms can cause endodontic post-treatment infections only if they continue to develop and are capable of reaching periradicular areas, inducing or maintaining periradicular disease. *E. faecalis* has been identified as the main bacteria that cause treatment failure. Coronal seal plays an important role in the success of treated teeth. Once the root canals are clean and obturated, coronal restorations can prevent bacterial entry into the root canal and help provide complete seal. Some studies suggest that filling of root canals that are hermetic but with inadequate restorations are at risk of endodontic treatment failure. Leakage restoration post root canal treatment causes saliva contamination and dissolution of root canal sealer, causing microorganisms to re-colonize in root canal and get nutrition intake [1, 3, 5, 6].

The main factors associated with endodontic treatment failure are persistent microorganism infections in the root canal and periradicular areas. Microorganisms in the root canal play an important role in periradicular infections. In most cases, endodontic treatment failure is the result of persistence of microorganisms in the apical root canal, even in well-treated root canals. Bacteria in the region of isthmus, ramifications, delta, dentine tubules can sometimes not be eliminated by disinfection procedures. Endodontic treatment has a high success rate if the infection is successfully removed completely before root canal obturation. If microorganisms survive in the root canal at the time of filling the root canal or enter the root canal after treatment is complete, then the risk of failure becomes higher. The risk of re-infection depends on the quality of root canal obturation and coronal seal [2, 5, 8]. In this case, it was decided to re-treat the root canal (non-surgical), but if after a good re-treatment, patients still feel pain, we can consider endodontic surgery [1, 2]. Root canal retreatment began with removal of the restoration and metal post and continued with access preparation. The removal of metal post should be done with appropriate techniques to prevent fracture of the roots and maintain the rest of the tooth tissue as much as possible. The obturation material in the root canal can be removed using a rotary retreatment instrument assisted with eucalyptol oil as a solvent. During root canal treatment, irrigation was done with *chlorhexidine* 2% that has been shown to kill E.faecalis bacteria and the medicament used was calcium hydroxide [1, 10]. The advantage of using fiber post is the biomechanical properties is similar to dentin and reducing the risk of root fracture [9, 10]. After re-treatment, appropriate restorations are required to protect the cusp of the tooth from functional load, preventing tooth fracture and to obtain a good seal so that the root canal will not be contaminated with oral or bacterial fluids. If in the control examinations of 6 months to 5 years, there are signs of healing, such as healing of periapical lesions, no symptoms, no signs of inflammation of the gingiva, intact post-retreatment restoration, we can consider the retreatment to be successful [11].

CONCLUSION

Success in root canal treatment depends on technique used when removing the rest of the restorations, posts, and obturation materials so that much of the remaining tooth tissues are intact. This can improve the prognosis of treatment. Root canal treatment can be performed non-surgically and techniques used as well as visualization have an important role in determining the success of the treatment. In this case, root canal treatment was done because the obturation of the root canal was precise, the appropriate use of post fiber, and the usage of crown restoration. Therefore, the goal of this treatment to remove the symptom and for restore the function of the oral health patient, could be achieved accordingly.

REFERENCES

[1] Ferlay, J., Soerjomataram, I., Dikshit, R., Eser, S., Mathers, C., Rebelo, M. et al. (2011). Cancer Hargreaves, K., Cohen, S. Cohen's Pathways of the Pulp. 11th ed. Missouri: Mosby Elsevier.

[2] Ingle, J. I., Bakland, L. K., Baumgartner, J. C. (2008). Ingle's Endodontics 6. Hamilton, Ontario: BC Decker Inc.

[3] Gillen BM, Looney SW, Gu LS, Loushine BA, Weller RN, Loushine RJ, Pashley DH, Tay FR. Impact of the quality of coronal restoration versus the quality of root canal fillings on success of root canal treatment: a systematic review and meta-analysis. J Endod. 2011 Jul;37(7):895-902.

[4] Siquera. (2011). Treatment of Endodontic Infections. Batavia, IL: Quintessence Publishing.

[5] Sadashiv, D. (2013). Endodontic Failures-A review. IOSR J. Dent. Med. Sci., 4(5):5-10.

[6] Borges, M. G. et al. (2015). Does the moment of fiber post cutting influence on the retention to root dentin. Braz. Dent. J., 26(2):141 - 5.

[7] Daokar, S., Kalekar, A. (2013). Endodontic Failures-A.Review. J. Dent. Med. Sci., 4(5):5-10.

[8] Harreaves, Kenneth M., Louis H. Berman. (2016). Nonsurgical Retreatment. Elevent edition. Elsevier Inc. doi: 10.1016/B978-0-323-09635-5.00008-7.

[9] Lamichhane A, Xu C, Zhang FQ. Dental fiber-post resin base material: a review. J Adv Prosthodont. 2014 Feb;6(1):60-5.

[10] John, G., Pavan, K. (2015). Enterococcus Faecalis, A Nightmare to Endodontist: A systematic review. Afr. J. Microbiol. Res. , 9(13):898-908.

[11] Sisthaningsih, E., Suprastiwi, E. (2006). Perawatan Saluran Akar Ulang Akibat Lepasnya Restorasi (Laporan Kasus), Journal of Dentistry Indonesia. Edisi khusus KPPIKG XIV.

In: Clinical Reports in Dentistry
Editor: Lisa R. Amir
ISBN: 978-1-53617-328-4

Chapter 27

ENDODONTIC RETREATMENT OF A MAXILLARY FIRST PREMOLAR WITH TYPE V VERTUCCI CANAL CONFIGURATION: A CASE REPORT

Pramodanti Jiwanakusuma[1] and Anggraini Margono[2,*]
[1]Conservative Dentistry Residency Program, Faculty of Dentistry, Universitas Indonesia, Jakarta, Indonesia
[2]Department of Conservative Dentistry, Faculty of Dentistry, Universitas Indonesia, Jakarta, Indonesia

ABSTRACT

Introduction: Successful endodontic treatment depends on knowledge of root canal morphology, interpretation of radiograph, biomechanical preparation and obturation of root canal system. The possibility of root/canal variation should be considered, although the maxillary first premolar is commonly a bi-rooted tooth with an uncomplicated endodontic anatomy. This case report described the non-surgical endodontic retreatment on a maxillary first premolar with type V Vertucci canal configuration. ProTaper next instruments were used to remove the old gutta percha and to clean and shape all root canals, followed by the complete obturation with *cold lateral condensation* technique with *gutta percha* and accessory cone of root canal system.

Case report: A 21-year-old female patient came to specialist clinic of conservative dentistry Universitas Indonesia with the chief complaint of dull pain in upper right middle region of jaw. The patient had her previous endodontic treatment approximately two years ago. The patient also complained on the unpleasant feeling when eating. Intra-oral examination revealed a large cavity on her 14 tooth. Intra-oral periapical radiograph confirmed that the tooth had a previous root canal treatment, with incomplete root canal filling and chronic apical abscess. The tooth was diagnosed with a chronic apical abscess

* Corresponding Author's Email: margonodewi@yahoo.com.

caused by inadequate endodontic treatment. Treatment planning was root canal retreatment and dowel crown restoration. The condition was a consequence of the failure of the first treatment, where the palatal canal was undetected and untreated.

Conclusion: This case highlight the need to understand, interpret the maxillary first premolar with a Vertucci type V canal configuration to achieve successful results.

Keywords: maxillary first premolar, root canal morphology, anatomical variation, retreatment, root canal therapy

1. INTRODUCTION

A thorough knowledge on the basic root canal anatomy, morphology and the use of various diagnostic imaging technique could help to locate the root canals and is necessary for successful endodontic treatment. An unshaped and unfilled root canal will lead to failure of the endodontic therapy [1]. Root canals if left untreated may harbor microorganisms, which has been reported as a major cause of failure [2]. Vertucci in 1984 has classified a root canal system into eight types [3]. According to Vertucci the maxillary first premolar very often (74%) has two or more canals, approximately 7% incidence for type V (one canal leaves the pulp chamber and divides at the apical third or middle third into two separate canals with separate apical foramen) [3, 4]. In 71% of type V cases, the canal formed two branches in the middle third of the root, and the remaining 29% in the apical third. This case report described the endodontic retreatment on a maxillary first premolar with type V Vertucci canal configuration, diagnosed with chronic apical abscess *e causa* inadequate root canal treatment. However, the incidence of a maxillary first premolar with a single root and two canals (Vertucci type V) is very rare (5-7%) [3, 5].

2. CASE REPORT

A 21-year-old female patient came to specialist clinic of conservative dentistry Universitas Indonesia with the chief complaint of dull pain in the upper right middle region of the jaw. The patient had her previous endodontic treatment approximately two years ago. The patient also complained about the unpleasant feeling when eating and a large cavity on her tooth. On clinical examination, Class II cavity was observed in 14 tooth (Figure 1A). The tooth was sensitive to percussion. Intra-oral periapical radiograph confirmed that the tooth had a previous root canal treatment, with incomplete root canal filling and chronic apical abscess (Figure 1B). The tooth was diagnosed with a chronic apical abscess caused by inadequate endodontic treatment with treatment plan of root canal retreatment and dowel crown restoration. The condition was a consequence of the failure of the first treatment, where the palatal canal was undetected and untreated.

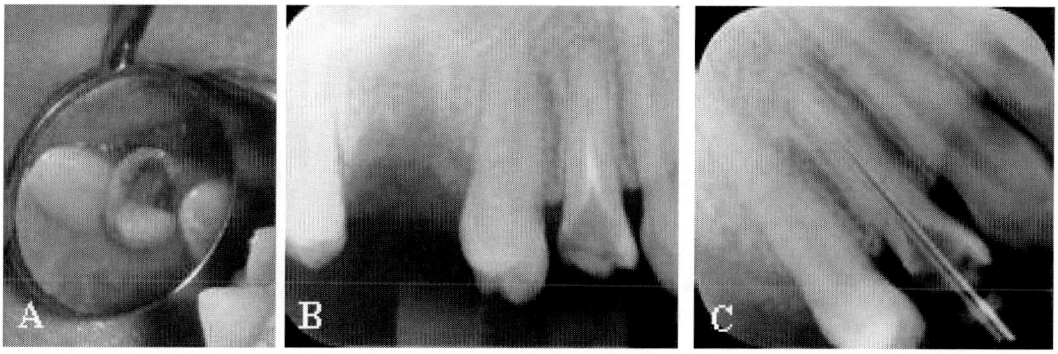

Figure 1. Preoperative photograph (A); and radiograph of tooth # 14 (B), Note the improper root canal fillings; Radiograph of the determination of the length of work (C).

2.1. Case Management

After providing information to the patient, all the remaining caries was removed and the artificial wall was made. When exposing the pulp chamber floor, a lot of debris, sealers and old gutta-percha were seen. The former *gutta percha* was removed using *eucalyptus oil* and protaper *rotary retreatment file* (*Dentsply* Maillefer, Switzerland). The removal of the former gutta percha allowed the clinician to discover one oval orifice was found on the pulp chamber floor. Canal was explored with a # 10 k file and clinician found that the file hitting towards bifurcation on the middle third of the canal. Two # 10 k file were inserted, and a working length radiograph was taken (Figure 1C). The working length radiograph confirmed bifurcation of the canal at middle third of the canal and also confirmed with apex locator. Apical enlargement was then performed with ProTaper Next instruments buccal X3/18 mm and palatal X3/20 mm. Instrument changes were carried out and subsequently the root canals were intermittently and copiously irrigated with 5 mL of NaOCl 5.25%. Irrigation with NaOCl was followed by 17% EDTA solution to remove the smear layer. Patency was assured on each of the root canals with a size 10 K-file. After the cleaning and shaping of the root canals was complete, final irrigation with sodium hypochlorite, sterile saline and 2% chlorhexidine solution for 5 minutes in each root canal was performed. The canals were dried with paper points and dressing with calcium hydroxide, then 2% chlorhexidine was placed as a medication in each root canal for a week.

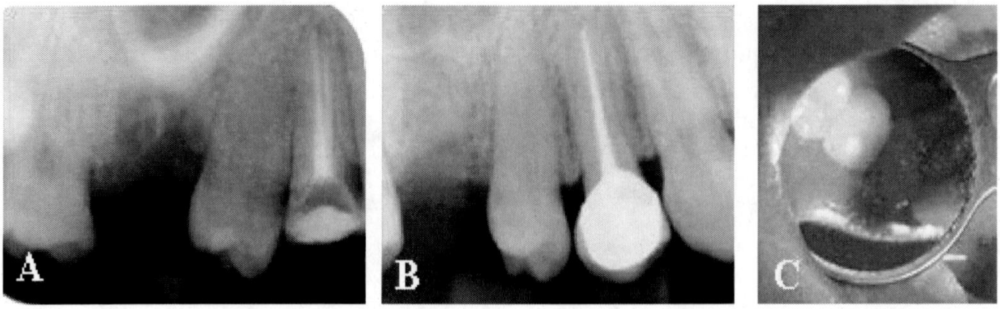

Figure 2. Post obturation radiograph of tooth #14 (A); Post core and crown restoration (B,C).

In the second visit, patient was not sensitive to percussion. Calcium hydroxide dressing was removed after that the canals were rinsed by using NaOCl 2.5% and dried with sterile paper points. The canals were obtured with cold lateral condentation technic with *gutta percha* (*Protaper®*, *Nippon Sika-Yakuhin, Shimonoseki, Japan*) and accessory cones. Temporary filling (Caviton, GC Corporation, Japan) was placed and a postoperative radiograph was taken to confirm the root canal system has been densely obturated laterally and vertically to the canal terminus (Figure 2A). On the 3 months follow up, the removal of obturation material was done followed by cementation of two fiber post and making a rubber base impression. In the next visit the crown was cemented to the teeth (Figure 2 B, C).

3. Discussion

This case presents chronic apical abscess *e causa* inadequate root canal treatment of 14 teeth based on the anamnesis, subjective, objective and radiographic examination. The inadequate root canal treatment was performed initially because the palatal canal was undetected and untreated. Treatment required in the case was endodontic retreatment followed by a dowel crown restoration (ceramage). The root canal system has a complex anatomy and has variations [7]. Ingle finds that one of the biggest causes of endodontic failure was the root canal that was not found [7-10]. Knowledge of root canal morphology and variations in tooth root canal systems and appropriate diagnostic imaging techniques is indispensable for achieving successful root canal treatment, especially in maxillary premolar [11].

Endodontic treatment of premolar is difficult and has a high rate of treatment failure, related to the fact that premolar has the most anatomical variation compared to other teeth [9, 12]. The present was on a maxillary first premolar with a Vertucci type V root canal classification. A tactile examination of all root canal walls was done with a small file tip #10, and the files could be moved from one orifice to another in the middle third of the root canal. Access preparation was done without difficulty. ProTaper Next was used because it has several advantages such as made from the latest type of NiTi material that is M-wire alloy with super elastic properties and resistant to cyclic fatigue [13]. Progressive taper will produce a good boost and improve efficiency when irrigation and debridement. Negative rake angle causes a scrapping movement that produces a smooth root canal surface [13]. The ProTaper Next cross-sectional design is off centered bilateral symmetrical rectangular so that the file has swaggering motion in order to reduce taper lock, screw in effect and stress thereby reducing the risk of broken files and initiating activation of irrigation materials [13]. The file will come into contact with two dentin points within the root canal making it possible to perform brushing motions for the oval root canal as in this case.

E. faecalis, which belongs to the class of gram-positive anaerobic facultative bacteria, play an important role in the incidence of re-infection case. *E. faecalis* can survive under conditions above 9.6 pH and nutritional deficiencies. Research by Distel et al. indicated that E. faecalis forms colonies of root canals that are medicated with calcium hydroxide and are able to form biofilms so they can survive in their environment and become resistant. The additional irrigation material used is 2% chlorhexidine which has strong antibacterial activity against gram positive, gram negative, facultative anaerob, aerob and fungi [14]. Chlorhexidine can diffuse into the dentine and its therapeutic effects are released gradually called residual effects or substantivity [14]. Several studies have suggested the use of 2% chlorhexidine as an effective irrigation agent in cases of root canal infections caused by gram-positive bacteria such as E. faecalis [14]. Calcium hydroxide has a good effect on abscess lesions because it releases calcium ions which can cause a blood vessel pre-capillary contraction resulting in reduced exudative accumulation and support for healing of lesions. The calcium ion can also activate calcium dependent adenosine triphosphate, which causes calcium to bind to carbon dioxide to form important calcium carbonate crystals for mineralization. In addition, hydroxyl ions also activate alkaline phosphatase which produces phosphate ions and will bind to calcium ions for bone mineralization process. Therefore, in this case the medicinal material of calcium hydroxide was used. The cold lateral condensation technique was used in root canal filling with oval root canal shape and single cone technique on a round root canal. AH plus sealer is a sealer that behaves very well with dentin. The sealer hardens and has a good density so it is able to prevent periapical leakage and can close communication between pulp and periodontal tissue.

CONCLUSION

This case report showed a successful endodontic retreatment of a maxillary first premolar with type V Vertucci canal configuration. The first treatment had failed because of missing canal variation. Untreated root canal, improper cleaning, shaping and filling of the root canal will lead to failure of the endodontic treatment. Deep understanding and knowledge of the tooth anatomy, morphology, and its variations, and accurate periapical X-rays technique and interpretation improves the predictability and the successful rate of root canal treatment.

REFERENCES

[1] Gutmann JL, Fan B. (2016). Pathways of the pulp.pdf. In: Hargreaves KM, Berman LH, eds. *Pathways of the Pulp*. 11th ed. Elsevier, 130-208.

[2] Hemanth S, Sujatha I, Vamshi K. (2017). Endodontic Management of Mandibular Second Premolar Having Type-V Vertucci Canal Configuration - Case Series, 76-80. doi:10.21276/sjodr.2017.2.3.5.

[3] Vertucci FJ. (1984). Root canal anatomy of the human permanent teeth. *Oral Surg. Oral Med. Oral Pathol.,* 58(5):589-599. doi:10. 1016/0030-4220(84)90085-9.

[4] Hepsenoglu YE, Ersahan S. (2018). Endodontic treatment of a mandibular premolar with Vertucci type V root canal morphology: a rare case report, 19-22.

[5] Vertucci FJ, Gegauff A. (1979). Root canal morphology of the maxillary first premolar. *J. Am. Dent. Assoc.*, 99(2):194-198. doi:10. 14219/jada.archive. 1979.0255.

[6] Shuman I. (2016). *A Clinical Review of Endodontic Posts*, 1-10.

[7] Castellucci A. (2001). Two canals in a single root: clinical and practical considerations. *Endodontic Practice*, 17-23.

[8] Hema BS, Chandu GS. (2011). Endodontic Management of Type II Canal in Mandibular Incisors: A Case Report. *Indian J. Stomatol.,* 2(4):270-272.

[9] Borisova-Papancheva T. (2015). Endodontic Management of an Uncommon Anatomic Variation of Mandibular Second Premolars: a Case Report. *J. IMAB - Annu. Proceeding* (Scientific Pap, 21(4):945-947. doi:10.5272/jimab.2015214.945.

[10] Muppalla JNK, Kavuda K, Punna R, Vanapatla A. (2015). Management of an Unusual Maxillary Canine: A Rare Entity. *Case Rep. Dent.,* 2015:1-3. doi:10.1155/2015/780908.

[11] Cleghorn BM, Christie WH, Dong CCS. (2008). Anomalous mandibular premolars: A mandibular first premolar with three roots and a mandibular second premolar with a C-shaped canal system. *Int. Endod. J.*, 41(11):1005-1014. doi:10.1111/j.1365-2591.2008.01451. x.

[12] Al-Mahroos SE, Al-Sharif A, Ahmad I. (2016). Mandibular premolars with unusual root canal configuration: A report of two cases. *Saudi Endod. J.,* 6(2):87. doi:10.4103/1658-5984.180622.

[13] Elnaghy AM. (2014). Cyclic fatigue resistance of ProTaper Next nickel-titanium rotary files, 1-6. doi:10.1111/iej.12244.

[14] T N A, Idris M, I B G, et al. (2015). Root Canal Irrigants and Irrigation Techniques: a Review. *J. Evol. Med. Dent. Sci.,* 4(27):4694-4700. doi:10.14260/jemds/2015/679.

In: Clinical Reports in Dentistry
Editor: Lisa R. Amir

ISBN: 978-1-53617-328-4

Chapter 28

CALCIUM HYDROXIDE $CA(OH)_2$ AS INTRACANAL MEDICAMANENT FOR TREATMENT OF CHRONIC APICAL LESIONS: A CASE REPORT

Luh Putu T. B. Utami[1] and Endang Suprastiwi[2,*]
[1]Conservative Dentistry Residency Program,
Faculty of Dentistry, Universitas Indonesia, Jakarta, Indonesia
[2]Department of Conservative Dentistry, Faculty of Dentistry,
Universitas Indonesia, Jakarta, Indonesia

ABSTRACT

Introduction: This was a case report on the usage of calcium hydroxide $Ca(OH)_2$ as an intracanal medicament for the treatment of chronic apical lesions caused by pulp necrosis. Chronic apical lesions generally are asymptomatic, sensitive to percussion, and often has established sinus tract. The purpose was to report the calcium hydroxide intracanal medicament for the treatment of chronic apical lesions.

Case report: Patient is female, 24-year-old, diagnosed with a chronic apical lesions e.causa pulp necrosis on tooth #16. Root canal treatment was performed using intracanal medicament calcium hydroxide/$Ca(OH)_2$. Six months after root canal treatment, there were no signs of infection clinically and decreased radiolucency on the mesial apex was observed. Post-core crown were applied as the final restoration.

Conclusion: Calcium hydroxide as intracanal medicament can induce regeneration process on chronic apical lesions cases.

Keywords: calcium hydroxide, chronic apical lesions, root canal treatment

* Corresponding Author's Email: esuprastiwi@yahoo.co.id.

1. Introduction

The bacterial colonies existing inside the root canals can spread to periapical areas within long-term. Bacteria and their products spread to periapical areas caused inflammatory responses. If no treatment is done, the inflammation will lead to acute or chronic apical periodontitis, acute or chronic apical lesions, periapical cyst or even celullitis [1]. Chronic apical lesions occur from an increased number of PMN (Polymophonuclear Neutrophil) killed by proteolytic and hydrolytic enzymes whose destruction exceeds the protective capacity of macrophage, resulting in liquid areas surrounded by PMNs, creating lesions. Chronic apical lesions generally are asymptomatic, sensitive to percussion and often have established sinus tract [2-4].

Calcium hydroxide/$Ca(OH)_2$ is a slow-acting antibacteria because it needs longer time to dissolve into tissue fluid. Leonardo et al. (2000) evaluated the antimicrobial activity of $Ca(OH)_2$ paste against seven bacterial strains using the diffusion method. The test showed that $Ca(OH)_2$ is effective in killing the tested bacterial strains, namely; Gram-positive cocci, Micrococcus luteus, Staphylococcus aureus, Staphylococcus epidermidis, Enterococcus faecalis, Streptococcus mutans and Gram-negative rod: Escherichia coli, Pseudomonas aeruginosa [5-7]. Pavelic et al. (1991) evaluated antimicrobial effect of $Ca(OH)_2$ using an agar diffusion method which succeeded in inhibiting microorganisms growth within 24 hours, with different level of sensitivity for each type of microorganisms. *Streptococcus mutans* was the most sensitive, while E. *faecalis* was the least sensitive [6, 7]. Another study using $Ca(OH)_2$ as an intracanal medicament for seven days showed 99.9% bacterial reduction [8]. This case report discusses the effect of $Ca(OH)_2$ as an intracanal medicament for the treatment of chronic apical lesions.

2. Case Report

In a 24-year-old female patient subject, the upper right tooth had been cavitated 5 years ago and the tooth causes pain when used to eat or bite and the gum surrounding the tooth had been swollen for one month. Gum swelling occurs a lot of times, and the tooth was temporarily medicated two weeks ago by a general dentist. Upon clinical examination, it was found that tooth #16 has 2 sites of caries, involving the pulp. The vitality test was negative, percussion test was insensitive, and sinus tract containing pus on buccal gingiva around tooth #15 and #16 (Figure 1A). Radiograph examination showed caries extending to the pulp chamber, widening of the periodontal space around mesial apex, discontinuity of lamina dura and radiolucency diffuse border with a diameter of 3 mm (Figure 1B). The result of the diagnosis came out with tooth #16 suffering chronic apical lesions e causa pulp necrosis followed with a treatment plan consisting of root canal treatment and post-core crown restoration.

2.1. Procedure

Cleaning necrotic tissues and caries alongside access opening were carried out using diamond round bur and endo access bur. The orifices was explored with the visual aid of dental loupe (magnification 3.5x) and four orifices on tooth #16 were located: 1 distobuccal, 2 mesiobuccal and 1 palatal orifice (Figure 2A).

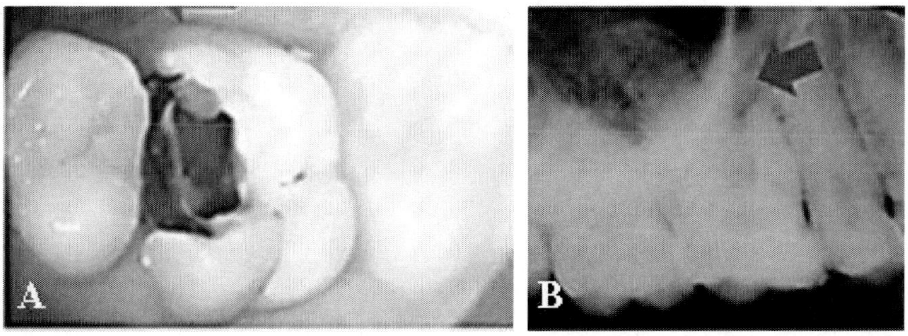

Figure 1. Clinical and radiographic condition pre-treatment periapikal lesion at mesial canal was indicated with red arrow (A,B).

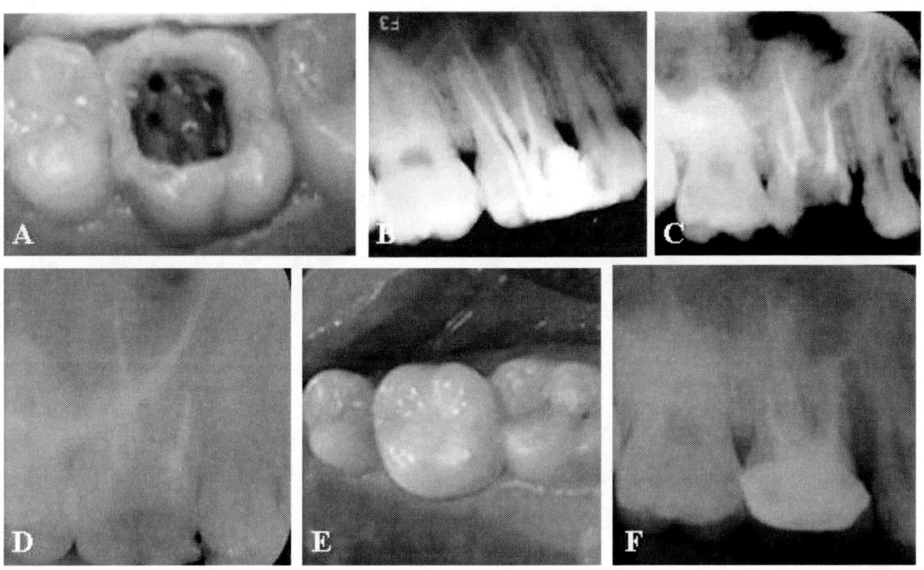

Figure 2. Four oriffices were observed in distobuccal, 2 in mesiobuccal and 1 in palatal (A); Radiographic view of master cones (B); after obturation (C); six months post-treatment (D); Clinical and radiograph view after crown cementation (E,F).

Establishing the glide path on all canals using K-file ISO #15 (Colorinox, Dentsply). Then root canal preparation on tooth #16 was started by creating *coronal flaring* by Protaper Hand-use (Dentsply/Maileffer) shaping files - S1 and SX - with clockwise and anticlockwise motion until 2/3 of working length. The definitive working length was established using apex locator and each canal has a different working length: palatal 22 mm, mesiobuccal canals 18 mm and 17 mm, distobuccal 16 mm. After working length was established, coronal preparation of the canals was done using Shaping files (S1 and S2) then continued by Finishing files (F1, F2, and F3) until established working length was achieved. After that, a radiograph was made to determine master cone according to the size of the last Protaper file that was used. Every file change was followed by irrigation using natrium hypochlorite (NaOCl) 2.5%, and flushed with saline, followed by irrigation using chlorhexidine 2%, and flushed with saline. Every file change was also followed by apical confirmation using ISO files. After preparation by F1, recapitulation was done using ISO file #20. After preparation by F2, recapitulation was done using ISO file #25. After preparation by F3, recapitulation was done using ISO file #30. The root canals were then dried using paper point, then $Ca(OH)_2$ (Calcipex Plain II, Nippon Shika Yakuhin Co. Ltd) was applied as intracanal medicament at working length, and the access cavity was sealed using temporary restoration.

After the patient was confirmed asymptomatic subjectively and objectively and the sinus tract was healed, the obturation of the root canals was commenced. Obturation was done through single cone technique using Protaper gutta-percha and AH Plus sealer (Figure 2B, C) and the tooth was restored using temporary restoration. Examination after 6 months post-treatment showed radiographic improvement, marked by a reduction in radiolucency on the apex of the root (Figure 2D). The next step was to create restoration for the tooth. Cementation fiber post in the palatal root using Breeze self-adhesive resin cement (Dental Pentron). The tooth was then prepared for a metal-porcelain crown. The crown was cemented using type 1 glass ionomer cement (GC Fuji I, GC Japan. Inc.) (Figure 2E, F).

3. Discussion

Bruder et al. (2000) defined chronic apical lesions as a lesion marked by intermittent pus discharge via sinus tract, also called as suppurative chronic periodontitis [9]. While Grossman (2015) defined chronic apical lesions as long-standing periradicular lesions with decreasing infection grade because of drainage of the lesions through sinus tract [3].

Apical lesions occur when the number of bacteria entering the lesion increases. The PMN rushes to the site of infection because of the chemotaxis, induced initially by bacterial lipopolysacharides (LPS). The number of dead PMNs is increased, caused by proteolytic and hydrolytic enzymes released by bacteria. This is a major cause for tissue breakdown in acute phases of apical lesions. Macrophages entering the site of inflammation is a chronic phase of apical lesions. If the change in the number of bacteria is temporary then lymphocyte, plasma, and macrophage cells is increased so that there is induced healing process [7, 10]. In this case, diagnosis on tooth #16 was chronic apical lesions, based on clinical examination of the following; caries on the occlusal-proximal surfaces extending to the pulp, negative vitality, negative percussion tests, sensitive to palpation and fistula containing pus on the buccal gingiva around tooth #15 and #16.

Based on the principle of endodontic treatment, on the first visit, after access opening and establishment of the root canal pathway, coronal flaring using Protaper hand-use (Dentsply) SX files and shaping files (S1) up to 2/3 of working length are required for good removal of the necrotic tissues and debris through irrigation. The preparation was continued until working length using Protaper hand-use up to size F3 so that the root canal has a flared shape.

The intracanal medicament used was calcium hydroxide/$Ca(OH)_2$, to sterilize root canals and to induce healing of the lesion. Calcium hydroxide was first introduced by Hermann (1920) as a useful material in dentistry, including as intracanal medicament [8, 11]. Calcium hydroxide is release as calcium ions and hydroxide ions (Ca^{2+} and OH^-) in an aqueous environment. Antimicrobial effect of $Ca(OH)_2$ is associated with a release of hydroxide ions, creating a highly alkaline environment which is bactericidal. Hydroxide ions destroy bacteria by damaging bacterial cytoplasmic membrane, denaturing bacterial proteins, damaging bacteria DNAs and hydrolysis of bacterial lipopolysacharides (LPS/endotoxin) [1, 7]. Calcium hydroxide has a long antimicrobial effect because of its low solubility, resulting in longer contact with tissue fluid [4, 8]. Estrella (2001) found the antimicrobial activity of Ca $(OH)_2$ is complete after 48 hours [8,12]. Lin et al. (2005) found that Ca $(OH)_2$ is effective up to 200-500μm within dentinal tubules for 7 days [8, 13].

Calcium ions from $Ca(OH)_2$ is important for healing and repair of periapical tissues. Calcium ions activated ATP for cells transportation, cells proliferation, cells differentiation, and mineralization process. Calcium ions bond with carbon dioxide from anaerobe bacteria, creating calcium carbonate ($CaCO_3$). Calcium ions stimulated peripheral vessel constriction, thereby decreasing exudate to the tissues. Calcium ions are also mitogenic against fibroblasts in the pulp and activate tissue enzymes such as alkaline phosphatase and fibronectin glycoprotein, which induce mineralization. These enzymes work on the alkaline environment (pH 9 to 10.5) hence calcium ions can be deposited on bones [14, 15].

The use of $Ca(OH)_2$ as the intracanal medicament for this case is good because of the weeping canals associated with the periapical lesion. Six months after obturation, the case showed improvement by reduction of radiolucent area on a mesial apex of the root. The most important step in the healing process is the formation of granulation tissues, which is marked histologically by blood vessel proliferation (neovascularization) and fibroblast growth stimulated by growth factors. Macrophage regulates the formation of granulation tissues by removing extracellular debris and fibrins, elaborates host mediators to induce fibroblast proliferation and production of extracellular matrix (ECM). In inflammatory areas, there are also mast cells, and chemotactic environments that correspond to lymphocytes may appear. Each of these cells may play a direct or indirect role in the proliferation and activation of fibroblasts. The formation of new blood vessels (angiogenesis) accelerates regeneration and normalization of tissues. Neovascularization of vitamins, minerals, glucose, and amino acids supply media for fibroblasts, to increase collagen formation and clear necrotic tissues, antigens, and infection, thus accelerating the healing process. Several factors that induce neovascularization are basic epithelial growth factors (bEGF) and vascular endothelial growth factors (VEGF) [16].

Final restoration of this case inserted fiber post to provide long-term resistance of the tooth. The non-rigid post was the chosen because the tooth still had plenty of remaining structures. Fiber post has a modulus of elasticity, compressive strength, flexural strength and thermal expansion similar to dentin. Fiber post will flex alongside the tooth under functional pressure, reducing a functional load to the root and the risk of root fracture [17, 18].

CONCLUSION

The use of calcium hydroxide as an intracanal medicament for the treatment of chronic apical lesions results in apical healing and rehabilitation within six months post-treatment. A long-term follow-up study of 1, 2, 3, and 4 years would provide the much-needed data pertaining to the efficacy of calcium hydroxide for endodontic treatment.

REFERENCES

[1] Hargreaves KMLH. (2016). *Cohen's Pathways of The Pulp 11th*. 11th ed. Elsevier.

[2] Harty. (2010). *Harty's Endodontics Clinical Practice*. 6th ed. (San CB, ed.).

[3] Grossman Louis. (2015). *Grossman's Endodontics Practice 12th Ed.*

[4] Siqueira J. Endodontic Infections. pdf. 2011.

[5] Leonardo MR, Da Silva LAB, Tanomaru Filho M, Bonifácio KC, Ito IY. (2000). *In vitro* evaluation of antimicrobial activity of sealers and pastes used in endodontics. *J. Endod.*, 26(7):391-394. doi:10.1097/ 00004770-200007000-00003.

[6] Pavelić B, Anić I, Najzar-Fleger D, Stilinović B T, K. (1991). The antimicrobial efficiency of aqueous solutions of calcium hydroxide on Streptococcus mutans, Streptococcus faecalis and Candida albicans, *in vitro*, *Acta Stomatol. Croat.* 25(4):207-212.

[7] Kim D. (2014). Antimicrobial effect of calcium hydroxide as an intracanal medicament in root canal treatment: a literature review - Part I. *In vitro* studies. *Restor. Dent. Endod.* 39(4): 241-252.

[8] Mohammadi Z, Shalavi S, Yazdizadeh. (2012). Antimicrobial Activity of Calcium Hydroxide in Endodontics: A Review, *Chonnam. Med. J.* 48(3): 133-140.

[9] Bruder GA, Chalian GG, Practice P, et al. (2000). *Color Atlas of Dental Medicine*. New York: Thieme Stuttgart.

[10] Graunaite I, Lodiene G, Maciulskiene V. (2012). Pathogenesis of Apical Periodontitis: a Literature Review. *J. Oral Maxillofac. Res.* 2(4):e1. doi:10.5037/jomr.2011.2401.

[11] Hermann. (1987). Calcium hydroxyd als Mittelzurn, Behandeln und Fullen von Wurzelkanalen [Calcium hydroxide as a central treatment, treatment and filling of root canals]. Wurzburg: (printed in: Malo PRT, Kessler Nieto F, Vadillo MVM (1987) Hidroxido de calcio y apicoformacioÂn [Calcium hydroxide and apicoformation]. *Revista EspanÄ ola de Endodoncia*, 1920,5:41-61.

[12] Estrela C, Bammann LL, Pimenta FC, Pécora JD. (2001). Control of microorganisms *in vitro* by calcium hydroxide pastes. *Int. Endod. J.,* 34(5):341-345. doi:10.1046/j.1365-2591.2001.00368.x.

[13] Lin S, Tsesis I, Zukerman O, Weiss EI, Fuss Z. (2005). Effect of electrophoretically activated calcium hydroxide on bacterial viability in dentinal tubules - *In vitro. Dent. Traumatol.*, 21(1):42-45. doi:10. 1111/j.1600-9657.2004.00293.x.

[14] Holland R, Gomes Filho JE, Cintra LTA, Queiroz ÍO de A, Estrela C. (2017). Factors affecting the periapical healing process of endodontically treated teeth. *J. Appl. Oral Sci.,* 25(5):465-476. doi: 10.1590/1678-7757-2016-0464.

[15] Misra P, Bains R, Loomba K, et al. (2017). Measurement of pH and calcium ions release from different calcium hydroxide pastes at different intervals of time: Atomic spectrophotometric analysis. *J. Oral Biol. Craniofacial Res.*, 7(1):36-41. doi:10.1016/j.jobcr.2016. 04.001.

[16] Mahmoud T, Walton RE, Fouad AF. (2015). *Mahmoun Torabinejad Endodontics.* Pdf. 5th ed. Missouri: Elsevier.

[17] Rosenstiel et al. 2016. *Contemporary fixed prosthodontics fifth edition*. Elsevier.

[18] Lamichhane A, Xu C, Zhang F. (2014). Dental fiber-post resin base material: a review. *J. Adv. Prosthodont.*, 6(1): 60-65.

In: Clinical Reports in Dentistry
Editor: Lisa R. Amir

ISBN: 978-1-53617-328-4

Chapter 29

ENDODONTIC MANAGEMENT FOR A VERTUCCI TYPE II J-SHAPED ROOT CANAL OF THE MANDIBULAR FIRST MOLAR

***Siti U. Dewi*[1] *and Anggraini Margono*[2,*]**
[1]Conservative Dentistry Residency Program, Faculty of Dentistry, Universitas Indonesia, Jakarta, Indonesia
[2]Conservative Dentistry Department, Faculty of Dentistry, Universitas Indonesia, Jakarta, Indonesia

ABSTRACT

Introduction: The *goal* of endodontic treatment is the prevention or cure of apical periodontitis. Biomechanically, this means cleaning, shaping and disinfection that enable three dimensional obturation of root canal systems. Evaluation of one or more periapical radiographs is mandatory. Here, we discuss the endodontic treatment of a Vertucci type II (2-1) J-shaped root canal identified radiographically.

Case report: A 29-year-old woman visited the Specialist Clinic of Conservative Dentistry University of Indonesia. The patient was referred there to continue dental treatment of the mandibular first molar. The mandibular first molar had undergone root canal treatment 9 months previously; however, the procedure had not been completed. One month previously, she started experiencing discomfort in the area while eating. A complete history was taken, and clinical and radiographic examinations were performed. She was diagnosed with a chronic apical abscess caused by inadequate endodontic treatment, and she underwent non-vital root canal treatment with post-endodontic onlay ceramage restoration.

Conclusion: Endodontic management in this case was successful because of adequate diagnosis, preparation, obturation and restoration. The treatment restored tooth morphology and function. Further evaluation are needed at 1, 3, 6 and months postoperatively.

* Corresponding Author's Email: margonodewi@yahoo.com.

Keywords: Vertucci's type II, J shape, endodontic treatment, root canal morphology, root canal curvature

1. INTRODUCTION

The goal of endodontic treatment is the prevention or cure of apical periodontitis [1]. Biomechanically, this involves cleaning, shaping and disinfecting the area, and these procedures enable three dimensional obturation of the root canal. One of the clinical challenges that can occur during root canal treatment is the complexity of the root canal anatomy [2]. Thorough knowledge of root canal anatomy may improve the prognosis. Thus, before endodontic treatment, the dentist should have thorough knowledge of the pulp chamber and root canal anatomy. Once access is achieved, the treatment outcome is related to the elimination and prevention of microbial contamination [2].

For the assessment of root canal anatomy, various techniques such as radiography, cleaning techniques and plastic resin injection, have been used [1]. CBCT also used to identify various configuration of root morphology. Evaluation of one or more periapical radiographs is mandatory in clinical practice. Periapical radiograph at different angle can provide information on root canal morphology [3,4]. Martinez-Lozano et al. (1999) stated that on altering the horizontal angle by 20-40 degree the number of root canals seen in radiograph of the first mandibular premolars and second premolars corresponds to the number of the root canals [5]. Chourasia et al. (2012) showed wide variation of mesial and distal roots of mandibular first molar. In mesial root, type IV configuration was most prevalent (54%) followed by type II (36.6%), type VI (8%), and type V (0.6%) [6]. This configuration incidence in mandibulary first molar has been reported quite high, at 41.87% [7].

In the present case report, we discuss the endodontic treatment of a Vertucci type II (2-1) J-shaped root canal identified radiographically. In this canal configuration, the mesial root canal of the mandibular first molar fuses into one canal from different orifices identified radiographically.

2. CASE REPORT

A 29-year-old woman visited the Specialist Clinic of Conservative Dentistry University of Indonesia. The patient was referred to continue dental treatment of the mandibular first molar. The mandibular first molar had undergone root canal treatment 9 months previously; however the procedure had not been completed. One month previously, she started to experiencing discomfort in the area while eating.

Clinical assessment showed caries at D6 on tooth 36 site 2 (Figure 1). We noted, temporary restoration on the tooth, percussion sensitivity, palpation negativity, and normal gingiva. A Preoperative radiographic examination revealed radiolucency features at the crown up to pulp chamber and radiolucency with unclear bounded at the mesial and distal canal (Figure 1). She was diagnosed with a chronic apical abscess caused by inadequate endodontic treatment and we planned non-vital root canal treatment and onlay ceramage restoration.

2.1. Case Management

At the first visit, complete was taken, a rubber dam was placed and the temporary restoration was removed. The access cavity was refined and caries tissue was removed. Then an artificial wall was created at the distal wall (Figure 2). After completion of access preparation, three orifices were visible (one in the distal and two in the mesial area). Then, scouting was performed using hand file instrument (K-file ISO #8, #10, #15 subsequently) with estimation oh the working length from preoperative radiographs. The working length was determined using an apex locator (Propex Pixi, Dentsply), and then radiographs were obtained to check the working length by using the SLOB technique with ISO file #15 (Figure 2).

Radiographs showed that the mesial canal fused at one-third of the apical end (Vertucci type II) with a J shape. The distal root canal working length was identified as 19.5 mm, and then, root canal preparation was attempted using Protaper Next (Dentsply Mailefer, Switzerland) up to file X3.

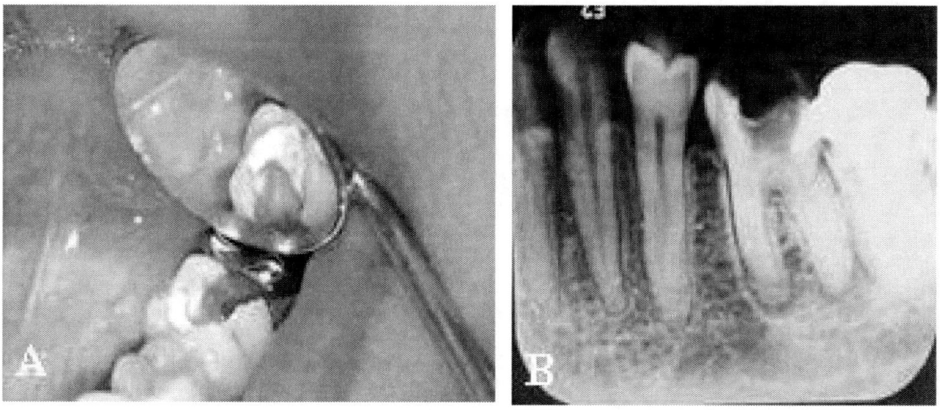

A B

Figure 1. (A) Preoperative clinical image of tooth 36. (B) Preoperative radiograph of tooth 36.

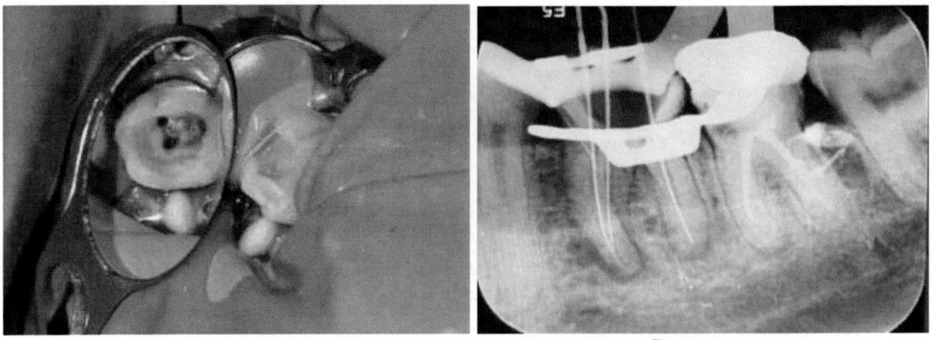

A B

Figure 2. (A) Access preparation. (B) Radiograph of working length determination.

Irrigation was performed with 2.5%, NaOCL 17% EDTA and finally 2% chlorhexidine. Irrigation was activated through sonic vibration (EndoActivator; Dentsply, Tulsa, OK). Owing to time limitation, the distal root canal was dried using a paper point. Additionally, intracanal $Ca(OH)_2$ was applied (Calcipex, Nippon Sika-Yakuhin, Shimonoseki, Japan) and a cotton pellet was placed with temporary restoration (*Caviton, GC Corporation, Japan*).

At the second visit, root canal treatment of tooth 36 was performed (followed by rubber dam placement, the temporary restoration was removed, $Ca(OH)_2$ was flushed out and the mesial canal was prepared.

The mesiolingual canal was prepared, and then mesiobuccal canal was prepared using Protaper Next (Dentsply Mailefer; up to file X2). Initially, tge mesiobuccal canal was prepared using Protaper Next; however, when file X1 was used, the system was locked. Thus, Protaper Next was changed to HyflexCM (Coltene Whaledent, Altstätten, Switzerland) because of its curvature up to file 30/0.4. Irrigation with NaOCL 2.5%, EDTA 17% and last using chlorhexidine 2%.

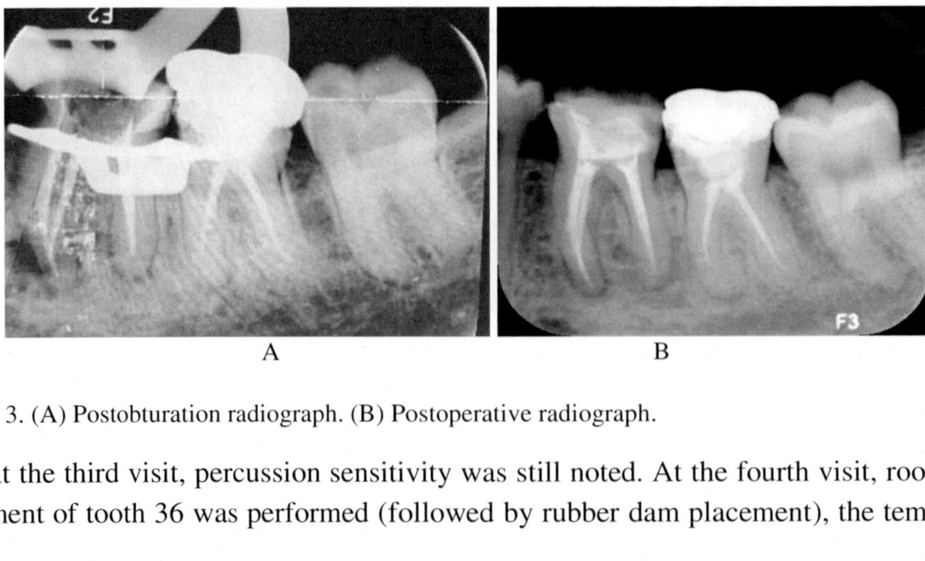

A B

Figure 3. (A) Postobturation radiograph. (B) Postoperative radiograph.

At the third visit, percussion sensitivity was still noted. At the fourth visit, root canal treatment of tooth 36 was performed (followed by rubber dam placement), the temporary restoration was removed, and $Ca(OH)_2$ was flushed out. The canal was filled by the single-cone technique using gutta-percha (Dentsply Maillefer and Coltene Whaledent) and AHPlus (Dentsply Maillefer) as root canal sealers. Temporary filling (Caviton, GC Corporation) was performed, and a postoperative radiograph was obtained to assess the quality of obturation (Figure 3).

At the fifth visit, onlay ceramage was prepared, a rubber base impression was sent to the laboratory, and temporary restoration was placed. At the sixth visit, the onlay ceramage was placed and resin cement (Breeze; Dentsply Maillefer) was applied (Figure 3).

3. Discussion

Based on the patient's history and the subjective, objective and radiographic findings, our patient was diagnosed with a chronic apical abscess caused by inadequate root canal treatment. She underwent non-vital root canal treatment followed by onlay ceramage restoration at site 2.

A thorough knowledge of the pulp chamber and root canal anatomy might improve the prognosis. An optimal cleaning, shaping and sealing would not have been achieved if the morphology of the root canal system had not been known before chemomechanical preparation started. A previous report mentioned that lack of knowledge of root canal morphology could cause many problems during treatment [4]. An unprepared root canal is one of the main problems than can cause root canal treatment failure [5].

Identification morphology of the root canal system is important before starting treatment, as it might influence cavity access [4]. Evaluations using multiple radiographs with different angles provides dentist with accurate information about the real anatomical state of a tooth. A tool that can aid in the identification of the location of the root canal is the dental operating microscope, which is intended to increase visibility [5]. The Vertucci type II canal configuration has been reported to be second most common configuration found in the mesial roots of mandibular molars, which is consistent with the situation in the present case [1]. The incidence of the Vertucci type II canal configuration in the mandibular first molar has been reported to be 41.87% [7].

The use of gutta percha for one of the root canals during preparation of another canal can prevent transportation and over instrumentation. In this case, Protaper Next was used initially, but the system locked in the mesiobuccal canal; thus HyflexCM was used. Protaper Next has a rectangular cross section in the center of the file that has a swaggering movement effect. This asymmetric movement enables Protaper Next to reach the end of the root canal with few files. This file system is suitable for use at the distal and mesiolingual roots that have a less crooked root shape [8].

HyflexCM can be used in the mesiobuccal canals that have a J shape. HyflexCM has a controlled memory effect that helps maintain the shape of the root canal even when the file has been removed. Its extreme flexibility and small size make it very useful for root canals *that* show severe curvature and it can help avoid issues, such as ledge formation, transportation and perforation [6].

In addition to 2.5% NaOCl and 17% EDTA, 2% chlorhexidine can be used as an irrigation material with an antibacterial effect on *Enterococcus E. faecalis. E. faecalis* is a facultative gram-positive anaerobe which found in small amounts in the root canal; however, it plays an important role in the etiology of persistent infection [9]. In this case the, infection was prolonged and the tooth had received incomplete treatment previously.

The obturation technique adopted in this case involved vertical condensation using gutta percha *non-ISO* according to the working length. This technique was selected because the master cone has tug back, feels and looks fit on the root canal and can be inserted at the same time. Thus, obturation could be performed simultaneously.

In this case, post endodontic restoration involved an onlay to prevent fracture. Onlay ceramage was placed at site 2 for final restoration. Ceramage was selected for aesthetic reason by the patient.

CONCLUSION

Our patient successfully underwent endodontic treatment of a Vertucci type II J-shaped root canal because of adequate diagnosis, preparation, obturation, and restoration. The treatment restored tooth morphology and function. The prognosis of our patient was good, since all root canals were accessible, systemic diseases were absent, and the patient was cooperative. Further evaluations are needed at 1, 3, 6, and 12 months post-operatively.

REFERENCES

[1] Keleş A, Keskin C. Apical root canal morphology of mesial roots of mandibular first molat teeth with vertucci type II configuration by means of micro-computed tomography. *Journal of Endodontics*. 2016,43,481-485.

[2] De Pablo ÓV, Estevez R, Sánchez MP, Heilborn C, Cohenca N. Root anatomy and canal configuration of the permanent mandibular first molar: a systematic review. *Journal of Endodontics*. 2010,36,1919-1931.

[3] Vertucci FJ. Root Canal Anatomy of the Human Permanent Teeth. *Oral Surgery Oral medicine Oral Pathology*, 1985,58,589-599.

[4] Aggarwal K. Mandibular Lateral Incisor with Vertucci Type IV Root Canal Morphological System: A Rare Case Report. E. *Journal of Natural Science Biology and Medicine,* 2016, 7: 101-104.

[5] Vertucci FJ. Root Canal Morphology and Its Relationship to Endodontic Procedures. *Endodontic Topics*, 2005, 10: 3-29.

[6] Chourasia HR, Meshram GK, Warhadpande M, Dakshindas D. Root Canal Morphology of Mandibular First Permanent Molars in an Indian Population. *Inter. J. Dent.*, 2012, 1-6.

[7] Akhlaghi NM, Khalilak Z, Vatanpour M, Mohammadi S, Pirmoradi S, Fazlyab M, Safavi K. Root Canal Anatomy and Morphology of Mandibular First Molars in a Selected Iranian Population: An In Vitro Study. *Iranian Endodontic Journal*, 2017, 12: 87-91.

[8] Patnana AK, Chugh A. Endodontic Management of Curved Canals with Protaper Next: A case Series. *Contemp. Clin. Dent.*, 2018, 9:168-172.

[9] Grossman LI. *Grossman's Endodontic Practice*. 12 ed. Philadelphia: Lippincott Williams & Wilkins; 2010

In: Clinical Reports in Dentistry
Editor: Lisa R. Amir
ISBN: 978-1-53617-328-4

Chapter 30

ENDODONTIC TREATMENT OF MAXILLARY CANINE WITH UNUSUAL LENGTH: A CASE REPORT

***Swesty Mahardhini*[1] *and Ratna Meidyawati*[2,*]**
[1]Conservative Dentistry Residency Program, Faculty of Dentistry,
Universitas Indonesia, Jakarta, Indonesia
[2]Department of Conservative Dentistry, Faculty of Dentistry,
Universitas Indonesia, Jakarta, Indonesia

ABSTRACT

Introduction: Permanent maxillary canines can present with an unusual length. This case report described a clinical case of endodontic treatment of a 32 mm upper cuspid, with the emphasis on the adjustments to the preparation and obturation steps of the root canal procedure.

Case report: A 66-year-old male patient presented to Conservative Dentistry Clinic, Faculty of Dentistry, Universitas Indonesia with pain sensation in his upper left canine upon biting on tooth #23. This tooth was previously restored with amalgam and has a secondary caries. During the root canal treatment, the tooth was found to have an unusual length of 32 mm. Adjustments of the instruments used, root canal preparation technique and fabrication of custom-made gutta-percha were needed to suit the working length of the tooth and obtain good root canal preparation and obturation results.

Conclusion: Successful endodontic treatment of an unusually long tooth can be achieved if adjustments are made to provide proper disinfection, preparation, obturation of the root canal as well as preservation of the remaining tooth structure.

Keywords: anatomy of the root canal, maxillary canine, unusual tooth length, root canal treatment

* Corresponding Author's Email: meidyawati58@gmail.com.

1. Introduction

A thorough knowledge of tooth anatomy, including the root canal system and morphological variation, is an important factor in root canal treatment. Clinicians should therefore have a thorough understanding of the detailed anatomy of the root canal in order to utilize the appropriate techniques and protocols to increase the rate of successful treatment [1]. Studies have reported that anatomical variation in permanent teeth can include a length above the average range. One tooth reported to show great variation in length is the maxillary canine [1, 2]. The average length of the maxillary canine is 26.5 mm, but it may reach various lengths exceeding 30 mm or longer [3].

In some cases, maxillary canines can have several anatomical anomalies which typically involve the root part rather than the crown. One example of such anomaly is radiculomegaly, a condition of teeth with extremely long roots. This unusual tooth appearance is strongly related with occulo-fascio-cardio-dental (OFCD) syndrome, a rare genetic syndrome related to the X chromosome. Radiculomegaly is also characterized by congenital cataracts, facial dysmorphy and congenital heart disease [4]. Patients with OFCD syndrome have been reported to have canines with lengths of 42.5 mm, 47 mm, and 47.5 mm [5-7]. Data presented in the literatures show endodontic treatment for maxillary canines with extreme lengths of 32 mm, 36 mm, 47 mm and 47.5 mm [6-9]. Root canals treatment for teeth with long roots can be quite challenging because endodontic instruments longer than 31 mm are not commercially available. As a result, clinicians may need to modify the standard treatment protocol in a way that is still in accordance with endodontic principles to achieve good root canal results in patients with long teeth [9]. The present article reported root canal treatment of a 32 mm long maxillary permanent canine and described the treatment steps and adjustments made during root canal preparation and obturation.

2. Case Report

A 66-year-old male patient with a non-contributing medical history was referred to the Conservative Dentistry Clinic, the Faculty of Dentistry, Universitas Indonesia, for a non-surgical endodontic treatment on maxillary left canine (tooth #23). The patient's chief complaint was a painful sensation in the tooth upon biting. Clinical examination revealed a large amalgam restoration on the mesio-occlusal part of the tooth with secondary caries in the occlusal margin (Figure 1A-B). In addition, the tooth showed attrition, as seen from the facet representation at the tip of the tooth surface where some portion of the cusp tip was flat, which was estimated to be 1-2 mm shorter than the original structure. The tooth was sensitive to percussion but revealed no response to the cold test. The soft tissue around the tooth was found to be normal.

Periapical radiography image revealed a diffused radiolucency feature in the periapical region (Figure 2A). A panoramic radiograph showed that the tooth had an irregular root morphology in the form of long crowns and root compared to the adjacent teeth (Figure 2B). In addition, the patient had multiple tooth loss, causing unstable occlusion and wanted removable dentures after completion of the root canal treatment. Based on clinical and radiographic findings and American Association of Endodontics guidelines, the dental diagnosis of tooth #23 was pulp necrosis with symptomatic apical periodontitis.

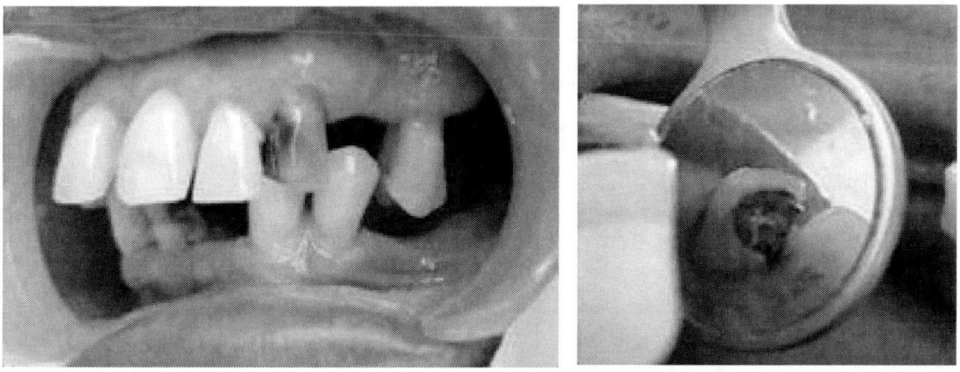

Figure 1. Clinical appearance of tooth #23.

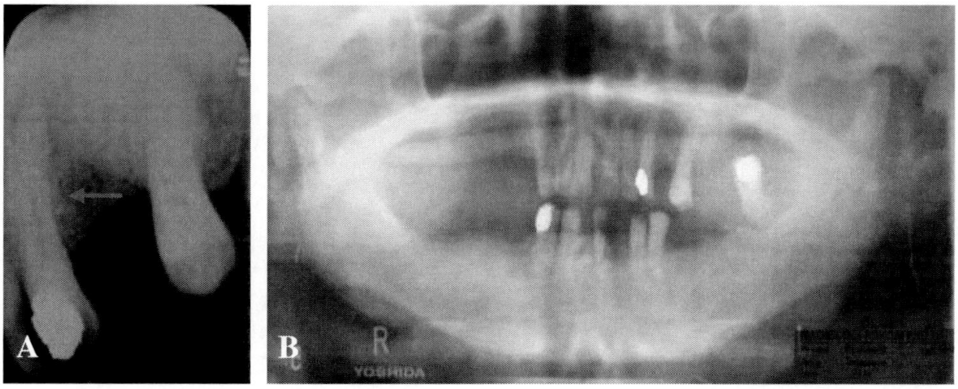

Figure 2. Preoperative radiographic image. Periapical image of tooth 23 (A); Panoramic image (B).

On the first visit, treatment started with placement of a rubber dam (KSK Clamp, Dentech, Japan) for isolation of the work area. The caries was removed, and an access opening was made using round diamond and metal burs (Mani, Japan) at high-speed rotation. Cavity preparation was done with Diamendo and Endo-Z burs (Dentsply Maillefer, Switzerland) to form and smooth a divergent access cavity wall, then an artificial wall of the mesial of the tooth was made. First, the cavity was closed with Teflon tape covering the orifice area. The cavity margin of the mesial wall area was then etched with 37% phosphoric acid (Scotchbond, 3M Espe USA) and coated with bonding liquid (Adper Single Bond 2, 3M Espe USA). The artificial wall was completed with the help of a sectional matrix using heavy high-flow filler composite resin (Grandioso Heavy Flow, Voco). After the composite was polymerized using a light-curing source, the sectional matrix and Teflon tape were removed and the cavity wall was smoothened using a Diamendo bur.

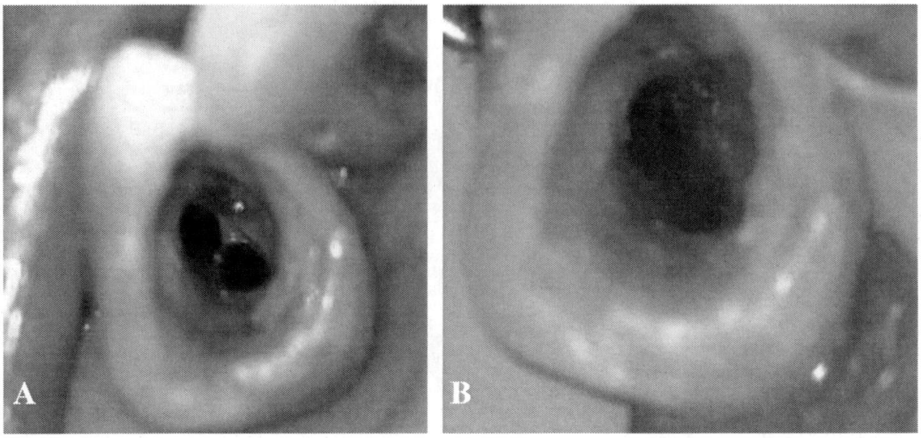

Figure 3. Clinical appearance after initial orifice pre-flaring (A); After smoothening and refining with ultrasonic tip, a large oval orifice with kidney-shaped root canal walls were observed (B); Photos taken using a dental microscope (OPMI PICO Dental Microscope, Carl Zeiss German) at 18X magnification.

At the initial access opening, two orifices were found on the labial and palatal parts of the coronal region separated by a thin dentin wall (Figure 3A). The orifices were pre-flared using the Protaper Hand-Use (Dentsply Maillefer, Switzerland) SX file. However, after confirming the access cavity using a dental microscope (OPMI PICO Dental Microscope, Carl Zeiss German) Zeiss), the thin dentin wall in the middle of the cavity was found to only separate one-third of the coronal part of the root so root canal actually consisted of one canal instead of two. An ultrasonic tip (Satelec P5 Newtron XS) was then used to remove the thin dentin wall between the previously-suspected orifices and refine the cavity access wall.

Soon after, it was found that the tooth had a large oval orifice with kidney-shaped root canal walls (Figure 3B). The large root canal was explored with a 25 mm long k-file size #15 (Dentsply Maillefer, Switzerland). Initial insertion was carried out with soft, slow movements towards the tooth apex. The initial work length radiographic image showed a 7 mm distance between the k-file tip and radiographic apex, confirming a root canal length of 32 mm for tooth #23 (Figure 4A). Assuming the apical foramen was located 0.5-1 mm from the radiographic apex, a definitive 31 mm working length was determined and reconfirmed by apex locator measuring and another radiographic image with a 31 mm k-file (Figure 4B).

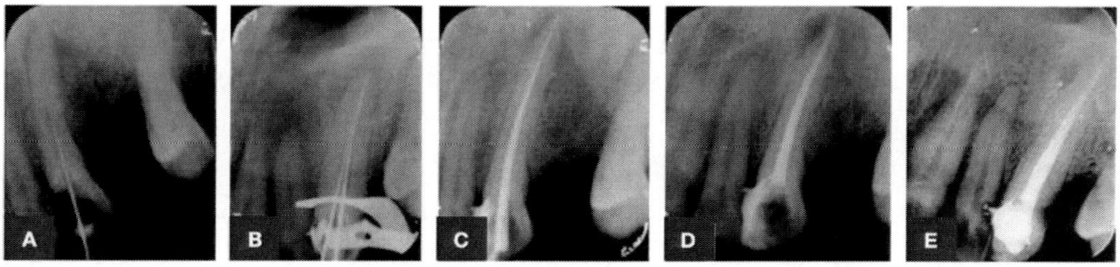

Figure 4. Initial file photo with 25 mm k-file #15, showing a 7 mm distance from the tip of the file to the root apex (A); Second initial file photo with 31 mm k-file #15; the end of the instrument corresponds to the actual root length (B); Radiographic image of the master cone placement inside the root canal (C); Root canal obturation (D); Radiographic evaluation three weeks after obturation of the root canal (E).

This working length corresponds to the length of the longest file instrument available after the rubber marker was removed. Because the canal wall was kidney-shaped, it was prepared as would be done for two root canals. Protaper Next rotary files were used to prepare the root canal by insertion from the labial and palatal direction with light brushing and circumferential filing motions by sequence according manufacturer's recommendation, done until X3 file. Root canal preparation was carried out under irrigation with 2.5% sodium hypochlorite (NaOCl) solution, followed by 17% ethylenediaminetetraacetic acid (EDTA) with the active sonic irrigation method using Endoactivator (Dentsply Maillefer, Switzerland), and then dried with sterile paper points. A calcium hydroxide paste (Calcipex II Nishika, Shimonoseki, Japan) was used as intra-canal medication to improve dentine tubular disinfection. Lastly, the cavity was closed with Caviton (GC Corporation, Japan) as temporary restoration. Since the 31 mm Protaper Next gutta-percha is not commercially available, adjustments were made by fabricating a custom-made gutta-percha with a length that corresponds to the actual working length of the tooth. The master cone was made by incorporating two Protaper Next X3 gutta-perchas using the rolled-up technique (Figure 5A-D).

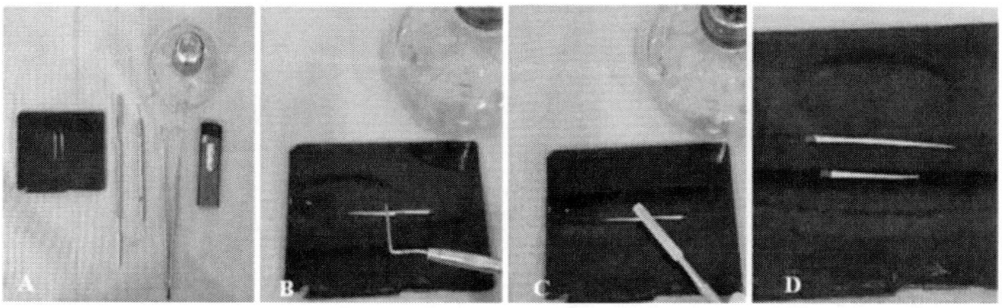

Figure 5. (A); Tools and materials used for the fabrication of custom gutta-percha using the rolled-up method (B); Both gutta perchas were aligned then softened with a warm plugger instrument (C); The gutta-perchas were then rolled with medium pressure using a warm metal spatula cement instrument until becoming a long sized gutta percha (D); Comparison of custom-made gutta-percha with standard size gutta percha.

The colored base point of the first gutta-percha was removed. The second gutta-percha was then placed beside the first one, warmed with a heated metal instrument tip (plastic filling or plugger), and then rolled together using a metal spatula cement instrument on a glass slab with medium pressure until both were combined into one long gutta-percha with a smooth surface. This rolled-up method was used to obtain a master cone corresponding to the actual working length, which was placed inside the root canal and confirmed by radiographic photograph.

Two weeks after the root canal cleaning and shaping procedures, the patient did not have any subjective complaints. Clinical examination showed normal gingiva conditions, and the tooth was not sensitive to percussion or palpation. After removal of the temporary restoration, the calcium hydroxide paste was cleaned away by copious irrigation of 2.5% sodium hypochlorite (NaOCl) solution and 17% EDTA and dried with sterile paper points. Next, the root canal was filled with custom-made gutta-perchas with AH-plus (Dentsply Maillefer, Switzerland) sealer packed by the lateral condensation method, with additional gutta-perchas to achieve solid and hermetic obturation (Figure 4D). The gutta-percha filling was cut at 1 mm below the orifice surface, condensed with a warm hand-plugger instrument, and then covered with resin modified-glass ionomer cement (Fuji II GC, Japan) as a base liner. The cavity was then closed with the temporary restoration using zinc-phosphate cement (Zinc Phosphate Elite Cement, GC, Japan).

Three weeks later, the patient returned for evaluation. He did not report any subjective complaints. Clinical examination showed normal gum conditions, and the tooth was not sensitive to percussion or palpation. Radiographic images revealed changes indicating tissue repair, and no new lesion in the periapical region was observed (Figure 4E). The patient was then referred to the Prosthodontic Department for a definitive restoration and removable dentures.

3. Discussion

A thorough knowledge of tooth anatomy, including its root canal system and morphological variation,is essential because the success of endodontic treatment is associated with thorough cleaning of the root canal system [1]. Clinical and radiographic examination from various angles, efficient use of exploratory instruments, adequate access opening, good illumination and magnification can help clinicians predict tooth condition so that they can determine the appropriate instruments and protocols for root canal treatment [10]. The maxillary canines are the longest teeth in the dental arch and usually present few anatomical variations. When variations do present, the root is more frequently affected than the crown. The root can be dilacerated or can have extreme variations in length [11]. Canines exceeding 30 mm in length, however, can cause technical difficulties during endodontic treatment. As a result, modification or adjustment may be necessary to enable available instruments to reach the working length without damaging the crown of the tooth [9]. Although uncommon, clinicians can prepare to treat long teeth by clinical examination and good pre-operative radiograph imaging [9].

The increasing use of dental operating microscopes (DOM) in the last two decades has improved the outcomes of both conventional and surgical endodontic treatments. Most DOMs can provide intense illumination and magnification of 3x-20x to provide a better view around the work area [12]. A clear and enlarged visual display allows the operator to recognize dentin covering the orifice, which can be accurately removed using ultrasonic unit and tips [13]. In the present case, two orifices were initially found and separated by a thin dentin wall. Even under observation at 3.2x magnification it was still difficult to ascertain whether the root of the tooth actually consisted of two ore one root canals. This difficulty was caused by the deep cavity chamber that obscured the orifices. As a result, re-observation and confirmation using a DOM was needed, which clearly showed that the walls between the two orifices were actually dentin that had not been completely removed.

The removal of the dentin covering, as well as refinement of the cavity walls and root canal, can be done using ultrasonic tips with abrasive surfaces, which are smaller and shorter than round burs. Hard tissue removal by ultrasonic tips is less aggressive than removal by burs, minimizing the risk of over-preparation or perforation of hard tissue [3]. In this case, this step was performed accurately and effectively because the working area was clearly visible under microscope observation.

The lack of commercial endodontic instruments longer than 31 mm may require clinicians to adjust their techniques to achieve the actual working length in a way that the instrumentation and cleaning still meet the biological and mechanical principles of root canal treatment [9]. There are several ways can be done. The first method is to change the reference point from the top of the dental cusp/tip to the cingulum/cervical area of the access cavity. This is a more conservative approach where the working length can be achieved without damaging the crown, maintaining as much healthy dental hard tissue as possible [9]. The second method uses special endodontic instruments designed for animal teeth. Some case reports describe preparation using endodontic instruments such as 40-60 mm long k-files or reamers that specifically designed for animal teeth [7, 14]. Such instruments include the Vetinox series manufactured by Dentsply Maillefer, but they are not widely available [7, 14]. The third method is by cutting the crown as much as needed, but this should be considered the last option because it involves damaging healthy tooth structures.

In this case, although estimated tooth length from radiographic assessment was 32 mm, but the working length of the treated tooth was 31 mm; after a 0.5-1 mm reduction which considered as the distance from apex foramen to apical constriction. This means although the tooth considered as longer than average, preparation using the longest rotary instrument available was still possible. Adjustment was done by simply removing the rubber stopper, without the need to cut the cusp/tip of the crown to maintain the remaining coronal hard tissue.

Another adjustment in this case was the fabrication of customized gutta-perchas using the rolled-up method. This technique can be used to make gutta-perchas longer than the standard length of 28 mm. Other method reported by Maden (2010), who made a customized gutta percha for a 47.5 cm long maxillary canine using an acrylic block prepared with master apical file used in patient's root canal preparation. The acrylic block used as a customized cast, injected with warm gutta percha, and then set cold [7]. Pace (2011) also reported other obturation method using modified Thermafil system (Dentsply Maillerfer). Adjustments were made by cutting obturator's plastic handle, then connect it to an adequate length stainless steel wire using a plastic micro-canule (extended obturator). This method allows gutta percha to obtain longer working length [14].

The rolled-up gutta percha method in this case was chosen because it was more simple, allowed better observation of the gutta-percha position to the tooth's reference point, more predictable placement of gutta-percha, used more commonly by clinicians, and was reported to give good obturation results in previous case reports [3]. The custom-made gutta-perchas were used together with resin-based sealer AH plus with additional cones and packed inside the root canal using lateral condensation techniques. This method was used because it is reliable and highly effective. Other obturation methods could not accommodate a long root canal system and, even if they could, the modification would have been more complex than customizing the gutta-perchas.

Regular clinical and radiographic examination is the best way to evaluate root canal treatment. In this case, the prognosis was good because clinical and radiographic evaluation three weeks post-obturation of the root canal showed changes indicating tissue repair. The patients did not report any subjective complaints, there were no clinical abnormalities, and the radiographic images showed increased density of the bone in the form of radiopacity around the periapical area. This case report and similar cases indicate that teeth with long root anatomy may be encountered in daily practice, even though their frequency is low. Thus, longer endodontic instruments are needed to facilitate root canal treatment while avoiding unnecessary removal of remaining hard tooth structures.

CONCLUSION

In the present case, a thorough knowledge of the anatomy and variation of the tooth and its root canal system, the use of a microscope for better illumination and magnification, proper selection of instruments, and custom gutta-percha fabrication allowed us to provide good root canal disinfection, preparation, and obturation while preserving the remaining tooth structure. Although longer periods of evaluation are needed, the good results and changes indicating healing and tissue repair. This was observed a few weeks after root canal obturation, indicated that the treatment was successful. Therefore, the technique used in this case report may be appropriate for similar treatments involving unusually long teeth.

REFERENCES

[1] Vertucci FJ. (2005). Root canal morphology and its relationship to endodontic procedures. *Endod. Top.*, 10(1):3-29.

[2] Nelson SJ, Ash MMJ. (2010). *Wheeler's Anatomy, Physiology and Occlusion.* 9th Ed - Ash.

[3] Gutmann JL, Fan B. (2016). *Tooth Morphology, Isolation and Access*. Eleventh E. Elsevier Inc.

[4] Iwase M, Nishijima H KGI. (2015). Radiculomegaly of permanent canines and first premolars: Report of two cases in conjunction with oculo-facio-cardio-dental syndrome. *Int. J. Case Reports*, 6(3):189-192.

[5] Larhant M, Sourice S, Grimaud F, et al. (2014). Giant canine with dentine anomalies in oculo-facio-cardio-dental syndrome. *J. Cranio-Maxillofac. Surg.*, 42(4):321-324.

[6] Marashi AH, Gorlin RJ. (1990). Radiculomegaly of canines and congenital cataracts - A syndrome? *Oral Surgery, Oral Med. Oral Pathol.,* 70(6):802-803.

[7] Maden M, Savgat A. (2010). Radiculomegaly of permanent canines: report of endodontic treatment in OFCD syndrome, 1152-1161.

[8] Al-Dahman YH, Al-hawwas AY, Al-jebaly AS. (2017). Root Canal Treatment of a 32-mm Length Maxillary Canine - A Case Report. *Int. J. Contemp. Med. Res.*, 4(11):2297-2299.

[9] Report C. (2010). Endodontic treatment of a 36-mm long upper cuspid: clinical case report. *Baseline*, 25(4):412-416.

[10] Shrivastava N, Nikhil V, Arora V, Bhandari M. (2013). Endodontic management of mandibular canine with two canals, 5(1):24-26.

[11] Ingle J, Bakland L, Baumgartner *J. Endod.*, 6. 2008:997-1018.

[12] Khayat BT, He U. (1998) Se of Magnification in Endodontic Therapy: *Pract. Periodont. Aesthet. Dent.*, 10(1):137-144.

[13] Yoshioka T, Kobayashi C, Suda H. (2002). Detection Rate of Root Canal Orifices with. *J. Endod.*, 6-7.

[14] Pace R, Giuliani V, Pagavino G. (2011). Endodontic management in oculo-facio-cardio-dental syndrome: A case report. *J. Endod.*, 37(4):558-561.

In: Clinical Reports in Dentistry
Editor: Lisa R. Amir
ISBN: 978-1-53617-328-4

Chapter 31

NON-SURGICAL TREATMENT OF APICAL EXTERNAL RESORPTION USING MINERAL TRIOXIDE AGGREGATE

Adeline Clarissa[1] and Nilakesuma Djauharie[2,*]
[1]Conservative Dentistry Residency Program,
Faculty of Dentistry, Universitas Indonesia, Jakarta, Indonesia
[2]Department of Conservative Dentistry Department,
Faculty of Dentistry, Universitas Indonesia, Jakarta, Indonesia

ABSTRACT

Introduction: External resorption of tooth may occur following dental trauma and pulp necrosis and result in loss of apical constriction. This will complicate the endodontic treatment since there is a risk of endodontic obturation material to extrude beyond the apex to the periodontal tissue. Mineral Trioxide Aggregate (MTA) has been known for its bioactivity, biocompatibility, antibacterial potential and ability to induce tissue regeneration and repair. This case report aimed to present the non-surgical treatment of apical external resorption using MTA.

Case report: A 23-year-old male came to Conservative Clinic Faculty of Dentistry Universitas Indonesia with a chief complaint of his discolored front tooth. The diagnosis of tooth #11 was chronic apical periodontitis e causa pulp necrosis with open apex due to external resorption. The treatment plan was non-vital root canal treatment, apical plug using MTA, internal bleaching using 30% hydrogen peroxide for the tooth discoloration followed with post-endodontic restoration using resin composite.

Conclusion: MTA is still one of the materials of choice that can be used for apical plug. At 3-months follow up, the tooth was asymptomatic and functional. No re-darkening of tooth color occured after internal bleaching. There were no signs of gingival inflammation. Radiographic examination showed lesion regression, increased alveolar

* Corresponding Author's Email: nila.setyopurnomo@gmail.com.

bone density and successful healing at tooth #11. In this case, MTA has successfully repaired apical external resorption and induced hard tissue formation in the apical area.

Keywords: non-surgical treatment, external resorption, apical plug, mineral trioxide aggregate

1. Introduction

External resorption is a pathologic condition which results in loss of external root surface due to several etiology factors. It may occur on tooth following dental trauma such as luxation and avulsion. Damage to pre-cementum and contusion to periodontal ligament due to trauma may precipitate external resorption [1]. Another factor that may cause external resorption is the presence of bacteria and its by-products inside the root canal system and dentin tubulus after the pulp necrosis occurred and the loss of pre-cementum as the protective layer. If this condition is not treated, it may cause rapid loss of tooth structure [2].

Successful endodontic treatment on teeth with open apex due to external resorption could be achieved through entire root canal debridement, root canal disinfection and optimal obturation. This could stop the resorption process and promote conducive environment for hard tissue repair of the resorbed root surface. Loss of apical constriction may occur due to external apical root resorption.

This communication may increase the risk of bacterial leakage from the pulp to the periapical region. Care should be taken to prevent over-instrumentation and over-filling during root canal treatment in such cases. Over-instrumentation might facilitate the extrusion of microbes and infected debris from the root canal system. Over-filling might cause mechanical and chemical inflammation of periapical tissue. Apical plug on tooth with open apex due to external resorption should be done to minimize the risk of root canal material extrusion [3].

Mineral Trioxide Aggregate (MTA) is one of the bioactive materials of choice for sealing the open apex. MTA has good biocompatibility, good sealing ability and also has the ability to promote periapical tissues regeneration such as cementum, periodontal ligament, and dental alveolar bone [4]. Due to the nature of its properties, MTA could be a good material for repairing tissue destruction that caused by external resorption [5]. Non-surgical treatment approach of sealing the apex is the treatment of choice compared to surgical approach [6]. MTA apical plug could be done using ortho-grade approach without the need to destroy the surrounding dental tissue due to the more invasive nature of surgical treatment [7]. The following case report presents a case about a discolored front tooth with open apex due to external resorption which was treated using MTA apical plug.

2. Case Report

Male patient, 23-year-old, came to Conservative Clinic Faculty of Dentistry Universitas Indonesia with a chief complaint of his discolored front tooth after motorbike accident 5 years ago (Figure 1A). There was no pain upon his first visit. Patient does not have any systemic disease. On 2013, patient suffered from maxillary dentoalveolar fracture due to the motorbike accident and the fracture was being treated with internal fixation using plate. Clinical examination presented that tooth #11 was intact with grayish-brown discoloration, no sensitivity to cold test, and sensitivity to percussion. Radiographic examination revealed that there was apical external resorption on tooth #11 with radiolucency sign on the periapical region (Figure 1B). The diagnosis of tooth #11 was chronic apical periodontitis e causa pulp necrosis with open apex due to external resorption.

After the patient's informed consent for treatment and publication has been obtained, access to the root canal of tooth #11 was done through the palatal side using round diamond bur and dental loupe (*Xenosys, Korea*) with 3,2x magnification as visualization aid. The whole pulp roof was removed using round diamond bur and the pulp chamber walls were smoothened using endo-z bur (Figure 2A). The root canal was then irrigated using 2.5% NaOCl due to its effective bactericidal effect. The 2.5% NaOCl has less cytotoxic properties than 5.25% NaOCl concentration therefore it is the most suitable concentration for endodontic treatment [8]. The working length determination was done using apex locator (*Morita Root ZX II*) and the readings showed that the estimated length was 20 mm. From the radiographic examination using k-file #25, it was confirmed that the definitive working length was 20 mm (Figure 2B).

Root canal preparation was done with crown down technique using Protaper Next (Dentsply, Maillefer, Switzerland). Glide path was made using Proglider (Dentsply, Maillefer, Switzerland) to help ensure straight line and smooth access for the subsequent files to reach full working length. Preparation using Protaper Next (Dentsply, Maillefer, Switzerland) was done until X5/20 mm. Recapitulation and gauging process was done each time the rotary files were changed. Then the root canal was irrigated using 2.5% NaOCl, 17% EDTA, and 2% Clorhexidine (OneMed) followed by the application of calcium hydroxide as intra-canal medicament (Calcipex®, Nippon Sika-Yakuhin, Shimonoseki, Japan). The irrigation process was done using #30gauge side-vented needle and activated using sonic wave EndoActivator (Dentsply, Maillefer, Switzerland). Copious irrigation with aquadest was done between the interchange of irrigants. The cavity was then sealed using temporary restoration (Elite Cement, GC Corporation, Japan).

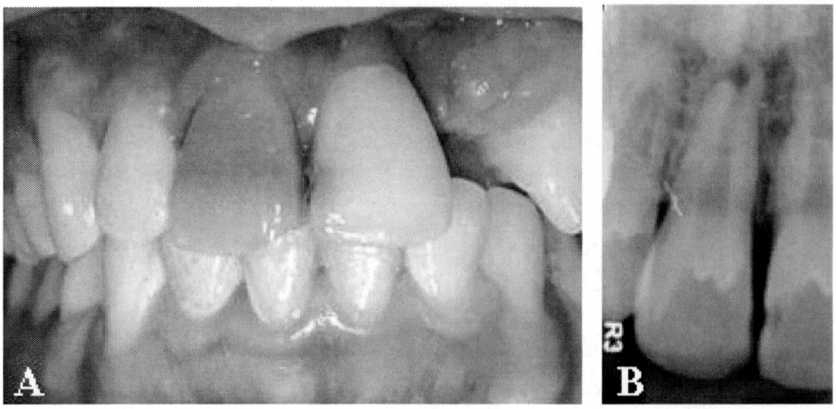

Figure 1. Clinical examination shows that tooth #11 is intact with grayish-brown discoloration (A); Radiographic examination of tooth #11 as diagnostic aid (B).

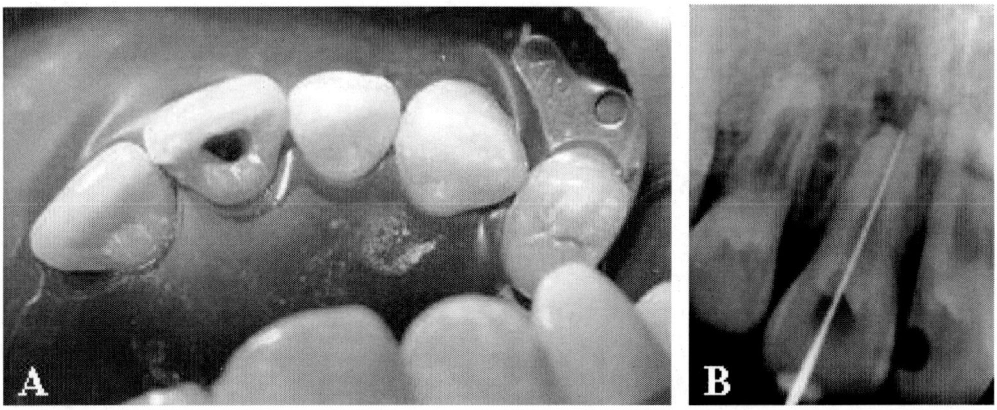

Figure 2. Access preparation of 11 (A); Radiographic picture of 11 to confirm the working length (B).

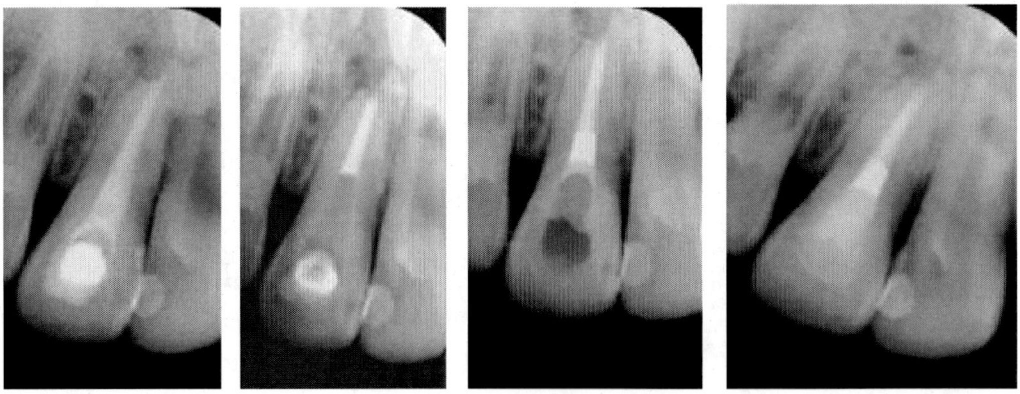

Figure 3. Radiographic appearance of tooth #11 after 2-week recall (A); Evaluation of MTA apical plug on tooth #11 (B); Obturation of the remaining root canal using gutta-percha and placement of RMGIC barrier (C); Radiographic evaluation of tooth #11 three months after *MTA Apical Plug* (D).

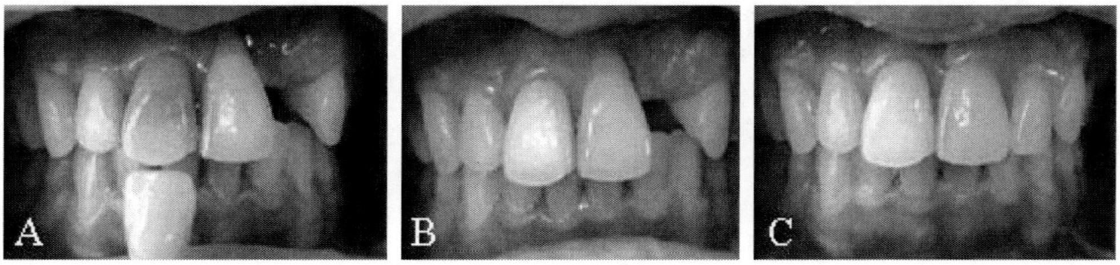

Figure 4. Clinical appearance of tooth #11 before internal bleaching (A); Clinical appearance of tooth #11 after internal bleaching (B); Clinical appearance of tooth #11 3 months after apical plug using MTA (C).

The patient was then recalled after two weeks, there was no subjective complaint. Tooth #11 showed no sign of hyperemia, sinus tract or swelling. There was no sensitivity to percussion and palpation (Figure 3A). Rubber dam was placed to isolate tooth #11. The temporary restoration was then removed, the calcium hydroxide medicament was cleaned from the root canal system (Figure 3B) and the irrigation process was done using NaOCl 2,5%. Root canal was then dried using paper points. Apical plug was done using MTA Angelus (Londrina, PR, Brazil) with approximately 6 mm thickness. The MTA was delivered incrementally using MTA Angelus applicator (Londrina, PR, Brazil) and condensed with hand plugger (Dentsply, Maillefer, Switzerland) gently. Radiographic imaging then was done to confirm the proper placement of the MTA (Figure 3C). Wet sterile cotton pellets were placed on top of the MTA within the root canal and then the cavity was sealed using temporary restoration (Elite Cement, GC Corporation, Japan).

After three days, temporary restoration and the cotton pellets were removed. The remaining root canal was then obturated using custom-made gutta-percha and AH plus sealer (Dentsply, Tulsa Dental, Tulsa, OK, USA). The gutta-percha was then cut until 2 mm below the orifice and Resin Modified Glass-Ionomer Cement barrier with approximately 2 mm thickness was placed on top of the obturation material. Internal bleaching was done using 30% hydrogen peroxide (Opalescence Endo, Ultradent) that was placed within the pulp chamber (Figure 4A). The cavity was sealed using cotton pellet and temporary restoration (Elite cement, GC Corporation, Japan).

After five days, the bleaching procedure had reached the desired shade (Figure 4B). The cavity was rinsed using aquadest. Cotton pellet was then placed in the pulp chamber. The cavity was sealed using temporary restoration (Caviton, GC Corporation, Japan) for 2 weeks in order to ensure all the remnants of peroxide or free oxygen were completely removed. Remnants of peroxide could inhibit the polymerization process of resin composite. These remnants could compromise the bond strength between resin composite to enamel and dentin. The patient was then recalled after two weeks. The temporary restoration and cotton pellet were removed from the cavity. The access cavity was subsequently restored using resin composite (Palfique LX5, Tokuyama, Japan). Three months after MTA apical plug, there was not any subjective complaint and tooth #11 was functional with no sensitivity to percussion and palpation. There were no signs of gingival inflammation (Figure 4C). Intra-oral radiograph showed regression in periapical lesion's diameter and there was an increase in alveolar bone density surrounding the apex (Figure 3D).

3. DISCUSSION

External resorption may be caused by injury following trauma, orthodontic movement, chronic pulp infection and chronic periodontal infection [9]. In the present case, there was an external root resorption on tooth #11 that could be resulted from dental trauma and pulp necrosis. Trauma may cause destruction to the root protective layer such as pre-cementum. Loss of pre-cementum on root surface would allow osteoclasts to attach onto the mineralized root surface and do resorption [6, 9]. Successful endodontic treatment of tooth with external resorption is affected by effective chemomechanical preparation [1]. In this case, before the MTA apical plug was done, calcium hydroxide as intra-canal medicament was applied into the root canal to help disinfecting the root canal system. This was done due to chemo-mechanical preparation alone could not ensure the entire elimination of microorganism within the root canal [7]. In addition to its antibacterial properties, calcium hydroxide can also induce hard tissue regeneration around the root to help reduce the lesion diameter. This could be helpful to reduce the risk of MTA extrusion during apical plug procedure. Application of calcium hydroxide as intra-canal medicament can also transform the neutral environment into base environment to stop the resorption process.

MTA is a bioactive and biocompatible material that has the ability to induce regeneration of supporting tooth structure [5]. One of the challenges in doing endodontic treatment on tooth with no apical constriction due to external resorption is the risk of obturation material to extrude from the root canal into the periodontal tissue [2]. Apical plug using MTA could reduce the risk of obturation material extrusion. Hermetic three-dimensional obturation will lessen the risk of infection due to bacterial leakage from the root canal to periodontal tissue. This will increase the possibility of successful endodontic treatment [1, 2].

Many researches showed that MTA could conduct and induce hard tissue regeneration and repair. This is attributed to its ability to release many ions from the material to the surrounding tissue. The monomer and polymer of silicate could increase osteoprotegerin expression and modulates the activity of osteoblasts and osteoclasts. The increased osteoprotegerin expression would inhibit the differentiation of osteoclast precursors and increase osteogenesis therefore MTA could inhibit the resorption process and induce hard tissue regeneration [4, 5]. The calcium ion that was released from the material will activate calcium receptor on osteoblast and increase IGF-I and IGF-II (Insuline Growth Factor I and II) expression. The antibacterial activity of MTA is attributed to the increasing initial pH from 10.2 to 12.5 after three hours MTA application was done. High base pH could inhibit almost all microorganism including *Enterococcus faecalis* [10].

Success rate of endodontic treatment using MTA in external resorption cases is 84% [3]. This is due to its biocompatibility and the ability of MTA to produce BMP-2 and TGF-β1 which may induce biological response on periapical tissue [5]. Stimulated production of interleukin by MTA could induce the growth of cementum and facilitates the regeneration and repair of the periodontal ligament and bone formation [6, 11]. One of the drawbacks of MTA is it may discolor tooth if the material left or trapped at the pulp chamber of the tooth. In this case, the apical plug was done carefully at the apical part only and the remnants of MTA on the coronal part of tooth was cleaned properly. Three months evaluation after bleaching showed no change of tooth color. MTA has long setting time which could be suitable for apical plug procedure since the proper placement of apical plug could not always be easily done within short time [4, 12, 13].

Periodical evaluation through clinical and radiographic examination should be done 1 month, 3 months, 6 months, 1 year and 2 years following endodontic treatment. Any signs of periodontal inflammation should be noted such as the presence of hyperemia, edema, sinus tract [11]. The present case report showed, the tooth was asymptomatic and functional clinically at 3 months follow up. The intra-oral radiographs showed positive outcome; there were signs of hard tissue repair on the tooth #11, the lesion had regressed and there was an increase of the surrounding alveolar bone density near the apex.

Conclusion

MTA is still one of the material of choice that can be used for apical plug. MTA has good biocompatibility, good sealing ability, easy handling and on top of that is still one of the most reliable bioactive material that can be used for apical plug in apical external resorption cases. In this case, MTA has successfully repaired apical external resorption and induced hard tissue formation in the apical area.

References

[1] Hargreaves K, Berman L. (2016). *Cohen's Pathway of Pulp*. 11th Edition. Mosby.

[2] Ashwini T, Hosmani N, Patil CR, Yalgi VS. (2013). Role of mineral trioxide aggregate in management of external root resorption. *J. Conservat. Dent.*, 16(6):579-581. doi:10.4103/0972-0707.120937.

[3] Mente J, Hage N, Pfefferle T, et al. (2009). Mineral Trioxide Aggregate Apical Plugs in Teeth with Open Apical Foramina: A Retrospective Analysis of Treatment Outcome. *J Endod.,* 35(10):1354-1358. doi:10.1016/j.joen.2009.05.025.

[4] Torabinejad M, Parirokh M, Dummer PMH. (2018). Mineral trioxide aggregate and other bioactive endodontic cements: an updated overview - part II: other clinical applications and complications. *Int. Endod. J.*, 51(3):284-317. doi:10.1111/iej.12843.

[5] Cehreli ZC, Sara S, Uysal S, Turgut MD. (2011). MTA apical plugs in the treatment of traumatized immature teeth with large periapical lesions. *Dent. Traumatol.*, 27:59-2.

[6] Utneja S, Garg G, Arora S, Talwar S. (2012). Nonsurgical endodontic retreatment of advanced inflammatory external root resorption using mineral trioxide aggregate obturation. *Case Rep. Dent.*, 624792.

[7] Güneş B, Aydinbelge HA. (2012). Mineral trioxide aggregate apical plug method for the treatment of nonvital immature permanent maxillary incisors: Three case reports. *J. Conservat. Dent.*, 15(1):73-76. doi:10.4103/0972-0707.92611.

[8] Marion J, Manhaes F, Bajo H, Duque TM. (2012). Efficiency of different concentrations of sodium hypochlorite during endodontic treatment. *Dent. Press Endod.,* 2:32-37.

[9] Fernandes M, de Ataide I, Wagle R. (2013). Tooth resorption part I - pathogenesis and case series of internal resorption. *J. Conservat. Dent.*, 16(1):4-8. doi:10.4103/0972-0707.105290.

[10] Macwan C, Deshpande A. (2014). Mineral trioxide aggregate (MTA) in dentistry: A review of literature. *J. Oral Res. Rev.,* 6(2):71. doi:10. 4103/2249-4987.152914.

[11] Asgary S, Ehsani S. (2012). MTA resorption and periradicular healing in an open-apex incisor: A case report. *Saudi Dent. J.,* 24(1):55-59. doi:10.1016/j.sdentj.2011.08.001.

[12] Kang SH, Shin YS, Lee HS, et al. (2015). Color Changes of Teeth after Treatment with Various Mineral Trioxide Aggregate-based Materials: An *Ex Vivo* Study. *J. Endod.,* 41(5):737-741. doi:10.1016/ j.joen.2015.01.019.

[13] Parirokh M, Torabinejad M. (2010). Mineral Trioxide Aggregate: A Comprehensive Literature Review-Part III: Clinical Applications, Drawbacks, and Mechanism of Action. *J. Endod.,* 36(3):400-413. doi:10.1016/j.joen.2009.09.009.

In: Clinical Reports in Dentistry
Editor: Lisa R. Amir
ISBN: 978-1-53617-328-4

Chapter 32

MANDIBULAR FIRST MOLAR TEETH WITH VERTUCCI'S TYPE II CONFIGURATION: A CASE OF ENDODONTIC RETREATMENT

***Anita Erdiani*[1] *and Munyati Usman*[2,*]**
[1]Conservative Dentistry Residency Program,
Faculty of Dentistry, Universitas Indonesia, Jakarta, Indonesia
[2]Department of Conservative Dentistry Department,
Faculty of Dentistry, Universitas Indonesia, Jakarta, Indonesia

ABSTRACT

Introduction: Knowledge on the anatomy of the root canals and an accurate interpretation of radiograph results are required before endodontic treatment. The mesial roots of the mandibular first molars commonly have two canals. These canals, however are merged in the apical root. This variation is called the Vertucci's type II configuration, and it has an incidence rate of 41.87%. Such variation was identified via clinical and radiographic examinations obtained using various angles. This study aimed to identify and manage the root canal treatment of the mandibular first molar with Vertucci's type II configuration.

Case report: A 25-year-old female patient complained of pain in the left mandibular molar. In tooth 36, filling and a metal post were observed, and radiographic results showed that the tooth has been initially treated. Moreover, a radiolucency was observed in the distal root. Based on history taking and clinical examination, chronic apical abscess caused by non-hermetic endodontic treatment was observed in tooth 36. Endodontic retreatment was provided and the removal of the gutta-percha and metal post, root canal treatment, adequate obturation and restoration with fiber post and porcelain fused to the metal crown were initiated.

Conclusion: Complex knowledge about the anatomy and morphology of the tooth is required for chemo-mechanical preparation to remove necrotic tissues and bacteria in the

* Corresponding Author's Email: munyati.usman@gmail.com.

root canal and to produce adequate obturation. Thus, adequate post-treatment restoration can prevent root canal failure and maintain teeth for as long as possible in the jaw.

Keywords: endodontic retreatment, Vertucci's type II configuration

1. Introduction

Root canal treatment is performed by removing infected pulp tissues from the pulp chamber and root canal, followed by filling with solid root canal sealer to prevent further abnormalities or recurrent infections. Root canal treatment aims to maintain the teeth as long as possible in the jaw; thus, the function and shape of the dental arch remain good [1-3]. The success rate of root canal treatment is 86%-98%. However, root canal failure can also occur and to maintain the tooth, retreatment is required. These failures occur due to improper root canal cleaning, persistence of bacteria in the root canal and apical region, poor obturation quality, such as non-hermetic filling, excess or lack of root canal sealer and leakage of the coronal. Bad root canal filling can occur due to the operator's lack of knowledge about the anatomy and morphology of the tooth [4].

Knowledge about common root canal morphology and anatomy, accurate interpretation of radiographic findings, and adequate access is a prerequisite for root canal treatment. There are several classifications of root canals, which include Vertucci, Gulabivala, and Weine [1]. The mandibular first molar commonly has two roots and three root canals, with variation of 40% of distal roots had two root canals [5]. According to Raed Hakem, the results of the study on mandibular first molar in Palestinian population have shown that the most common canal configuration in the mesial roots was Vertucci type IV (53.8%) followed by type II (38.8%). In the distal roots, the most prevalent canal configuration was Vertucci type I (57.5%) followed by type II (22.5%) and type III (10.6%) [6]. Razmi et al. have shown that the distal root mandibular first molar teeth may vary according to the following Vertucci's classification: type I, 54.9%; type II, 19%; type III, 1.9%; type IV, 14.2%; type V, 4.2%; type VI, 1%; type VII, 0.3%; and type VIII, 0%. Meanwhile, based on the Vertucci classifications, the possibilities of varying mesial roots with two canals are as follows: type II, 41.87%; type III, 0.49%; type IV, 53.69%; and type V, 3.94% [7]. A proper understanding of the tooth anatomy and morphology is important before performing root canal treatment since this may affect the success of treatment. Vertucci type II represents that two canals join at the apical root to form one root canal. Vertucci stated that this anatomy is best treated by preparing and obturating the main canal to the apex and the other canal to the point of juncture [8]. This case report will discuss about root canal treatment on the mandibular first molar tooth with Vertucci's type II configuration.

2. Case Report

A 25-year-old female patient came to the Endodontic Clinic Faculty of Dentistry Universitas Indonesia with a chief complaint of lower left back tooth pulsed pain lasting for a few days. The patient took analgesic and antibiotic to reduce the pain. However, the pain did not completely disappear. The patient avoided chewing on the left side due to the pain. Based on the clinical examination, the 36 tooth was sensitive to percussion and palpation and had been previously treated with the presence of rough filling and a metal post. Moreover, no swelling on the gingiva was noted. Radiographic findings revealed a previously treated tooth with incomplete and non-hermetic root canal treatment, post in the distal root canal, normal root, widening periodontal membrane, discontinuation of the lamina dura and radiolucency with unclear boundary on the distal root with a diameter ±4 mm. Chronic apical abscess caused by non-hermetic endodontic treatment as shown in Figure 1A.

During the first visit, the tooth was isolated with a rubber dam, the base was removed, and the glass ionomer cement (GIC) around the metal post until the orifice that was clearly visible was cleaned. After the removal of the GIC from the pulp chamber, an unprepared disto-buccal root that was made by the previous operator was observed, and this caused the periradicular infection on the root. Removal of the GIC from the metal post area was carried out using an ultrasonic scaler, and the metal post was cleaned until it can be held with an instrument, such as tweezers or needle holders. When the metal post can be held with the needle holder, it was turned counterclockwise and then pulled out [9]. The gutta-percha can be removed with rotary or manual instrument, such as the Hedstrom file. However, removal of the gutta-percha using hand files is time consuming. The use of NiTi rotary retreatment system has been proposed because of its safety, efficiency, and speed in removing gutta-percha and the sealer [10].

To remove the gutta-percha, rotary instrument, such as the ProTaper Universal Retreatment, D-Race, and Mtwo Retreatment, can be used. However, ProTaper Universal Retreatment is more efficient in removing the gutta-percha from the root canal. It has a triangular convex cross-section; thus, it has a larger internal mass than Mtwo Retreatment and D-Race. According to current studies, every method and instrument cannot perfectly remove the gutta-percha and sealer materials [11]. In relation to this, further root canal preparation is required [10]. Using the solvent can help remove the gutta-percha from the inside of the root canal because the solvent can effectively dissolve such material. In this case, the solvent was only used in the early stages of cleaning the gutta-percha, and eucalyptus oil was used to dissolve the gutta-percha at coronal 1/3 to help penetrate the D1 file [2].

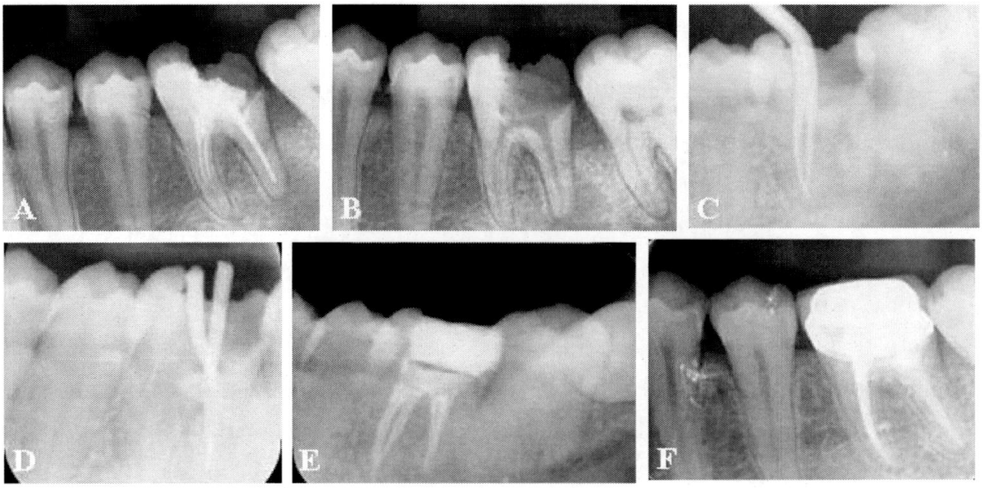

Figure 1. Radiographic Images. Pre-operative radiographic findings. (A); post gutta-percha removal (B); Gutta-purcha placement in the mesial root canal (C); and distal root canal (D) post obturation of the root canal (E); post insertion of fiber post and porcelain fused to metal crown (F).

Removal of the gutta-percha was conducted using eucalyptus oil at coronal 1/3 and ProTaper Universal Retreatment with the crown-down technique. The removal started from the disto-lingual root. First, the cavity was immersed in eucalyptus oil, and then, the gutta-percha was cleaned in the order of D1 (#30/.09) for coronal 1/3, D2 (#25/.08) for medial 1/3, and D3 (#20/.07) for apical 1/3 at 400-500 rpm and 3 Ncm torque. After the root canal was cleaned, it was irrigated with 2.5% NaOCl and dried with a paper point. Then, removal of the gutta-percha from the mesio-buccal and mesio-lingual was continued with the same technique. A radiograph was conducted to validate if the root canals were completely clean from the sealer and gutta-percha (Figure 1B).

Preparation of the root canals started from the mesial root, and a root canal exploration was carried out with k-file #10 throughout the estimated work of 17 mm that was measured based on the radiographic image. The initial file on the mesial root was #20/17 mm. When entering k-files simultaneously on the mesio-buccal and mesio-lingual roots, k-files in one root could not enter the length of the estimation work. When k-files are entered separately, however, each k-file can be entered according to the length of the estimation work, and radiograph was then performed to determine the actual working length. Based on the radiographic results, the working length was -3 mm, and it can be determined below the actual working length of 20 mm.

Moreover, the measurement of the working length using an apex locator and the length of each mesial root canal was 20 mm. The root canal was irrigated with 2.5% NaOCl and dried with a paper point. Assessment of the root canal was performed at the distal root with k-file #10 along the estimated work of 18 mm.

Then, radiograph was performed to determine the actual working length by entering k-file #25/18 mm on both distal roots. Based on the radiographic results, the working length was -2 mm, and this was also confirmed by measuring the length of work using the apex locator. The actual working length was 20 mm.

Mesio-buccal root canal preparation was conducted using the ProTaper Next X3/20 mm. After the mesio-buccal root canal was prepared, apical gauging with k-file #30/20 mm was performed, and it feels snug fit. The main gutta-percha X3 cone was inserted into the mesio-buccal root canal, and then, k-file #20 was inserted into the mesio-lingual root canal. The main gutta-percha cone gains were marked at the location of the meeting point between the two root canals. The mesio-lingual root working length was measured from the reference point to the mark on the main gutta-percha, which was 16.5 mm. Thereafter, mesio-lingual root canals were prepared using the ProTaper Next X3/16.5 mm. Each instrument was always lubricated with EDTA gel, and every change of instrument was irrigated with 2.5% NaOCl and dried with a paper point.

Next, the disto-buccal and disto-lingual root canals were prepared using the ProTaper Next X4/20 mm. Once the distal root canal preparation is completed, apical gauging was conducted with k-file #40/20 mm, and it feels snug fit. The main X4 gutta-percha cone was inserted into both the distal root canals throughout the work, and radiograph was conducted to assess whether the preparation was suitable for the actual working length (Figure 1C,D). The four root canals were irrigated with 2.5% NaOCl and 17% EDTA and rinsed with Aqua Bidest and CHX 2%. Each change of irrigation fluid was always dried first with a paper point. Then, $Ca(OH)_2$ medicament was poured into the root canal and covered with a temporary filling.

During the next visit, the patient did not have subjective complaints and the percussion and palpation were negative. Moreover, the gingiva was normal; therefore, the root canal can be filled. Isolation of the work area was carried out with a rubber dam, and the temporary filling was removed, cleaned with $Ca(OH)_2$ by irrigating with 2.5% NaOCl, and dried with a paper point. The root canal was re-irrigated with 17% EDTA, washed with Aqua Bidest, and dried. Then, it was irrigated with CHX 2% and dried with a paper point. Root canal filling was conducted using a single cone technique at the mesio-buccal root using the gutta-percha X3/20 mm cone, mesio-lingual root X3/16.5 mm, and disto-buccal and disto-lingual X4/20 mm. The sealer was AH plus. The gutta-percha was cut with a heated excavator to the orifice boundary and condensed with a plugger.

The RMGIC base is then applied and covered with a temporary filling. Radiograph was conducted to evaluate for obturation (Figure 1E). A fiber post and porcelain fused to the metal crown were used for the post-treatment of the root canal in tooth 36 (Figure 1F).

3. DISCUSSION

In this case report, tooth 36 had been previously treated. However, the obturation was not hermetic and underfilled, and this can be observed based on the radiographic and clinical examination results showing the untreated disto-buccal canal. Post-endodontic restoration from the previous treatment was composite resin. However, it was broken. A defined radiolucency was found on the distal root of the tooth indicating a chronic apical abscess. Inadequate root canal obturation and restoration and untreated root canal can cause post-endodontic infection or root canal treatment failure [4].

Retreatment is a procedure to remove root canal filling material from the tooth, followed by cleaning, shaping and obturation of the canals [12]. Complete removal of gutta-percha from root canal walls, reestablishing working length, promoting disinfection and re-obturating the root canal are the main goals of non-surgical retreatment to reestablish healthy periapical tissues and obtain predictable success [13]. The main goal of root canal treatment is to clean and shape the root canal system and seal it in three dimensions to prevent reinfection and retain the tooth with durable outcome [14]. In addition, teeth with inadequate obturation and unfilled or untreated root canals contain bacteria and necrotic tissues. With the intake of nutrients, the bacteria can continue to grow and cause periradicular tissue infections [4]. In this case, there were four root canals, and the mesial root canals joined into 1 on the apical 1/3 area, a variation called the Vertucci's type II configuration. This type of configuration is one of the most commonly encountered configurations on the mesial root of the mandibular first molars. There are controversial approach regarding the instrumentation of these canals. Vertucci believes that this anatomy is best treated by preparing and obturating the main canal to the apex and the other canal to the point of juncture. If both canals are enlarged to the apex, an hourglass preparation may results; the point where the two canals join is more constricted than the preparation at the apex [8].

Removal of the previous obturated material is important before chemo-mechanical preparation. The obturation material of the root canal blocked the entrance of the instrument to the apical region, and the last gutta-percha inside the root canal can be a place for bacterial retention. Thus, root canal cleaning, which is conducted from the gutta-percha, has a higher success rate for the retreatment of root canal [15]. A mesial root canal preparation on tooth 36 that has a configuration root similar to Vertucci's type II configuration must be cautiously treated to prevent damage in the apical foramen and overtreatment of the canal walls. If these two canal roots enlarge until the apical portion, hourglass preparation, which is the narrowing of the meeting point of the two canals, is preferred rather than the apical preparation, and the filling in this situation is not usually hermetic because there will be a blank space on the apical 1/3 [15]. The NiTi rotary instrument has been used cautiously on this type of anatomy because the instrument can break and it will go to the inside part of the root canal. A comprehensive chemo-mechanical preparation is sometimes challenging to achieve because of the several variations in the shape and direction of the root canal [1]. The long line of mesio-buccal root canals is measured from the reference point until the apical foramen. However, the mesio-lingual root canal is measured from the reference point until the meeting point between these two root canals.

Tooth 36 had lost the disto-buccal wall, and it have a thin disto-lingual root. Thus, we chose the restoration after root canal treatment using fiber post and a porcelain fused to the metal crown. This treatment done in four visits until obturation. Two weeks after obturation, treatment continued with insertion of the fiber post and crown preparation for artificial crown. This patient has been followed up three times after treatment was completed, specifically at one month, three months and six months after treatment.

CONCLUSION

In this case, endodontic retreatment was successfully conducted as evidence by the removal of previous obturation material, metal active post, and identification of Vertucci's type II configuration on the mesial root. Clinicians must know the variations in the clinical and radiographic anatomy of the root canals before initiating root canal treatment. Thus, adequate chemo-mechanical preparation and obturation can be performed. An important factor in a successful root canal treatment also involves post-endodontic restoration that can provide good coronal seals and support the remaining tooth structure.

REFERENCES

[1] Hargreaves KM, Cohen S. (2011). *Cohen's pathways of the pulp* 10th ed. St Louis: Mosby.

[2] Ingle JI, Bakland LK, Baumgartner JC. (2008). *Ingle's Endodontics 6*. Hamilton, Ontario: BC Decker Inc.

[3] Torabinejad M, Walton R. (2009). *Endodontics Principles and Practice*. 4th ed. Missouri: Saunders Elsevier.

[4] Tabassum S, Khan FR. (2016). Failure of Endodontic treatment: The usual suspects. *Eur. J. Dent.*, 10:144-7.

[5] Carrote P. (2005). 21st Century Endodontics Part 2. *Inter. Dent. J.*, 55:162-167.

[6] Mukhaimer, Raed Hakam. (2014). Evaluation of Root Canal Configuration of Mandibular First Molars in a Palestinian Population by Using Cone-Beam Computed Tomography: An *Ex Vivo* Study. *Inter. Scholar Res Notices.*

[7] Akhlaghi NM, Khalilak Z, Vatanpour M, Mohammadi S, Pirmoradi S, Fazlyab M, Safavi K. (2017). Root canal anatomy and morphology of mandibular first molars in a selected Iranian population: An in vitro study. *Iran. Endod. J.*, 12:87-91.

[8] Moradi Saeed, Maryam Gharechahi, Fatemeh Bonyadimanesh. (2018). Influence of Two Preparation Techniques on Transportation of Simulated Type II Root Canals. *Iran. Endod. J.*, 13(3):385-389.

[9] Radeva EN. (2015). Removal of metal posts in retreatment of teeth with failed endodontic treatment (clinical cases). *Inter. J. Sci. Res. (IJSR)*, 4:2084-2088.

[10] Dixit S, Kumar P, Agarwal S, Dixit A. (2014). Comparative Evaluation of Effectiveness of Protaper Universal Rotary Retreatment System and Mtwo Retreatment System for Gutta-percha Removal with or without Solvent - an *in vitro* Study. *Ind. J. Dent. Sci.,* 3:12-15.

[11] Marques da Silva B, Baratto-Filho F, Leonardi DP, Henrique Borges A, Volpato L, Branco Barletta F. (2012). Effectiveness of ProTaper, D-RaCe, and Mtwo retreatment files with and without supplementary instruments in the removal of root canal filling material. *Inter. Endo. J.*, 45:927-932.

[12] Bodrumlu E, Uzun O, Topuz O, Semiz M. (2008). Efficacy of 3 techniques in removing root canal filling material. *J. Can. Dent. Assoc.*, 74(8):721-721e.

[13] Somma F, Cammarota G, Plotino G, Grande NM, Pameijer CH. (2008). The effectiveness of manual and mechanical instrumentation for the retreatment of three different root canal filling materials. *J. Endod.*, 34(4):466-69.

[14] Uezu MK, Britto ML, Nabeshima CK, Pallotta RC. (2010). Comparison of debris extruded apically and working time used by protaper universal rotary and protaper retreatment system during gutta-percha removal. *J. Appl. Oral Sci.*, 18(6):542-45.

[15] Vertucci FJ. (2005). Root canal morphology and its relationship to endodontic procedures. *Endod. Topics*, 10:3-29.

In: Clinical Reports in Dentistry
Editor: Lisa R. Amir

ISBN: 978-1-53617-328-4

Chapter 33

MANAGEMENT OF FRACTURED INSTRUMENT IN VERTUCCI'S TYPE V CANAL MAXILLARY LATERAL INCISOR: A CASE REPORT

Cut Thysa[1] and Nilakesuma Djauharie[2,*]
[1]Conservative Dentistry Residency Program, Faculty of Dentistry,
Universitas Indonesia, Jakarta, Indonesia
[2]Department of Conservative, Faculty of Dentistry,
Universitas Indonesia, Jakarta, Indonesia

ABSTRACT

Introduction: The aim of this paper was to present the management of the fractured instrument on curvature of the Vertucci's type V canal in a maxillary lateral incisor by means of bypass techniques.

Case report: A-50-year-old male was referred with a history of lingering pain mainly at night in the upper left front teeth. The examination revealed secondary caries beneath the composite restoration, sensitive to vitality test, insensitive to percussion, and the tooth was confirmed radiographically to have a single root canal with curvature in the apical third. The patient was diagnosed with Irreversible pulpitis e causa secondary caries. The treatment plan was a vital root canal treatment combined with fiber post and direct composite restoration. During instrumentation, there was a fractured instrument due to a narrowed canal, and the dental radiograph confirmed the root canal has divided into 2 canals in the curvature. The fractured instrument was successfully bypassed with K-File, and the obturation was done using the GuttaCore obturation system.

Conclusion: The bypass technique is a favorable alternative to remove the fracture instruments in the apical third and the GuttaCore obturation system can be used to reach both canals branches in Vertucci's type V canal.

* Corresponding Author's Email: nila.setyopurnomo@gmail.com.

Keywords: fractured instrument, Vertucci type V, maxillary lateral Incisor, bypass, gutta core

1. Introduction

Effective root canal treatment requires an excellent knowledge of anatomy and root canal morphology. In human teeth, the anatomical variations of each tooth are numerous, specifically for numbers and shapes of the root and root canals [1]. In general, the endodontic literature suggests that maxillary lateral incisors have one root and one canal. This statement is not entirely true because several reports found that the lateral incisors could possibly have two or three root canals [2]. On the other hand, during endodontic treatment or retreatment, fracture of the instruments may occur in the root canal. Clinical studies reported that the incidence of these complications may vary from 0.39% to 5% [3]. The prevalence of fractured endodontic stainless steel hand instruments has been reported to be in the range of 0.7 – 7.4% [4]. The probability of removing a fractured instrument is closely related to the visibility of the instrument, whereas visibility itself depends on the location of the fractured instrument. When the instrument is inside the curvature, the root canal must be straight in order to gain good visibility. This can lead to unnecessary dentin retrieval, thereby weakening the tooth structure. An alternative technique that can be done without clear visibility is "bypass", where files are inserted between fracture instrument and root canal walls to achieve working length and allow instrumentation and obturation with the fractured instrument remaining on the root canal [5]. This case report explains the treatment of fracture instrument on curvature in Vertucci's type V using the bypass technique. The root has one canal and is separated into two canals in the apical third, and this morphology is called Vertucci type V.

2. Case Report

A 50-year-old male was referred with a history of lingering pain mainly at night at the upper left front tooth. The patient was taken medications to reduce the pain. Prognosis of this case is good because all the root canals are accessible and the patient is cooperative. The selected treatment plan was a vital root canal treatment and fiber post with direct composite restoration. Examination revealed a composite resin restoration site 2 size 2 at the tooth #22, sensitive to vitality test and unresponsive to percussion test. Radiographic examination showed a radiolucent appearance on the proximal portion and below the restoration indicating secondary caries occurrence. In the apical third, the root of the tooth forms a curvature, with one root and one canal (Figure 1). The diagnosis of this tooth is Irreversible Pulpitis e cause secondary caries. The treatment plan is a vital root canal treatment and fiber post combined with direct composite restoration.

At the first visit, mepivacaine 2% with 1:100.000 epinephrine was delivered and a rubber dam was placed. Access preparation was done by using a round bur diamond, and orifice identification was conducted by using endodontic explorer and found one orifice. Then pulp extirpation was performed with NaOCl 2,5% as an irrigant.

The apex was located by using an electronic apex locator (Propex Pixi, Dentsply).

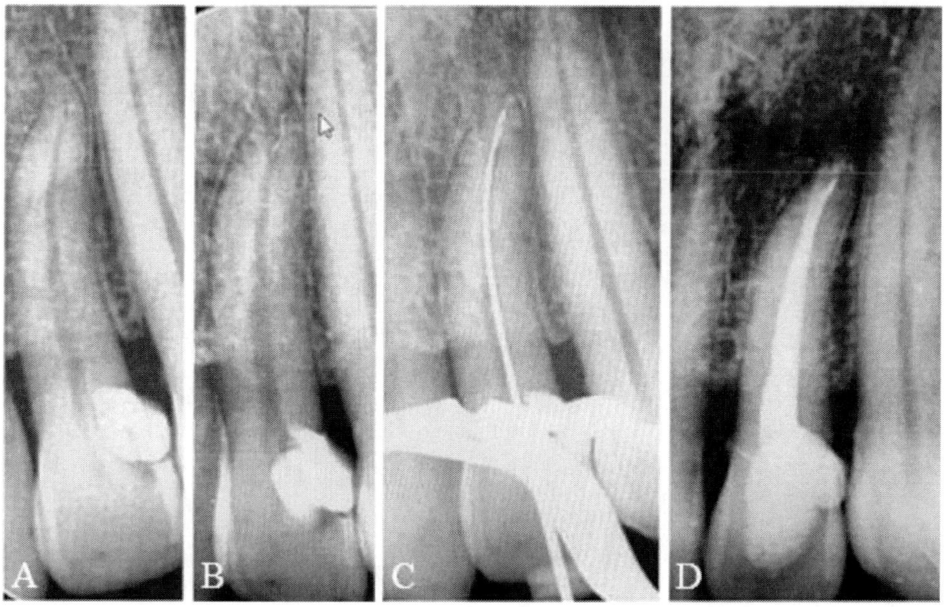

Figure 1. Radiographic Images. Pre-operative (A); Fractured Instruments on Root Canal Branch (B); Bypassing the Fractured Instrument using Size 25 K-File (C); Post Obturation (D).

Preparation was done carefully with K-File (Dentsply Maillerfer, Switzerland) to avoid ledge, but once it reaches the apical third, K-File no #15 failed to reach the apex. Attempts were carried out to reach the apical third using K-File no #10, and then no #8, but also failed to reach the apex. Because the root canal was estimated to be extremely narrow, K-File no #6 was used. When the K-file no #6 was pulled out, the measured length of the file was reduced. Radiographic evaluation was performed and the image showed a part of fractured instrument on root canal branch (Figure 1B).

Dental microscope (Carl Zeiss Meditec, Germany) with 10x magnification was used to see the fractured instrument in the root canal. However, there was no visual confirmation on its location. Because the fractured instrument was located on the apical third and no visual was available, the bypass technique was chosen as the treatment plan. Bypass was started by utilizing pre-curved K-file no #10 and EDTA gel 17% was used as the chelating agent. The K-file no #10 was successfully reach the working length and laid beside the fractured instrument. The preparation continues until reach K-File no #25 (Figure 1C).

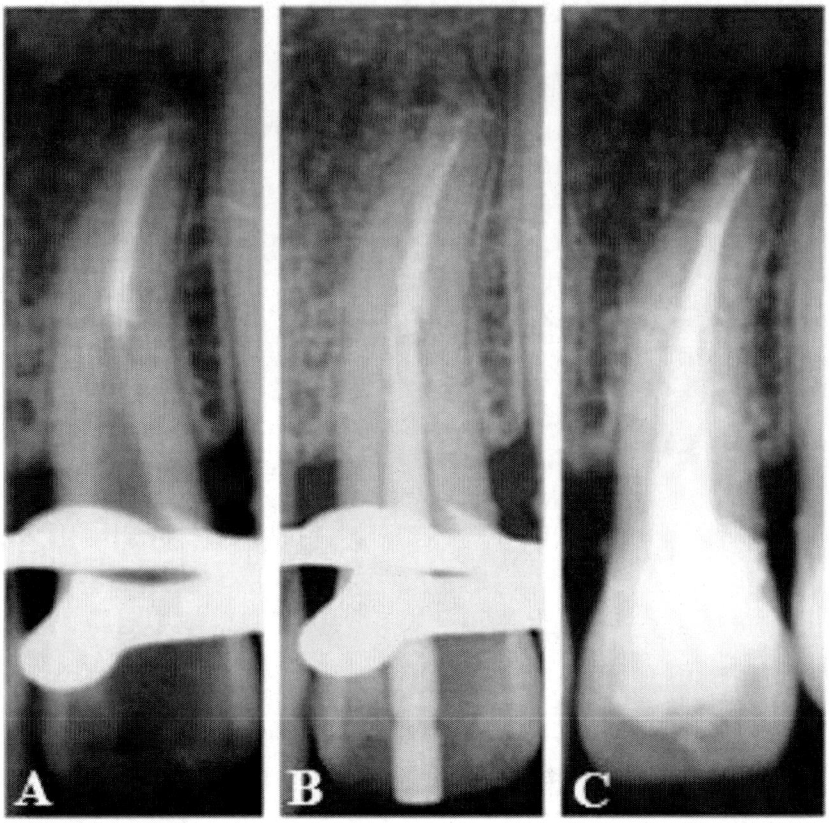

Figure 2. Radiographic Images. Gutta Percha Removal (A); Fiber Post Trial (B,C)

On the other hand, preparation on the mesial canal was done using Protaper Next (Dentsply, Maillerfer, Switzerland) until reach X3. During preparation, NaOCl 2,5%, EDTA 17% and distilled water was used alternately. The irrigation was done by using a side vented needle and activated by sonic wave EndoActivator (Dentsply, Maillerfer, Switzerland). $Ca(OH)_2$ was selected as a medicament, and the cavity was closed by using temporary restoration afterward.

On the second visit two weeks after, temporary restoration was removed and root canal was irrigated. Then, the root canal was obturated with carrier-based system (Gutta Core) to reach both canals. MTA Fillapex sealer was placed on the coronal with paper point and Gutta Core was placed on oven obturator (Thermaprep 2 Oven, Dentsply). After the heating process, Gutta Core was placed into the canal and condensation was done with plugger. After the working length was evaluated by radiograph confirmation, RM-GIC (Resin Modified Glass Ionomer Cement) was applied then continued with temporary closure (Figure 1D).

On the third visit two weeks after, temporary restoration was removed, and gutta percha was removed using the Gates Glidden Drill (Figure 2A). After the post working length is reached, Fibre Kleer drill was used to form root canals. Once it is formed, the fiber was cemented to the root canal using Breeze Self-Adhesive Resin Cement and the cavity was covered with a composite restoration (Figure 2B,C). On the last visit, 2 months after the first visit, post-treatment evaluation was conducted. There was no subjective complaints from the patient and clinical examination showed no abnormalities, insensitive on percussion and palpation test. The patient was educated that he has to do a routine follow up every 6 months.

3. Discussion

The diagnosis and management of additional root and root canals is undeniably an endodontic challenge, and in most situations, the tooth is advised to be extracted due to failure to identify other root canals [6, 7]. More than one root canal in the central and maxillary lateral incisors is a very rare finding. In fact, based on the morphological and anatomical studies of maxillary anterior teeth performed by Vertucci in 1984, 100% of these teeth showed a root canal. Contrary to a study conducted by Vertucci, in 1992, DeDeus conducted a survey and reported that about 3% of the maxillary lateral incisors had two root canals [7].

The possibility of these variations in the maxillary lateral incisor is a result of its highrisk location in the embryo. During the fourth and sixth weeks of human embryonic development, the maxilla, where the lateral incisors are located, is formed by the fusion of the medial nasal processes (MNP) and maxillary processes (MP). When the MNP fuses with each other, they form premaxilla, including the medial part of the upper lip (philtrum) and the primary palate. The exact source of the maxillary lateral incisor associated with the MNP/MP fusion site and the premaxilla/maxilla suture is still a question. The MNP/MP fusion area may be in the medial part of the lateral incisor or in the medial or middle third of the lateral incisor. The premaxilla/maxillary sutura lies between the lateral and canine incisors or in the middle third of the canines. Therefore, maxillary lateral incisors are often exhibiting diverse morphologic root canals [2]. On the other hand, the incidence of fractures of various types of instruments is a caution for clinicians and researchers. Ingerechts et al. conducted a study to assess the incidence, location and impact of fracture instruments on treatment prognosis. In 3854 root canals, 38 fractured instruments were observed in different groups. The higher incidence of fractured instruments is in the apical third of molar teeth with curvature and/or constricted root canals [3].

The presence of fractured instrument could seriously affects the outcome of root canal treatment and usually prevents access of other instruments to the apex, inhibits cleaning and shaping of root canal, drainage from the periapical area and prevents the three-dimensional obturation of root canal system. When the instrument is broken on the root canal, the clinician has two options, to remove the instrument or to perform a bypass procedure. To remove the fractured instrument, good visibility is required thus straight access is mandatory. However, if the fractured instrument is located in the curvature area, obtaining visibility requires much dentine retrieval to gain straight access, thereby weakening the dentin structure or actually making perforations. An alternative technique that does not require visibility is a bypass procedure, in which a file is inserted between the fractured instrument and the root canal wall. By this technique, working length can be achieved and allows the instrumentation and obturation of the root canal with fragment of the fractured instrument remained in the root canal. Unifying fractured instrument with obturation material will increase the prognosis of this cases [5].

In this procedure, the used of a chelating agent of 17% EDTA was associated with its action to create an active tip passes through a broken instrument. By doing such action, the instrument can be easily bypassed. With this technique, tooth structure can be avoided from unfavorable events like deviation or perforation which can make the prognosis worse. This treatment option is consistent with the previous study and found that if the fractured instrument is located on apical third, it is unlikely that instrument to be possibly removed, so this bypass procedure is a viable alternative [3].

The most common techniques used for root canal obturation are cold lateral compaction, warm vertical compaction and core-carrier system [8]. The core-carrier system is easy to do and has the ability to fill the root canals in three dimensions, with much less gaps than the lateral condensation method [9]. Recent development of Thermafil (Dentsply Tulsa Dental Specialties, Tulsa, OK) as a carrier-based obturation that uses a crosslinked gutta-percha core instead of using plastic carriers [10]. Cross-linked thermoset gutta-percha was used to replaced the Vectra (a liquid crystal polymer) or polysulphone plastic carriers in Thermafil Plus (Dentsply Tulsa Dental Specialties), which enables the carrier to be removed more easily if retreatment is needed [11]. In this case, GuttaCore system was used because the root canal have a split in the apical third and the cold lateral compaction can not resolve both canals. To reduce the possibilities of tooth fracture due to the weakening of the tooth structure caused by endodontic treatment, fiber post was chosen to be the next treatment. Because there was still considerable amounts on the corona, direct composite restoration was selected as final restoration.

CONCLUSION

A good knowledge of root canal anatomy is very important to achieve a successful endodontic treatment. Clinician should be aware of possibly more than one canal in maxillary lateral incisor. The dental microscope and Cone Beam Computed Tomography are favorable in identifying the anatomic complexity of the pulpal spaces. In this case, a successful treatment was achieved because fractured instrument was managed to be bypassed. Thus, steps of preparation, obturation and restoration was done adequately.

REFERENCES

[1] Ahmed, H. M. A. (2018). A new system for classifying accessory canal morphology. *Int Endod J.* 51(2):164-176.

[2] Lee, M., Ha, H., Kim, Y., Kim, S. (2013). Endodontic treatment of maxillary lateral incisors with anatomical variations. *Restor Dent Endod.* 38(4): 253–257.

[3] Machado, R., Donato, E., Engelke, E., Tomazinho, L. F. (2014). Bypassing separated iles in the apical third : A case series using the same technique. *Dent Press Endod.* 4(3):76-80.

[4] Mcguigan, M. B., Louca, C., Duncan, H. F. (2013). Endodontic instrument fracture: causes and prevention. *Nat. Publ. Gr.* 214(7): 341 - 348.

[5] John, P., M. R. K., Jayasree, S. (2016). Bypassing Separated Instruments in the Root Canal – Two Case Reports. J Dent Med Sci 15(6):8 - 13.

[6] Hemanth, S., Sujatha, I., Vamshi Krishna, D. J. K. (2017). Endodontic Management of Mandibular Second Premolar Having Type-V Vertucci Canal Configuration – Case Series. 76 - 80. doi: 10.21276/sjodr.2017.2.3.5.

[7] Singh, S., Rapsang, E., Mirdha, N., Sharma, Y., Tiwari, R. V. C. (2019). Endodontic treatment of rare anatomical complexity, two canals in maxillary lateral incisor: A case report. *IP Ind J Conservat Endod.* 1(c):29 - 30.

[8] Whitworth, J. (2005). Methods of filling root canals : principles and practices. *Endod Topics* (13):2 - 24.

[9] Marques-ferreira, M., Abrantes, M., Ferreira, H., Caramelo, F. (2017). Sealing efficacy of system B versus Thermafil and Guttacore obturation techniques evidenced by scintigraphic analysis. *J Clin Exp Dent.* 1;9(1):e56-e60.

[10] Beasley, R. T., Williamson, A. E., Justman, B. C. (2013). Time Required to Remove Gutta Core, Thermafil Plus, and Thermoplasticized Gutta-percha from Moderately Curved Root Canals with ProTaper Files. *J. Endodon.* 39(1):125-128.

[11] Li, G., Niu, L., Selem, L. C. et al. (2014). Science Direct Quality of obturation achieved by an endodontic core-carrier system with crosslinked gutta-percha carrier in single-rooted canals. *J. Dent.* 42;9:1124-1134.

In: Clinical Reports in Dentistry
Editor: Lisa R. Amir
ISBN: 978-1-53617-328-4

Chapter 34

Managing Iatrogenic Pulp Exposure with Biodentine: A Case Report

***Stefani A. Dewi*[1] *and Dewa Ayu N. P. Artiningsih*[2,*]**
[1]Conservative Dentistry Residency Program, Faculty of Dentistry, Universitas Indonesia, Jakarta, Indonesia
[2]Department of Conservative Dentistry, Faculty of Dentistry, Universitas Indonesia, Jakarta, Indonesia

Abstract

Introduction: This case report described the management of iatrogenic pulp exposure with Biodentine as direct pulp capping material.

Case report: A 19-year-old female patient complained about discomfort associated with thermal stimulation on the permanent mandibular left first molar. Pulp sensitivity was confirmed by thermal pulp vitality tests. The radiograph revealed a deep caries lesion close to the pulp and a lack of periapical radiolucency and periodontal ligament widening. Based on the examinations, the treatment plan was to cover the left dentine with pulp capping material indirectly, but iatrogenic pulp exposures occurred. Clinical procedures were taken consisted of caries removal, bleeding control, the Biodentine application as a direct pulp capping material, and resin composite application as the overlying restoration. Biodentine was the choice of treatment because of its high biocompatibility and bioactivity that can encourage protective hard formation and healing on the site of injury.

Conclusion: Clinical success for six months follow-up was confirmed by sensitivity over vitality test and lack of radiographic pathological findings.

Keywords: biodentine, pulp capping, iatrogenic pulp exposures

*Corresponding Author's Email: dewaayunpa@yahoo.co.id.

1. Introduction

The current principle of caries removal is to leave soft dentine or infected dentine adjacent to the pulp, which prevents it from pulp exposure [1]. However, an iatrogenic error sometimes unavoidable in the case of deep caries lesion [2]. Following the pulp exposure, the pulp experiences an inflammation response a spread of infection, and immediate procedure is taken to preserve the vitality of the pulp. Direct pulp capping is one of the procedures to preserve tooth vitality, in which a material is placed directly over the exposed pulp and aimed to encourage protective hard tissue formation after injury. The success rate of this procedure ranges from 30-80% and depends on the material used. Material biocompatibility is not sufficient enough as a qualification for direct pulp capping material, hence its bio-activity for the regeneration of the pulpo-dentinal complex are mandatory [3]. Historically, Calcium Hydroxide (CH) has been used as the gold standard, but recent development of calcium silicate materials such as Mineral Trioxide Aggregate (MTA) and Biodentine showed positive clinical outcomes. Calcium silicate-based materials have been applied for various dental treatments such as dentine replacement, pulp capping, pulpotomy, perforation repair, apexification and also root-end filling in endodontic surgery without adverse of clinical or radiographic symptoms [4]. These materials can be applied on an exposed pulp and overcome the shortcomings of CH, specifically it can dissolve beneath the restoration, cause tunnel defects and induce inflammation of the underlying pulp tissue [5].

Although MTA has successful treatment outcomes and a wide range of applications, it has some disadvantages such as tooth discoloration potential, handling difficulties, and long setting time [6]. Thus, calcium silicate-based material like Biodentine (Septodont, Saint-Maur-des-Fosses, France) has been introduced to conquer MTA's drawbacks. Biodentine, formulated with MTA-based technology, claims superior properties such as physical qualities, handling, setting time and bioactivity. Its compressive and flexural strength are higher than MTA according to studies, followed by its high biocompatibility and excellent bioactivity [7]. The efficiency of Biodentine as pulp capping material also has been reported with positive outcomes on a clinical basis [4]. Biodentine has two components, powder and liquid. The powder is composed of tricalcium silicates as a main core, dicalcium silicate as a second core material and calcium carbonate and oxide as a filler. The liquid contains calcium chloride as a setting accelerator and a water reducing agent. When the powder and the liquid of Biodentine are mixed, it leads to the setting and hardening of the cement. The hydration of the tricalcium silicate is then subjected to the formation of a hydrated calcium silicate gel on the cement particles and calcium hydroxide nucleates. This hydrogel will settle on the surface of the remaining silicate particles and in the space between particles which causes a significant reduction in material porosity and an increase in compressive strength over time. The complete reaction can be summarized as [8]: $2(3CaO.SiO_2) + 6H_2O \rightarrow 3CaO.2SiO_2.3H_2O +$

$3Ca(OH)_2$. This article reported a good clinical success on an iatrogenic pulp exposure in a permanent lower left first molar treated with Biodentine as a direct pulp capping material.

2. CASE REPORT

A 22-year-old woman was referred to Conservative Dentistry Clinic at the Universitas Indonesia with a history of pain which was caused by cold drinks and stuck food in the tooth's cavity of her permanent lower left first molar. The pain disappeared after the stimuli was removed. History of spontaneous and lingering pain was not confirmed. Clinical examination showed an extensive carious lesion in the occlusal site of her first permanent left lower molar without signs of extra-oral or intra-oral swelling or sinus tract formation (Figure 1A). The tooth was insensitive to percussions and palpations. Cold test, using cotton pellet sprayed with ethyl chloride which was inserted into the cavity, elicited the pain but it disappeared quickly after the stimulus was removed. Radiographic examination showed a mature tooth with a large carious lesion, leaving a thin layer of dentine in the occlusal site of the tooth. There were not radiolucencies appeared at the periapical area or widening of the periodontal ligament on the periapical radiograph (Figure 2A).

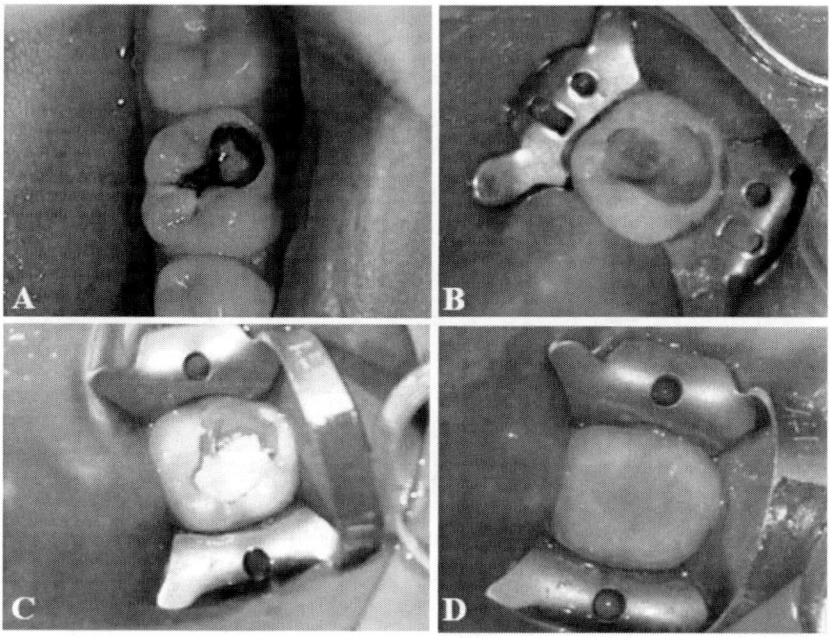

Figure 1. Permanent first lower molar with extensive carious lesion (A); View of the cavity floor after infected dentine removal. Note that there is one pinpoint of an exposed pulp 1mm in diameter (B); Biodentine as pulp-dressing material on the cavity (C); Resin composite restoration (D).

Based on the clinical and radiographic examination, the pulpal status of the lower left first molar was determined as vital with pulpitis reversible caused by caries. The treatment plan was to remove caries lesion partially, leave the infected dentine near the pulp, and preserve tooth vitality with indirect pulp capping. Direct pulp capping was performed in case of pulp exposure occurs.

2.1 Procedure

Local anesthesia was administered, and the tooth was then isolated with a rubber dam. Caries lesion in the margin area was removed by diamond bur at low-speed handpiece with water spray. Infected dentine near the pulp was removed with an excavator. The excavation was performed carefully to remove the wet dentine, but the roof of the pulp was exposed and showed a pinpoint. Moderate bleeding was observed, nevertheless hemostasis was obtained by cotton pellet soaked with NaOCl 2.5% for a few minutes. (Figure 1B). The cavity was rinsed using sterile water and then dried with sterilized cotton pellets. Biodentine (Septodont, Saint-Maur-des-Fosses, France) was mixed according to the manufacturer's instruction and a layer of it was applied directly over the exposed pulp on the cavity floor with 1-2 mm thick (Figure 1C).

Resin composite was applied after the setting of Biodentine as a liner for 12 minutes. The outline of the cavity was etched with 35% phosphoric acid gel for 30 seconds (Scotchbond™ Etchant, 3M/ESPE), rinsed and dried with a moistened cotton pellet. Following the bonding agent application (Single Bond™, 3M/ESPE), it was light-cured according to the manufacturer's instructions. Resin composite (Filtek Z250™, A3 shade, 3M/ESPE) was applied with incremental technique (Figure 1D). Each increment was polymerized with a light-cure for 40 seconds and occlusion was checked.

After a 6 months interval, a new examination was recorded. Spontaneous pain was not reported during this period and response to cold and hot stimuli was consistent with a normal vital pulp.

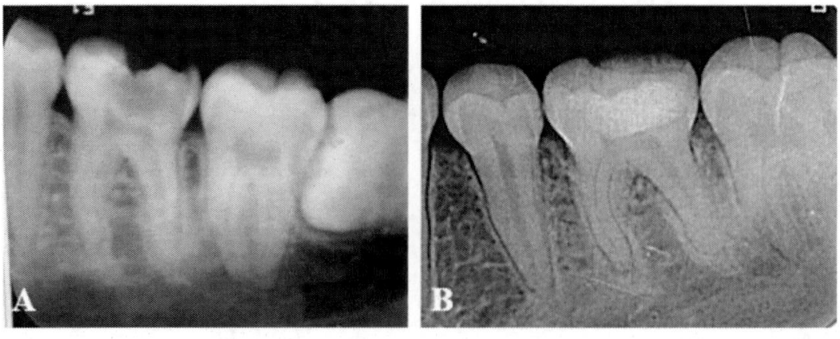

Figure 2. Initial periapical radiograph showing deep carious lesion and normal periapical status (A); Radiograph of 6 months follow-up after Biodentine application (B).

Radiolucency on the apical and widening on the ligament periodontal were not detected in the periapical radiograph (Figure 2B).

3. DISCUSSION

Partial caries removal is the latest concept of minimal intervention, in which the infected dentine is left to cover the pulp [2]. This procedure is completed using hand instruments subjectively, an explorer and tactile sense to differentiate soft from hard dentine. However, this method might have shortcomings because clinicians may unnecessarily remove the dentine that still has the potential to remineralize under a sealed restoration. The pulp could got exposed in iatrogenic means which is not consistent with the current concept of minimal intervention [9]. If this happens, preserving vitality of the pulp by vital pulp therapy should be considered as the first choice of treatment because it will encourage the formation of protective hard tissue barrier after injury. The process is initiated by materials that can induce odontoblast-like cells proliferation, recruited from the cell-rich zone and sub-odontoblastic layer, hence advance the repair of pulpo-dentinal defects after migration of highly vascularized tissue to the site. The treatment options for iatrogenic exposed pulp on permanent teeth include direct pulp capping and partial or complete pulpotomy [9]. Direct pulp capping is defined as placing a dental material directly on a mechanical or traumatic vital pulp exposure and sealing the pulpal wound to facilitate the formation of reparative dentine and maintenance of the vital pulp. The procedure is indicated for pulp exposures as a result of caries removal, trauma, or tooth preparation [10]. Following hemostasis with NaOCl, if the hemorrhage control cannot be accomplished after 10 minutes contact with 3% NaOCl, the pulp is in danger to be irreversibly involved, hence a partial or complete pulpectomy is required. After successful hemostasis, pulpal repair and reparative dentine formation can proceed normally in the absence of microbial, and thus rubber dam isolation is mandatory [11].

Sodium hypochlorite established effective hemostatic and antiseptic properties in humans without altering pulp repair, healing, and tertiary dentinogenesis. A study of pulp-capped human third molars, examined pulps histologically at 30 and 60 days after the use of 2.5% NaOCl for hemostasis and showed no impairment of the repair process [11]. Current data support the use of 1.25% to 6% NaOCl solutions in humans as a safe and appropriate hemostatic agent for direct pulp capping and pulpotomies [11, 12]. Calcium hydroxide (CH) is known as the gold standard for vital pulp therapy materials. Although the material has many advantageous properties, long-term study outcomes in vital pulp therapy have been inconsistent. CH has initial high alkaline pH release, which is important for stimulating fibroblasts, enzyme systems, and also good antibacterial properties. The weakness of CH includes inferior marginal adaptation to dentine, degradation and dissolution over time. Reparative dentine bridge formation after CH can also be attributed to tunnel defects. Histologically, CH established cytotoxicity in cell cultures and showed pulp cell apoptosis [5]. MTA has been reported with higher biocompatibility and better bioactivity than CH. However, it also has some disadvantages such as tooth discoloration, handling difficulties, and long setting time [13]. Since the introduction of MTA, new bioactive silicate-based cement materials are becoming more advance. Biodentine is one of the most recently launched bioactive material, based on tricalcium silicate cement technology that might conquer MTA's drawbacks. The study showed the biocompatible and bioactive properties of MTA with the capacity of releasing silicon, calcium, and alkaline ion. Previous study reported Biodentine has higher compressive and flexural strength, followed by lower porosity, solubility, and microleakage compared to MTA [4]. The other advantages include easier to manipulate, fast setting, has stable color and non-genotoxic nor cytotoxic when measured with the Ames mutagenicity test [6].

After the application of Biodentine and composite resin, the patient had no more complaints about thermal induced pain or lingering spontaneous pain associated with irreversible pulpitis. This could be a sign that inflammation has stopped, and the pulp is expected to be reversible at the normal state and started to heal after the loss of irritants. This could happen because Biodentine provides a good seal that covers the pulp from the further irritants and facilitates the dentinal bridge formation as a characteristic of repair process after pulp capping [8]. Biodentine releases Calcium ions and Alkaline ions with high pH which can induce odontoblast-like cell differentiation, stimulate biomineralization, and promote hard tissue formation when used as pulp capping material [7]. According to a study, the release of these ions induce reparative dentine bridge formation after application and culturing of Biodentine for 14 days. Calcium ions are needed to modulate osteopontin and BMP-2 for calcification, increase proliferation of human dental pulp cells, and aid the activity of pyrophosphatase which are responsible for the formation and mineralization of dentinal bridge [5]. The application of Biodentine in pulpotomy was also investigated in primary pig teeth and compared to formocresol and white MTA. The results of this study showed a thick dentin bridge by Biodentine that was formed in 90% of the cases without inflammation [14].

Mineralized structures appeared in the form of foci adjacent to the material is more likely associated with Biodentine as some cement particles was seen within the mineralized structures. This mineralized tissue resembles an early form of the reparative dentinal bridge as cells sequestered within these mineralization express odontoblastic markers such as nestin and dentine sialoprotein. This mineralization appeared due to the release of a transforming growth factor beta 1 (TGF-b1) from pulp cells incubated with Biodentine. This growth factor has been shown to be involved in odontoblast differentiation and also in the recruitment of pulp stem cells to TGF-b1 production site [14]. Faster setting time of 12 minutes and improvement with its handling properties and strength on Biodentine are due to the accelerator contained in the liquid. A study by

Torabinejad M et al. revealed a delayed setting time led to an increased risk of partial material loss and alteration of the interface during the finishing phase of the procedure [15].Therefore, Biodentine has better setting time compared to MTA that leads to a single visit for restoration application.

For the composite restoration on Biodentine, an interesting study compared the shear bond strengths of different adhesive systems to Biodentine. This study showed that the shear bond strengths were the same for different adhesive systems to Biodentine especially whencomposite resin applied after its setting. However, the highest shear bond strength was achieved on the application at the second week [16]. The adhesion mechanism is a micromechanical retention formed by etching that can cause crystalline structures mild loss of Biodentine [17]. The microleakage capabilities of Biodentine was also tested at the interface with composite resins and the result revealed an excellent seal against microleakage due to surface preparation of the material with phosphoric acid for 15 seconds [8]. A tentative diagnosis of tooth survivability can be made at the 3-month recall. One study demonstrated that the prognosis for long-term pulp survival was revealed at an observation period of 21 to 24 months. However, in the case of normal vitality during cold testing, recall reviews can be scheduled at 6 weeks and at 6 and 12 months depending on patient compliance [18].

CONCLUSION

The use Biodentine material for an iatrogenic pulp exposure case with direct pulp capping procedure has proven to be clinically successful. Nevertheless, the successful results in the presented case is still required to be observed in a yearly follow-up.

REFERENCES

[1] Barthel, C. R., Rosenkranz, B., Leuenberg, A. (2000). Pulp Capping of Carious Exposures : Treatment Outcome after 5 and 10 Years : A Retrospective Study. *J. Endod.*, (2):8-11.

[2] Bjørndal, L. (2008). Indirect Pulp Therapy and Stepwise Excavation. *J. Endod.,* 34(7):29-33.

[3] Cho, S., Seo, D., Lee, S. (2013). Prognostic Factors for Clinical Outcomes According to Time after Direct Pulp Capping. *J. Endod.*, 39(3):327-331.

[4] Rajasekharan, S., Martens, L.C., Cauwels, R.G.E.C. (2018), Anthonappa, R.P. Biodentine material characteristics and clinical applications: A 3 year literature review and update. *Eur. Arch. Paediatr. Dent.,*19(1): 1-22. 2019, 1-22.

[5] Gandolfi, M. G., Siboni, F., Botero, T., Bossù, M., Riccitiello, F., Prati, C. (2015). Calcium silicate and calcium hydroxide materials for pulp capping: biointeractivity, porosity, solubility and bioactivity of current formulations. *Appl. Biomater. Funct. Mater.,* 13(1):43-60.

[6] Nowicka, A., Lipski, M., Parafiniuk, M., Kosierkiewicz, A., Kaczmarek, W. (2013). Response of Human Dental Pulp Capped with Biodentine and Mineral Trioxide Aggregate. *J. Endod.,* 39(6):5-8.

[7] About, I. (2016). Biodentine: From biochemical and bioactive properties to clinical applications. *G Ital. Endod.,*30:1-8.

[8] Bachoo, I. K., Seymour, D., Brunton, P. (2013). A biocompatible and bioactive replacement for dentine : is this a reality ? The properties and uses of a novel calcium-based cement. *Br. Dent. J.,* 214(2):1-7.

[9] Bogen, G., Kuttler, S., Chandler, N. (2016). Vital Pulp Therapy.In Berman, L. and Hargreaves, K. (Eds.), *Cohen's Pathways of the Pulp, 11th Edition* (pp.849-876). St. Louis, MO: Elseveir.

[10] *Guide to Clinical Endodontics*, Sixth Edition. In www.aae.org. 2016:1-40.

[11] Silva, A. F., Tarquinio, S. B. C., Demarco, F. F., Piva, E., Rivero, E. R. C. (2006). The influence of haemostatic agents on healing of healthy human dental pulp tissue capped with calcium hydroxide. *J. Endod.*, 309-316.

[12] Garcia-Godoy, F., Murray, P. E. (2005). Systemic evaluation of various haemostatic agents following local application prior to direct pulp capping. *Braz. J. Oral Sci.,* 4(14):791-797.

[13] Kaur, M., Singh, H., Dhillon, J. S., Batra, M., Saini, M. (2017). MTA versus biodentine: Review of literature with a comparative analysis. *J. Clin. Diagnostic Res.,* 11(8):ZG01- ZG05.

[14] Laurent, P., Camps, J., About, I. (2012). Biodentine TM induces TGF- b 1 release from human pulp cells and early dental pulp mineralization. *J. Endod.,* 439-448.

[15] Torabinejad, M., Chivian, N. (1999). Clinical applications of mineral trioxide aggregate. *J. Endod.,* 25(3):197-205.

[16] Odabaş, M. E., Bani, M., Tirali, R. E.(2013). Shear bond strengths of different adhesive systems to biodentine. *Scientific World J.*, 2013:626103.

[17] Koubi, G., Colon, P., Franquin, J.C., Hartmann, A., Richard, G., Faure, M.O. (2013). Lambert, G. Clinical evaluation of the performance and safety of a new dentine substitute, Biodentine, in the restoration of posteriorteeth-A prospective study. *Clin. Oral Investig.,* 17, 243-249.

[18] Asgary, S., Ehsani, S., Hassanizadeh, R., Shirvani, A. (2016). Management of Carious Pulp Exposure in Vital Permanent Teeth : An Evidence-Based Clinical Practice Guideline. Management of Carious Pulp Exposure in Vital Permanent Teeth : An Evidence-Based Clinical Practice Guideline. *Journal of Regeneration, Reconstruction and Restoration,* 1(2):36-46.

In: Clinical Reports in Dentistry
Editor: Lisa R. Amir
ISBN: 978-1-53617-328-4

Chapter 35

A COMPOSITE RESIN ONLAY FOR FIRST PERMANENT MOLAR POST PULPECTOMY IN A 9-YEAR-OLD GIRL

Mochamad F. Rizal[1,*] ***and Cahyanti W. Susilo***[2]
[1]Pediatric Dentistry Department, Faculty of Dentistry,
Universitas Indonesia, Jakarta, Indonesia
[2]Pediatric Dentistry Residency Program, Faculty of Dentistry,
Universitas Indonesia, Jakarta, Indonesia

ABSTRACT

Introduction: The first permanent molar has a very high rate of caries in children with mixed dentition mostly due to deep pits and fissure of the occlusal surface, morphological features and developmental enamel defects. In case of deep caries lesions, the pulp can become infected leading to irreversible pulpitis. The managements of irreversible pulpitis include pulpectomy, root canal treatment, and tooth restoration. Adhesive restoration with an indirect resin composite onlay, offers many advantages for endodontically treated teeth. The case report aimed to present an indirect composite resin restoration onlay for a broken-down molar tooth of a pediatric patient.

Case Report: This paper described the clinical management of irreversible pulpitis in a first permanent molar of a 9-year-old girl from pulpectomy to placement of a composite resin onlay as a definitive restoration. On follow-up, the resin composite restoration remained in place with no fracture or subjective complaints.

Conclusion: Functional and aesthetic restoration of an endodontically-treated first permanent molar tooth of a pediatric patient can be achieved with the use of an indirect composite resin onlay and will directly impact the success of the root canal treatment and the longevity of the restoration.

Keywords: caries, first permanent molar, pulpectomy, endodontically treated teeth, composite resin onlay

* Corresponding Author's Email: levipedo@gmail.com.

1. INTRODUCTION

Dental caries is a common chronic infectious microbiologic disease in children that results in the dissolution and destruction of calcified tissues [1]. Several studies have reported a high prevalence of dental caries in the first permanent molar teeth of children aged 6-13 years [2-4], and the prevalence of caries of the first permanent molar in children between the age of 6 and 7 years is 40.19%, with the occlusal surface most commonly affected [3]. While another study observed that 75.5% of children had one or more caries of the first permanent molars and that the prevalence of caries increases significantly with age [5]. A study conducted in Indonesia reported that the prevalence of caries of the first permanent molar was 68.1% in children aged 6-9 years [6].

The first permanent molars are the most susceptible permanent teeth to caries due to the morphological features of deep pits and fissures, developmental enamel defects, lack of interest in oral hygiene in the early stages of tooth eruption, and there are often being mistaken by the parents as primary molars due to the positions of these teeth [2, 3, 7]. Special care must be given to the first permanent molars because of the important roles of these teeth in establishing occlusion and good functionality of the dental-maxillary anatomy [3].

The first permanent molars have large-sized crowns, are the strongest of all teeth, and are very important in mastication and guiding the eruption of other posterior teeth [8].

Pulpal inflammation caused by deep caries infection can be clinically managed by preserving the pulp tissue or by removing the pulp tissue and root-filling the tooth, depending on the diagnosis of the tooth [9]. In 2012, the American Association of Endodontics described the pulp diagnostic classifications of reversible pulpitis, symptomatic irreversible pulpitis, asymptomatic irreversible pulpitis, pulp necrosis, and previously treated (pulpless) [10].

Pulpectomy is a preliminary root canal treatment for the management of symptomatic irreversible pulpitis that involves complete pulp removal and total cleaning of the root canal [11]. The main goals of pulpectomy are to prevent infection in the pulp chamber, ensure asymptomatic condition, and maintain the health of the periapical tissue [9].

After completion of the root canal treatment, the normal form and function of the tooth are restored. The tissue of the endodontically-treated tooth has different physical characteristic and is more prone to fracture than vital teeth due to the use of medicaments and irrigation agents during root canal treatment. Therefore, it is important to emphasize coronal restoration and cuspal protection to reduce the risk of tooth fracture [9]. Beside gold onlay, a composite resin onlay is a viable option for restoration of endodontically treated posterior teeth. Studies have demonstrated that the weakening effect of tooth preparation can be alleviated with the use of adhesive materials to bind cusps and decrease flexion.

Moreover, composite resin has a lower elastic modulus than gold or amalgam and, thus, may transmit less stress to the remaining tooth structure [10]. In this report, an example of an indirect composite resin restoration onlay is described involving a pediatric patient with a broken first permanent molar.

2. Case Report

A 9-year-old girl and her mother presented to the Pediatric Dental Clinic of Universitas Indonesia, with a chief complaint of pain in the permanent mandibular left first molar. The child reported a lingering pain induced by cold food and beverages but no spontaneous pain. Her mother explained that the child was born prematurely at a very low birth weight. An intra-oral clinical examination showed a deep occlusal carious lesion of the permanent mandibular left first molar. There was no tenderness to percussion, and a radiographic examination revealed occlusal caries nearing the pulp. The tooth was first diagnosed with reversible pulpitis. On the initial treatment, the caries was excavated with a low speed metal bur and temporarily sealed. Yet, the next day, the patient reported sharp and spontaneous pain. The tooth was then diagnosed with irreversible pulpitis, and the proposed treatment included pulpectomy followed by endodontic treatment and restoration with a composite resin onlay.

Under local anesthesia, access preparation was performed using a high-speed round diamond bur with continuous irrigation with water spray. Pulpectomy followed by root canal treatment was performed, and the root was filled with gutta-percha (Figure 1).

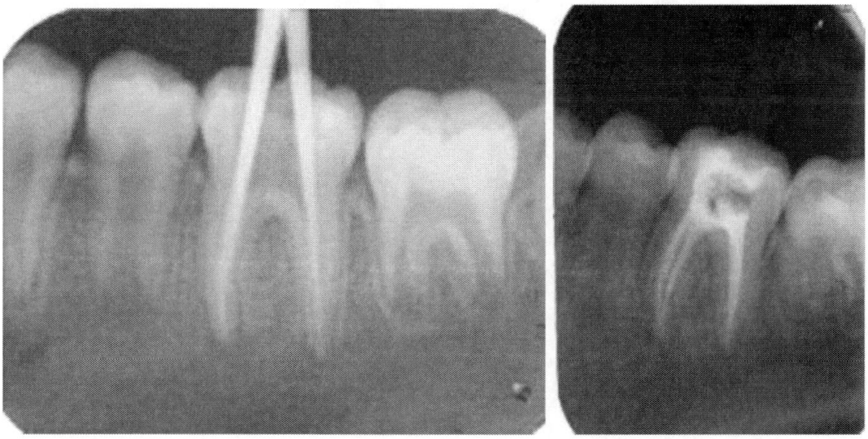

Figure 1. Radiograph after root canal treatment of a permanent mandibular left first molar.

Subsequently, a glass ionomer restoration was placed directly over the gutta-percha. Following the principles of tooth preparation to receive a composite resin onlay, the cavity was prepared. The cavity walls were made divergent with rounded internal line angles, and an interocclusal space of 2mm was prepared (Figure 2A). After final tooth preparation, the cavity was cleansed and dried. An impression was made with a polyvinylsiloxane material (Figure 2B). Afterward, a direct provisional restoration was placed using zinc phosphate cement. The shade of the restoration was selected using the Vita shade guide (Figure 2C). and the casts and shade prescription were sent to the laboratory for fabrication of the onlay.

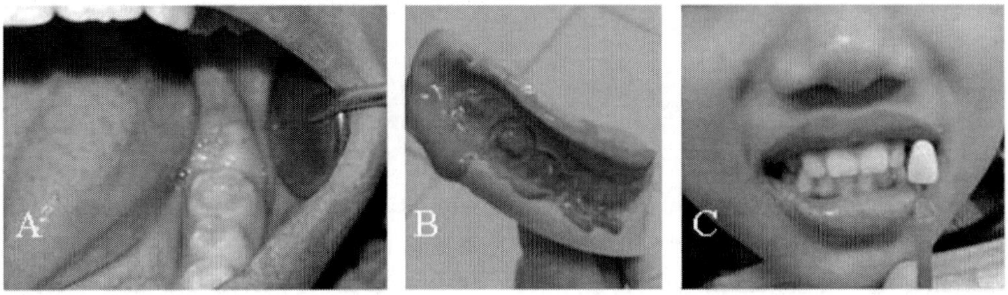

Figure 2. A procedure at dental office to produce a well-fitted onlay: A. Final preparation and impression of a permanent mandibular left first molar; B. An impression a polyvinylsiloxane material; C. Shade selection using the Vita shade guide.

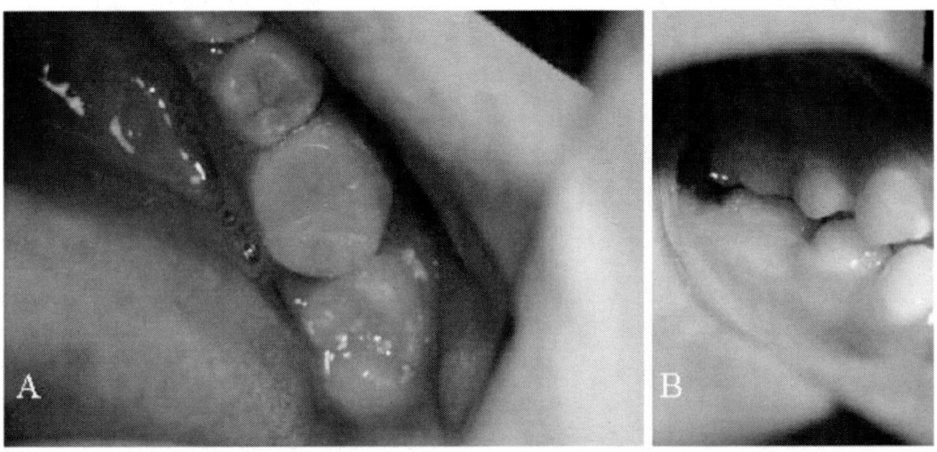

Figure 3. Placement of the composite resin onlay.

On the next visit, the provisional restoration was removed, and the cavity was cleansed by water rinsing followed by drying. Then cementation was carried out by applying a thin layer of self-adhesive resin cement on the cavity and the internal aspect of the composite onlay. The excess resin luting cement was removed, and the restoration was light-cured from the occlusal, lingual, and buccal sides for 40s. After cementation, the occlusion was evaluated (Figure 3). On follow-up, the restoration remained in place with no fracture or subjective complaints.

3. Discussion

It is important to maintain the first permanent molars in growing children because of the role of these teeth in guiding the eruption of other posterior teeth and establishing occlusion with good functionality of mastication [3, 8]. Deep caries infection of the first permanent molars is highly prevalent in children with mixed dentition from the age 6 to 13 years [2]. Such infections may be due to morphological features of the corona, deep pits and fissures of the occlusal surface and the developmental enamel defects, such as hypomineralization and hypoplasia [4]. Untreated caries can cause inflammation of the dental pulp, such as reversible pulpitis and symptomatic or asymptomatic irreversible pulpitis. Teeth with symptomatic irreversible pulpitis exhibit spontaneous, intermittent, and prolonged pain even after the stimuli has been removed [11]. These symptoms were applicable in our case as the patient was a 9-year-old girl with deep occlusal carious lesions of the permanent mandibular left first molar with a complaint of spontaneous and lingering pain.

Management of pulpal inflammation is dependent on the diagnosis of the tooth. In this case, the initial complaint of the patient was a lingering pain induced by cold food, and then the pain became sharp and spontaneous. The clinical diagnosis of tooth 36 was irreversible pulpitis. Pulpectomy as a preliminary root canal treatment was performed on as soon as possible to prevent further severe pain. In cases with irreversible pulpitis, the vital pulp is unable to self-heal; thus, management consists of the removal of the entire pulp and replacement with a root filling. Pulpectomy is mainly performed to prevent infection of the pulp chamber and to ensure an asymptomatic condition of the tooth, which can be achieved by proper asepsis during treatment, effective removal of the pulp tissue, and hermetic root canal fillings [12].

Long-term survival of an endodontically treated tooth is dependent on adequate root canal treatment and appropriate restoration. In this case, after the root canal treatment, a resin composite onlay was made to restore form and function. The main objectives of restoration are to prevent bacterial micro-leakage into the root canal that can cause future failure and to restore form and function [13]. There are several differences between endodontically treated teeth and vital teeth such as altered tissue characteristics, tooth composition, loss of tooth structure due to preparation of an access cavity, and chemical use during endodontic treatment. Such alterations affect tooth resistance to fracture [11]. The type of restoration of endodontically treated teeth is dependent on the remaining hard tooth structure. There is a direct relationship between the remaining structure and fracture resilience of the tooth, as the greater the remaining tooth structure, the greater longevity of the tooth [13]. For a medium-sized cavity limited to the occlusal surface as in this case, bonded indirect restoration (onlay) is acceptable as a final restoration to limit the removal of healthy dental tissue due to full crown preparation. Occlusal coverage by an onlay reduces stress to the remaining tooth structure, thereby reducing the risk of tooth fracture [9, 10].

Before cementation the cavity was rinsed with water and dried thoroughly. This is because composite resin is a sensitive restoration and its manipulation requires a dry and clean operative area in order to obtain adequate bonding strength [14]. The use of adhesive restorations for posterior endodontically treated teeth has been reported in several studies [10, 15, 16]. The adhesive feature of a composite allows bringing of the cusp and decreased flexion.

Composite has a lower elastic modulus than porcelain and metal; thus the load is mainly absorbed within the composite and less transmitted to the underlying tooth structure [10]. The higher resilience of resin composite restoration can also reduce the risk of periodontal bone resorption because less stress is transferred to the root dentin [11]. This is advantageous considering that pediatric patients are still undergoing growth and development. In this case, an indirect onlay was fabricated from a resin composite material in the laboratory. The combination of light, pressure, and vacuum polymerization of an indirect resin composite create a better polymerization with greater mechanical properties of the restoration which can overcome the major problem of polymerization shrinkage when placing a direct resin composite.

CONCLUSION

The clinical management of irreversible pulpitis of a first permanent molar includes pulpectomy, root canal filling, and placement of an onlay as a definitive restoration. Physical alteration of the tooth structure due to endodontic treatment renders the tooth more prone to fracture. Therefore, the selection of an appropriate restoration material will directly impact the success of the root canal treatment and the longevity of the restoration. Functional and aesthetic restoration of an endodontically treated first permanent molar of a pediatric patient can be achieved with the use of an indirect composite resin onlay.

REFERENCES

[1] Roberson, T., Heymann, H. O., Swift, E. J. (2006). *Sturdevant's Art and Science of Operative Dentistry*. 5th ed. Missouri: Elsevier Health Sciences.

[2] Serban, V., Maxim, A., Balan, A. (2009). Study on The Caries of First Permanent MolarsIn Children Aged Between 6 and 13 Years. *J. of Roman Med. Dent.*, 13(4):138-141.

[3] Chirca, E. M., Luca, R., Georgescu, D. (2015). The Prevalence of Caries in First Permanent Molar in A Group of School Children Aged 6 to 7 Years in Pitesti. *The Publishing House of The Romanian Academy*, Series B (Suplement 1):41-44.

[4] Chen, J., Leggitt, V. L. (2012). Pulp treatment for young first permanent molars: To treat or to extract ? *Endodontic Topics*, 23(1):34-40.

[5] Al-samadani, K. H. M., Ahmad, M. S. (2012). Prevalence of First Permanent Molar Caries in and Its Relationship to the Dental Knowledge of 9 – 12-Year Olds from Jeddah, Kingdom of Saudi Arabia. *International Scholarly Research Network*, 1-6.

[6] Mintjelungan, C. N., Gunawan, P. N. (2015). The prevalence of caries for permanent first molars in children aged 6 - 9 years in elementary school. *Journal e-GiGi*, 3(2):416-420.

[7] Seow, W. K. (2014). Developmental Defects of Enamel and Dentine: Challenges for Basic Science Research and Clinical Management. *Australian Dental Journal*, 59(1 Suppl):143-154.

[8] Azad, A. A. L. I., Ibrahim, M. W. (2011). Reasons and Pattern of First Molar Extraction – A Study. *Pakistan Oral and Dental Journal*, 31(1):51-54.

[9] Mannocci, F., Cowie, J. (2014). Restoration of endodontically treated teeth. *Nature Publishing Group*, 216(6):341-346.

[10] Torabzadeh, H., Ghasemi, A., Dabestani, A., Razmavar, S. (2013). Fracture Resistance of Teeth Restored with Direct and Indirect Composite Restorations. *Journal of Dentistry, Tehran University of Medical Sciences*, 10(5):417-426.

[11] Hargreaves, K. M., Cohen, S., Berman, L. H. (2011). *Cohen's Pathways of the Pulp*. 10th ed. Mosby Elsevier.

[12] Bergenholtz, G., Axelsson, S., Davidson, T. et al. (2013). Treatment of pulps in teeth affected by deep caries – A systematic review of the literature. *Singapore Dental Journal*, 34(1):1-12.

[13] Polesel, A. (2014). Restoration of the endodontically treated posterior tooth. *Giornale Italiano di Endodonzia*, 28(1):2-16.

[14] Putri, A. M., Suprastiwi, E., Usman, M. (2018). Effects of Cleansing Methods on Shear Bond Strength of Nanohybrid Composite Resin to Enamel after Saliva and Blood Contamination during Bonding. *Journal of International Dental and Medical Research*, 11(3):888-892.

[15] Scotti, N., Andrea, F., Borga, C. et al. (2012). Is fracture resistance of endodontically treated mandibular molars restored with indirect onlay composite restorations influenced by fibre post insertion ? *Journal of Dentistry*, 40(10):814-820.

[16] Brunton, P. A., Cattell, P., Burke, F. J. T., Wilson, N. H. F. (1999). Fracture resistance of teeth restored with onlays of three contemporary tooth-colored resin-bonded restorative materials. *The journal of Prosthetic Dentistry*, 82:167-171.

In: Clinical Reports in Dentistry
Editor: Lisa R. Amir

ISBN: 978-1-53617-328-4

Chapter 36

DELAYED REPLANTATION OF AVULSED ANTERIOR MAXILLARY TEETH: A CASE REPORT

Ike D. Maharti**, Aditya W. Putranto and Shalina Ricardo

Department of Conservative Dentistry, Faculty of Dentistry,
Universitas Indonesia, Jakarta, Indonesia

ABSTRACT

Introduction: We reported a case of delayed replantation of two avulsed maxillary central incisors.

Case Report: A 12-year-old boy attended the dental clinic because of avulsed teeth due to a bike accident. The accident occurred while the child was cycling on paved roads. His parents brought the avulsed teeth to the clinic 2 h later in dry condition as they kept the teeth in a plastic bag after they cleaned the teeth using detergent. Intra-oral examination showed the blood was continuously discharged from the tooth socket and the maxillary permanent central incisors were avulsed. Radiograph revealed no alveolar bone wall fracture or other hard tissue injuries. The avulsed teeth showed large canals with closed apex and endodontic treatment was extra-orally performed just before they were replanted into the sockets.

Conclusion: Six-month observation after the replantation showed no pathological symptoms such as no mobility, negative palpation test and different sound in percussion test on the avulsed teeth.

Keywords: tooth replantation, avulsed tooth, root canal, trauma

* Corresponding Author's Email: ike_efendi@yahoo.com.

1. Introduction

An avulsed tooth is defined as a tooth that is completely out of its socket and may also be referred to an exarticulation or total luxation [1, 2]. An avulsed permanent tooth is an emergency case in dentistry and dentists should always be ready to give first aid advice for avulsed teeth to the public as these injuries could happen anywhere and at any time [3]. The most common causes of dental trauma and supporting structures include falling while running, traffic accidents, acts of violence and sports [4, 5]. Among all dental injuries, avulsions and intrusions are the most common sequelae [1, 2].

Treatment aim is to replant the avulsed tooth for as long as possible. While this treatment may save teeth, it is important to be aware that some replanted teeth have lower chances of long-term survival and may be lost or extracted at a later stage. The success of avulsed tooth treatment depends on the extra-oral time prior to replantation. The better prognosis is observed when the avulsed tooth is replanted in "golden hour" aftermath the accident [5]. Quality and timing of initial care contribute to a desirable outcome by promoting healing [1]. Contraindications of this treatment include severe caries or periodontal disease, non-cooperative patients and severe medical conditions such as immunosuppression, and autoimmune and severe cardiac conditions [1]. Replantation of a tooth more than 5 minutes is defined as delayed replantation [6]. Early resorption increases in teeth that have additional damages or contamination or are kept in dry conditions for longer than 15 minutes [7]. A follow-up evaluation and care are important for long-term successful outcomes. Here, we presented a case of delayed replantation of two avulsed maxillary central incisors after a 2-hour dry period and six months of observation.

2. Case Report

A 12-year-old boy suffered from an accident when he was cycling on paved roads two hours before he attended our dental clinic. The accident resulted avulsed maxillary teeth. His parents spent two hours seeking information about treatment for avulsed teeth before they decided to go to the dental clinic. The parents brought the dry avulsed teeth to the clinic in a plastic bag after cleaned them using detergent (Figure 1A).

An extra-oral examination revealed no clinical symptoms and intra-oral examination showed the blood was continuously discharged from the tooth socket and the maxillary permanent central incisors were avulsed (Figure 1B). The root surfaces were very clean and without any remnants of periodontal tissue. The adjacent teeth showed a positive response in a vitality test. The periapical area revealed no alveolar bone wall fracture or other hard tissue injuries (Figure 1C). No panoramic radiograph was recorded. The avulsed teeth showed large canals with closed apex. After an informed consent was obtained, the sockets of avulsed teeth were rinsed with saline solution under local anesthesia (*Pehacain*, Phapros Tbk, Indonesia). The avulsed teeth were soaked in saline while the sockets were rinsed. An extra-oral endodontic treatments were performed on the avulsed teeth. The cleaning and shaping phase were carried out using a Master Apical File #80/24 mm and 2.5% NaOCl as the irrigation agent. The root canals were then filled using the cold obturation technique (lateral condensation) with gutta percha and resin-based sealer (*AH Plus*, Dentsply) (Figure 2A).

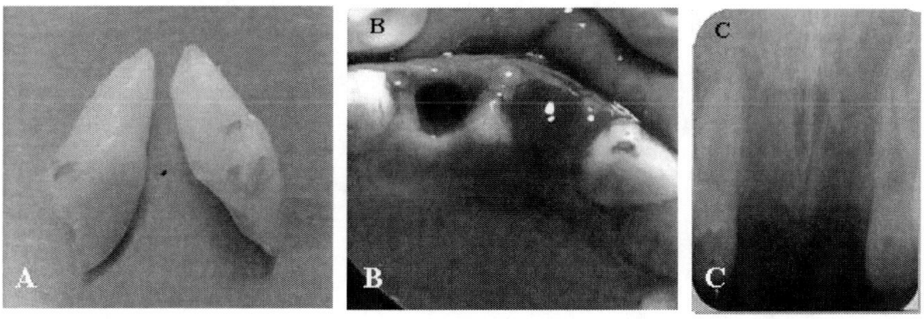

Figure 1. Two avulved maxillary central incisors (A); the tooth socket and bleeding, but no fracture was detected (B); Periapical radiograph showed no alveolar bone wall fracture or other hard tissue injuries (C).

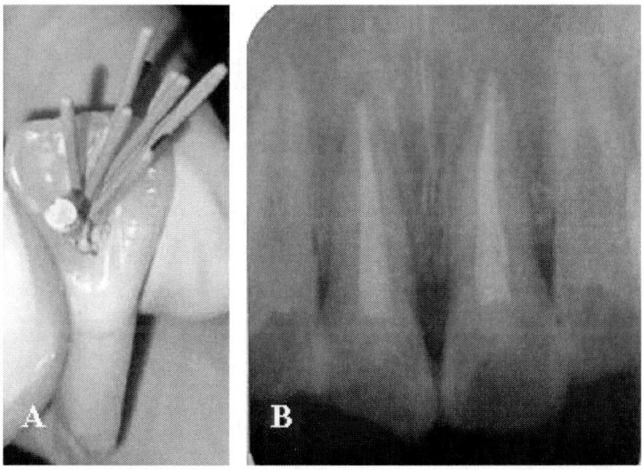

Figure 2. Extra-oral endodontic treatment of the avulsed teeth. The lateral condensation technique was used for obturation (A); The avulsed teeth were replanted into their original position that was confirmed radiographically (B).

The cavities were sealed with resin-modified glass ionomer cement (*SDR*, Dentsply). The replantation phase was carried out just after the extra-oral endodontic treatment was completed. The teeth were replanted gently into the sockets, and the patient was instructed to close their mouth to obtain a centric occlusion. The position of the replanted teeth was verified clinically as well as radiographically (Figure 2B). The teeth were subsequently stabilized using a splint with fiber strip and composite resin (*Z350*, 3M ESPE, USA) (Figure 3A). The patient was then given oral hygiene instructions to clean the teeth and splint, eat a soft diet, avoid using the anterior teeth during the stabilization period and use mouth rinse (*Minosep*, Minorock, Indonesia). Prophylactic antibiotic therapy of amoxicillin (*Amoxsan*, Caprifarmindo, Indonesia) at a dose of 750 mg/day for five days. The patient was referred for an anti-tetanus booster. The parents were requested to return regularly with the patient for clinical and radiographic follow-up.

The first observation was carried out two weeks after replantation without splint removal and showed no clinical or pathological changes (Figure 3B-C). The examination revealed no symptoms, well-adapted splint, good oral hygiene, and negative palpation and percussion test. The patient returned six months after replantation and the splint was finally removed. The examination demonstrated no pathological symptoms, no mobility, negative palpation test, and different sound in percussion test on the avulsed teeth (Figure 4).

3. Discussion

The maxillary central incisors are the most frequently avulsed teeth, while the lower jaw is seldom affected [2]. The level of the attachment apparatus of the avulsed tooth is essential when considering whether or not to replant the tooth. Radiographs and clinical examination are necessary to help detect possible alveolar fractures. In the present case, no panoramic radiograph was recorded but clinical examination showed there were no hard tissue injuries. The conditions of the avulsed tooth should be noted, such as contamination of the root surface, extra-alveolar period and storage condition. In the present case, the avulsed teeth had 2-hour extra-alveolar time and were cleaned using detergent and left dry. Although the incidence of dental trauma in the population aged 6 to 50 years is quite high, some are unaware of their dental injuries and choose to not seek dental treatment. This is the most common reason why immediate replantation cannot be carried out.

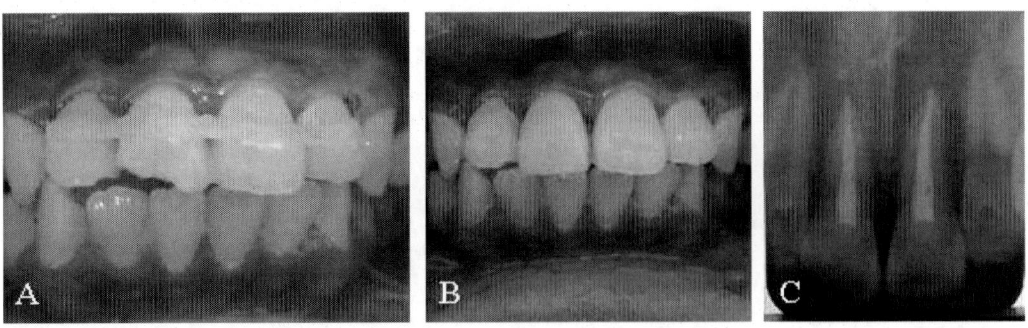

Figure 3. The teeth were stabilized using fiber strip splinting following replantation (A); 2-weeks follow-up (B); Radiograph showed no periapical lesion, no lamina dura appeared along the roots, and no ankylosis symptoms were detected (C).

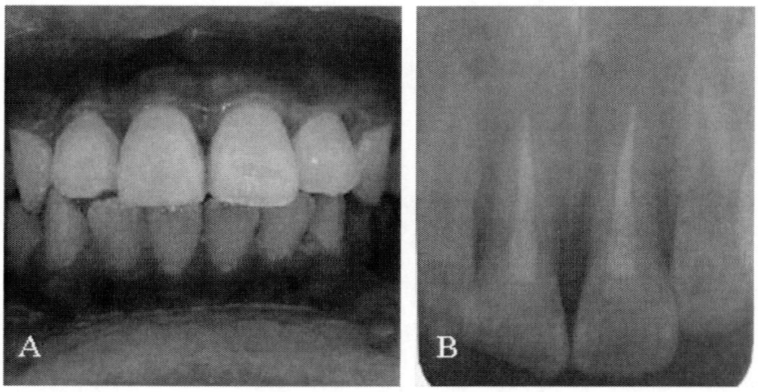

Figure 4. 6-months follow-up. The splint was finally removed (A); Radiograph revealed no periapical lesion, thin lamina dura was appeared along the lateral, and media canal 11 and 21, but not on the apical area (B).

According to treatment guidelines, scrubbing the avulsed tooth should be avoided to preserve the cells and fibers. Despite the unfavorable conditions in the present case, delayed replantation was still the treatment of choice due to the parents 'insistence and the young age of the patient. Early permanent tooth loss leads to severe arrest of alveolar bone development in a growing child. The alveolar ridge becomes narrow, making it difficult for prostheses/bridge/implant in the future. Andreason reported that there was a 95% chance of external resorption in teeth that had been out for more than 2 hours. A previous case report of an 11-year-old boy with 3-h delayed replantation highlighted the importance of replanting avulsed teeth even when conditions are not favorable. This case report showed that the absence of the infection is essential in the healing process. In this case, triple antibiotic paste containing ciprofloxacin, metronidazole and minocycline mixed with propylene glycol was used for root surface treatment and showed no evidence of resorption radiographically at 2-year follow-up [8]. However, this case did not use triple antibiotic paste because not available in the area. A similar case report of delayed replantation in a 22-year-old young adult with avulsed maxillary central incisors showed replacement resorption at the end of a nine-month observation period; however, the teeth remained functional and esthetically acceptable. The avulsed teeth had an extra-alveolar dry time of 24 hours and triple antibiotics treatment was not used [9].

The present case reports 2-hour delayed replantation because the parents did not know what to do. The availability and quality of the emergency services system, as well as information for traumatic dental injuries are necessary as the prognosis of these cases are decided at the scene of accident, in the first hours after the injury has occurred [3]. According to Ersin et al. (2013), there was a lack of knowledge of dental trauma and emergency procedures even among university student of School of Physical Education and Sports [10]. A replanted avulsed tooth may show excellent healing; however, if there is bacterial contamination or additional injury after the trauma incident, the resultant tooth resorption will lead to loss of the tooth [1]. This case demonstrated asepsis and sterile conditions as the basic principles of treatment. However, when severe damage cannot be avoided and osseous replacement is considered necessary, it is essential to slow the root replacement process by maintaining the tooth in the mouth as long as possible [11]. The possibility of ankylosis should be taken into consideration. Previous study reported despite of age, ankylosed incisors are frequently associated with infra-position and lack of physiological mobility [12].

In this case, the patient was prescribed a five-day course of amoxicillin to reduce bacterial contamination. The absence of bacteria could improve the periodontal healing. Fiber strip with composite resin was chosen to stabilize the replanted teeth in their original positions and allow the physiological movement of the teeth during healing. At the six-month evaluation we found a different sound in percussion test as root resorption character; however, no symptoms in subjective examination, and radiographic showed no periapical lesion. Nevertheless, the patient is still being followed up to determine the prognosis of the replanted teeth.

CONCLUSION

The avulsed teeth with delayed replantation technique may retain the dental arch and return functionality as long as it is performed in sterile conditions and follows comprehensive procedures. In cases of delayed replantation with no feasible storage, replantation should be performed, despite the risk of progressive replacement resorption and tooth loss. While this case report showed that this technique was successful after a six-month observation period, the patient still requires long-term periodic observation.

REFERENCES

[1] Trope M. (2008). *Endodontic considerations in dental trauma*. In: Ingle JI, Bakland LK, Baumgartner JC, editors. Ingle's endodontics 6. Hamilton: BC Decker Inc; p. 1330-1357.

[2] Andreasen JO, Andreasen FM. Avulsions. (2007). In: Andreasen JO, Andreasen FM, Andersson L, editors. *Textbook and color atlas of traumatic injuries to the teeth*. 4th Ed. Blackwell Munksgaard; p. 444-480.

[3] Alnaggar D, Andersson L. (2015). Emergency management of traumatic dental injuries in 42 countries. *Dent. Traumatol.*, 31:89-96. doi: 10.1111/edt.12155.

[4] Savas S, Kucukyilmaz E, Akcay M, Koseoglu S. (2015). Delayed replantation of avulsed teeth: two case reports. *Case Rep. Dent.*, Article ID 197202. doi: 10.1155/2015/197202.

[5] Andersson L, Andreasen JO, Day P, Heithersay G, Trope M, Diangelis AJ, et al. (2012). International association of dental traumatology guidelines for the

management of traumatic dental injuries: 2. Avulsion of permanent teeth. *Dent. Traumatol.*, 28:88-96. doi: 10.1111/j.1600-9657.2012.01125.x.

[6] Andreasen JO, Borum MK, Jacobsen HL, Andreasen FM. (1995). Replantation of 400 avulsed permanent incisors: 4. Factors related to periodontal healing. *Endod. Dent. Traumatol.,* 11:76-89. PMID: 7641622.

[7] Donaldson M, Kinirons MJ. (2001). Factors affecting the time of onset of resorption in avulsed and replanted incisor teeth in children. *Dent. Traumatol.*, 17:201-205. PMID: 11678538.

[8] Ravi KS, Pinky C, Kumar S, Vanka A. (2013). Delayed replantation of an avulsed maxillary premolar with open apex: A 24 months follow-up case report. *J. Indian Soc. Pedod. Prev. Dent.,* 31:201-204. doi: 10.4103/0970-4388.117971.

[9] Keshava Prasad BS, Praveen P. (2011). Delayed replantation of avulsed teeth: a case report. *Indian J. Dent. Sci.,* 3:26-28.

[10] Ersin N, Ertugrul F, Oncag O, Menderes M, Uzel I. (2013). Evaluation of high risk university students' knowledge about dental trauma and emergency procedures. *J. Int. Dent. Med. Res.,* 6(3):100-104.

[11] Trope M. (2002). Clinical management of the avulsed tooth: Present strategies and future directions. *Dent Traumatol.,* 18:1-11. PMID: 11841460.

[12] Bendoraitiene E, Zemgulyte S, Borisovaite M. (2017). Reasonable outcome of avulsed permanent upper incisor after seven years follow-up period: a case report. *J. Oral Maxillofac. Res.,* 8(4):e6. doi: *10.5037/jomr.2017.8406.*

In: Clinical Reports in Dentistry
Editor: Lisa R. Amir

ISBN: 978-1-53617-328-4

Chapter 37

DELAYED REPLANTATION OF AVULSED TEETH WITH 8-HOUR EXTRA ORAL TIME

Iffi Aprillia**[*] **and Munyati Usman
Department of Conservative Dentistry, Faculty of Dentistry,
Universitas Indonesia, Jakarta, Indonesia

ABSTRACT

Introduction: Dental avulsion is defined as a complete removal of tooth from the alveolar socket resulting in the complete disruption of blood supply to the pulp. Dental replantation is indicated for avulsed teeth with viable and aseptic periodontal ligament cells. Replantation is associated with the insertion and temporary fixation of avulsed teeth and aims to prevent tooth loss, so the function and aesthetic value of the tooth can be maintained as well as the height of alveolar ridges.

Case report: A 9-year-old male patient with the chief complaint of the first maxillary incisor having been released due to a fall. The avulsed tooth was carefully replanted in its original position after an extra oral root canal treatment, and a semi rigid splinting was consequently performed using the Ivy eyelet wiring ligation technique.

Conclusion: The risk of root resorption in replantation case is relatively high and relays on the clinical conditions of the periodontal ligament, apical foramen closure, duration of extra oral time and the age of patient.

Keywords: replantation, dental avulsion, root resorption

1. INTRODUCTION

Avulsion can be defined as a form of trauma that results in the complete removal of teeth from the socket, particularly maxillary incisors, and is very common in children

[*] Corresponding Author's Email: aprillia.iffi@gmail.com.

aged 7 – 14 years [1]. Replantation is an alternative treatment for tooth avulsion that can restore the physiological and aesthetic functions of tooth. The success of replantation is not measured by whether the tooth will remain vital and functional over the lifespan of patient; instead, maintaining the tooth and the height of the alveolar bone for the following few years can be a benchmark for treatment success and will be very influential for the prognosis of subsequent treatments [1]. The success of a replantation treatment is strongly influenced by several factors, such as the time that the tooth is outside the mouth, medium used for storage prior to replantation and systemic condition of the patient. Furthermore, an interesting and valid concern is dental avulsion often occurs in location that is far from the health centers; thus, it is essential to educate the public in regard to the emergency handling of an avulsed tooth as it may increase the percentage of successful treatments.

2. CASE REPORT

A 9-year-old male patient visited the dental conservation specialist clinic of Universitas Indonesia Dental Hospital with his chief complaint of his first maxillary incisor that avulsed when he fell on a train from Surabaya to Jakarta in about 8 hours at prior to his arrival at hospital. There was no history of unconsciousness or vomiting upon injury. During the trip to the hospital, the detached tooth was washed and stored in fresh milk at room temperature.

An extra-oral examination revealed no abnormalities. An intra-oral examination revealed a fracture in the labial alveolar wall, but there were no residual tooth fragments in the socket. Radiographic examination was performed to ensure that no fracture fragments of bone and tooth in the tooth socket were subjected to the avulsion (Figure 1A). The buccal area was anesthetized using infiltration techniques prior to the cleaning of the socket to remove any blood clot so it may not inhibit the replantation process. Simultaneous to the preparation of patient for replantation, the avulsed tooth was carefully cleaned using saline and prophylactic. An opening access and extirpation of the pulp was extra-orally performed, followed by a root canal preparation and obturation using gutta-percha and MTA-based sealer.

Subsequently, an incision was made in the apical third of the socket, and the tooth was carefully replanted in its original position. A Semi-rigid splinting to the adjacent teeth was performed using the Ivy eyelet wiring ligation technique (Figure 1B).

The patient's occlusion was checked and no premature contact on the tooth was found. To restore aesthetics, the incisor was repositioned parallel to the incisal line of the adjacent tooth.

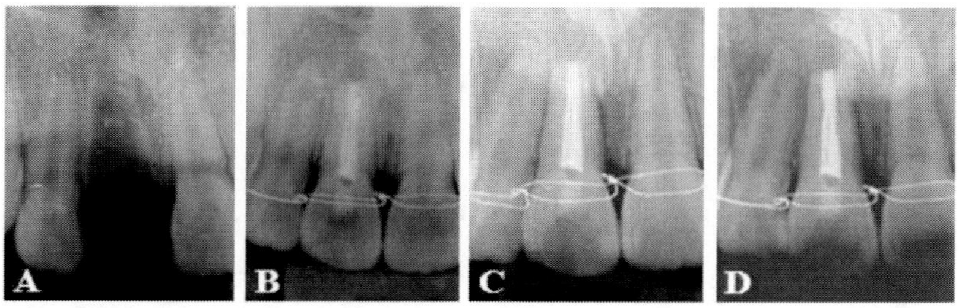

Figure 1. A radiograph at prior to replantation (A); Following replantation and splinting (B); 1-month post-replantation (C); C) 3-month post-replantation (D)

The patient was prescribed 500mg amoxicillin, 500mg metronidazole, and 500mg mefenamic acid three times a day for 5 days and was recommended soft diet during splinting. The patient was also advised to maintain oral cavity cleanliness to prevent secondary infection and to return for 1- and 3-month follow-ups. Splinting was released at the 3-month follow-up appointment, but the patient was encouraged to attend regular follow-ups in the fourth and sixth months.

One month after replantation, a radiolucent feature appeared on the mesial root surface from the direction of the gingival margins to two thirds apical (Figure 1C) but this feature was reduced at the 3-month follow-up (Figure 1D). The radiolucent is dissapeared in the sixth month Clinically, the patient did not complain of pain or mobility of the tooth following the release of splinting; however, the patient will continue to be monitored and may be given further treatment as needed.

3. Discussion

According to the International Association of Dental Traumatology, the performance of a permanent dental treatment procedure to repair avulsed teeth depends on two conditions, namely apical edge maturation (open or closed apex) and the condition of the periodontal ligament cells (Table 1) [2].

The success rate of replantation is closely related to the patient's medical history, apical edge maturity, duration of time that the tooth is outside the oral cavity and the storage medium prior to replantation. Following tooth avulsion, the periodontal ligament (PDL) and pulp tissue will be damaged; the PDL becomes disconnected, leaving behind a number of cells on the surface of the root, and the pulp tissue will experience necrosis in conjunction with the breakdown of blood supply through the apical foramen.

If the PDL cells remaining on the root surface do not dehydrate and die, then the success rate of dental replantation is very high because these cells can trigger the healing process by regeneration from the PDL without causing excessive inflammation [1].

Table 1. Dental protocols to repair permanent teeth undergoing avulsion [4]

Clinical Situation	Treatment
Teeth are immediately replanted following avulsion	Clean the wound area with water, saline, or chlorhexidine. Suture the part that experienced laceration. Confirm the clinical position of the tooth by radiography. Perform splinting for 2 weeks. Prescribe antibiotics. Perform root canal treatment 7 – 10 days following replantation before the splint is removed
Teeth replanted in <60 min following avulsion after being stored in special media	Clean the root surface and apical foramen using a flow saline and soak the teeth in saline. Irrigate the sockets using saline to remove any blood clot that have formed. Reposition the walls of the alveolar bone in case of fracture. Carefully replant the teeth back in the socket. Perform gingival suture if there is laceration. Confirm the clinical position of the tooth by radiography. Perform splinting for 2 weeks. Prescribe antibiotics. Perform root canal treatment 7 – 10 days following replantation before the splint is removed.
Teeth replanted >60 min following avulsion	Eliminate all necrotic tissues from the root surface. Perform root canal treatment prior to replantation, but it can also be performed 7 – 10 days following replantation. Irrigate sockets using saline to remove any blood clot that may have formed. Reposition the walls of the alveolar bone in case of fracture. Carefully replant the teeth back in the socket. Perform gingival suture if there is laceration. Confirm the clinical position of the tooth by radiography. Perform splinting for 4 – 6 weeks. Prescribe antibiotics.

The viability of PDL cells may still be possible if dental replantation is immediately performed following the occurrence of avulsion or within 60min but is considered unlikely when the tooth has been outside the socket for a longer period of time, even if it was stored in a proper media [2]. The condition of the PDL is highly dependent on the storage medium while the tooth is outside the oral cavity. The recommended storage media in case of avulsion are milk, saliva, saline, or Hank's Balanced Salt Solution [3]. In this case, the patient used milk, which has an osmolarity and pH suitable for the survival of PDL for over 8 hours [3]. The duration of time that a tooth is outside the oral cavity also greatly affects the viability of the PDL; perfect healing can be obtained if the avulsed tooth is immediately replanted within the first 5min, but if the length of time exceeds 60min before it is inserted into storage medium, then the PDL will likely be no longer viable [1]. The pulp tissue of an avulsed tooth will undergo necrosis. If no endodontic treatment is performed, then this necrotic pulp tissue will cause an inflammatory response. Such an inflammatory response caused by the necrotic pulp tissue and PDL cells can cause aggressive external resorption, which will continue to occur until the bacteria in the pulp and root canal are removed. As a result, there will be alveolar bone loss that will eventually cause tooth loss [1].

In this case, the tooth had been washed prior to its immersion in storage media and had been outside the oral cavity for more than > 60min; thus, the possibility of a viable PDL was very small. The operator, therefore, cleaned all necrotic tissues from the root surface to minimize an excessive inflammatory response following replantation. Extra-oral endodontic treatment was also performed to remove the necrotic pulp tissue. Obturation using a sealer containing MTA was performed because it stimulates the regeneration of hard tissues around the apical end. The calcium hydroxide released by MTA has an antibacterial effect and renders the environment around the apex more alkaline [5]. An alkaline pH stimulates cell activation for the resorption of necrotic and bacterial tissues and triggers alkaline phosphatase for the formation of hard tissues.

An incision in the apical third of the socket was performed, considering that there are several ramifications that can increase the probability of necrotic tissue in this area and inhibition of the healing process. The tooth socket was carefully cleaned to ensure the removal of any bone or tooth fragment that may reduce the efficiency of replantation. In this case, the operator repositioned the labial alveolar wall using a blunt instrument from inside the socket. The existing blood clot was slowly irrigated with sterile saline and aspirated using suction.

In this case, semi-rigid splinting was performed using the Ivy eyelet wiring technique, which allows the teeth to physiologically move under little pressure and facilitates the maintenance of oral health. Splinting used in the case of replantation of avulsed teeth should not exert excessive pressure because this increases the risk of resorption [6]. Composite splinting was attempted first, but the presence of blood made it difficult for the composite to properly adhere. The recommended length of fixation ranges from 7 to 10 days; however, 1 week is sufficient time for the periodontal ligament to support the tooth in position. Shorter fixation durations will decrease the rate of ankylosis; nevertheless, in cases in which there is a fracture on the alveolar wall, the length of fixation time may be extended to 8 weeks [1].

There exist four scenarios of periodontal tissue healing in cases of replantation [7]: 1) healing with the formation of a normal periodontal ligament. This radiographic feature of healing shows a normal dura lamina with no resorption on either the surface of the root or the adjacent alveolar bone; 2) healing accompanied by resorption of the root surface. This radiographic healing shows the appearance of superficial resorption surrounded by a newly formed cementum. This process is usually self-limiting, and dental clinical conditions look normal without complaints; 3) healing accompanied by the occurrence of ankylosis. This type of healing is associated with the loss of viability of the periodontal tissue on the surface of the root. This radiographic healing is characterized by resorption on the root surface due to osteoclast activity, which is replaced by the formation of the surrounding bone and loss of the lamina dura; and 4) healing accompanied by inflammatory resorption. The radiographs show a radiolucent area located between the alveolar bone and the root surface.

In this case, the resorption on the surface of the mesial root was seen in the first month following replantation, and the lamina dura in the mesial part of the root wasalso disappeared. However, in the third until sixth month, the radiolucent image was diminished and replaced by an image of new alveolar bone. The lamina dura remained invisible. The patient was advised to attend follow-up appointments at 6, 12, and 24 months for further evaluation.

Conclusion

Replanted teeth that have been delayed for longer than an hour still have a promising level of treatment success. In this case, keeping the tooth in a good position to maintain the height of the alveolar bone until the patient is old enough, thus, it may provide a good prognosis for subsequent treatment.

References

[1] Trope, M. (2011). Avulsion of permanent teeth: theory to practice. *Dental traumatology*, 27 (4): 410 - 427.

[2] Anderson, L., Andreasen, J. O., Day, P. et al. (2012). Avulsion of permanent teeth. International Association of Dental Traumatology guidelines for the management of traumatic dental injuries (2). *Dental traumatology*, 28 (2): 88 - 96.

[3] Tufenkci, P., Canbolat, F., Celikten, B., Sevimay, S. (2017). Reimplantation of an avulsed tooth after five hours of storage in milk: One-year follow-up case report. *Case report in internal medicine*, 4 (4).

[4] Flores, M. T., Andersson, L., Andreasen, J. O. et al. (2007). Avulsion of permanent teeth. Guidelines for thr management of traumatic dental injuries (II). *Dental Traumatology*, 23 (3): 130 - 106.

[5] Savas, S., Kucukyilmaz, E., Akcay, M., Koseoglu, S. (2015). Delayed replantation of avulsed teetht: two case reports. *Case Rep. Dent.*, 2015:197202.

[6] Sardana, D., Goyal, A., Gauba, K. (2014). Delayed replantation of avulsed tooth with 15 hours extra-oral time: 3-year follow-up. *Singapore Dent. J.*, 35:71 - 76.

[7] Johnson, W. T. (2002). *Color atlas of Endodontics*. Philadelphia: WB Saunders Company. p. 180 - 186.

In: Clinical Reports in Dentistry
Editor: Lisa R. Amir

ISBN: 978-1-53617-328-4

Chapter 38

CASE SERIES MANAGEMENT OF ENDO-PERIO LESIONS WITH CONVENTIONAL ROOT CANAL TREATMENT

Shalina Ricardo[1,*], Astinah[2], Kamizar[1] and Nurmeisari[2]
[1]Department of Conservative Dentistry, Faculty of Dentistry,
Universitas Indonesia, Jakarta, Indonesia
[2]Conservative Dentistry Residency Program, Faculty of Dentistry,
Universitas Indonesia, Jakarta, Indonesia

ABSTRACT

Introduction: Pulp inflammation can extend to the periodontium causing damage to the periodontal tissue. The relationship between pulp and periodontium occurs due to their interconnected vascularization and their close proximity to each other. Diagnosing endo-perio lesions can be challenging because pulp tissue and periodontium previously have been studied separately, and one primary disease had characteristics similar to the other.

Case report: This case reported two cases of endo-perio lesions that were performed in a conventional root canal treatment via sequential endodontic and periodontal treatments. Follow-up radiographs demonstrated the complete healing of the hard and soft tissue lesions.

Conclusion: Endodontic treatment performed with proper cleaning and shaping and specific medication, followed by periodontal treatment could be successful in treating endo-perio lesions.

Keywords: endo-perio lesion, conventional root canal treatment, scaling root planing

* Corresponding Author's Email: shalinaricardo@gmail.com

1. INTRODUCTION

Inflammation of the pulp can extend to the periodontium causing damage to the periodontal tissue. This is referred as retrograde periodontitis as well as retrograde pulpitis. Periodontal lesions can occur due to inflammation radiating from the periodontal tissue due to the pulpal inflammatory response [1].

The proper diagnosis and careful treatment are necessary in cases involving the pulp tissue and periodontium. The relationship between pulp and periodontium occurs because of their interconnected vascularization and close proximity to each other. Diagnosing endo-perio lesions is often challenging because pulp tissue and periodontium were previously studied separately, and one primary disease had characteristics similar to the other [2, 3, 5].

The root structure of the tooth separates pulp tissue from the periodontium. Normally, the periodontium is not affected by pulp disease. However, the presence of acute inflammation of the pulp can increase intrapulpal pressure so that inflammatory products could be pushed out through the apical foramen and accessory canals [3]. Periapical abscesses pass through the periodontal ligament to the gingival sulcus and periodontal pockets gradually over time.

Endodontic infection causes inflammatory changes in the periodontal tissue and can damage the epithelium attached to the tooth surface. Conversely, pulp disease can also affect the periodontium. According to the most studies, periodontal disease involves the pulp, manifesting as inflammation, calcification, secondary dentine deposition and root resorption [4, 8, 10].

Cohen classified combined endo-perio lesions as a combination of pure and concomitant lesions. As previously explained, both of these lesions have an etiology and course of endodontic and periodontal disease, respectively. The difference is the endo-perio concomitant lesions have not been united [2]. Proper diagnosis and preliminary consideration are very important prior to determining a treatment plan. Diagnosis can be established by recording the history of the disease from the patient, performing a clinical examination, and obtaining a history of illnesses including trauma and pain. The diagnosis of primary and periodontal-endodontic lesions is typically quite easy. Primary endodontic lesions have infected pulp and non-vital status, whereas primary periodontal lesions have vital pulp that is sensitive to vitality tests [5].

But diagnosing other lesions is difficult because they have similar clinical and radiographic features. Primary endodontic lesions usually resolve with endodontic treatment alone. Sinus tract that travels toward the gingival sulcus or furcation area disappears immediately after root canal treatment. At 4-6 months after PSA, healing usually occurs, periodontal pockets disappear, and bone formation occurs [6].

Although large radiolucent lesions and periodontal abscesses may be present, surgical procedures are not necessary in this case, and invasive periodontal treatment should be avoided as it may further damage the epithelial attachment and delay healing [4]. Healing of primary endodontic lesions with secondary periodontal involvement will not occur perfectly with endodontic treatment alone [7, 8].

2. Case Report

2.1. Case 1

A 27-year-old female patient presented to the Department of Conservative Dentistry, Universitas Indonesia, with the chief complaint of pain, swelling and mobility from the lower right premolar within the previous 2 weeks. The patient was uncomfortable while eating and chewing. Clinical evaluation identified 45 tooth has vitality (−), percussion (+), palpation (+), grade 2 mobility, gingival edema and fistula at the buccal region. Periodontal probing depths were 5 mm mesiobuccal and 4 mm mesiolabial. The periapical radiograph revealed widening of the periodontal ligament in the periapical area with an infrabony defect on the mesial aspect of the tooth. She was diagnosed with an endo-perio lesion associated with the mandibular second premolar.

We prepared an access cavity, cleaning and shaping the root canal using ProTaper in the first session with 2.5% sodium hypochlorite and 17% EDTA as irrigant. The canal was dressed temporarily with calcium hydroxide ($Ca[OH])_2$ and the access cavity sealed with temporary fillings. Scaling and root planing were done immediately following the root canal treatment. The patient returned after 2 weeks with no pain or signs of inflammation indicating that the final filling could be placed. Obturation was completed with gutta-percha and a root canal sealer (Figure 1A-B). The tooth was restored with composite onlay 1 week later. Follow-up at 1 month revealed a stable situation and no pain.

2.2. Case 2

A 50-year-old female patient presented to Department of Conservative Dentistry, Universitas Indonesia, with the primary complaint of loose front teeth. The upper left front teeth had been restored in the previous year due to caries in the front near the gum. Two weeks prior to her visit, her teeth suddenly experienced radiating, throbbing pain, swelling in the back part of the gum and the teeth felt loose. Finally, the patient went to a private dental clinic for treatment where she was examined for swelling behind the back of the teeth, and she was given temporary fillings, prescribed antibiotics and pain reliever and referred to a conservative dentistry specialist for further treatment. She worried that her teeth would fall out due to their mobility. Her attitude was cooperative and she desired to maintain her teeth. The patient had a temporary palatal restoration with the cavity reaching the pulp. There was grade 3 mobility, 2.5 mm gingival recession, abnormalities when teeth were dislodged sensitivity to percussion testing, palpation of the palatal gingiva, and clinically appearing red and swollen gingiva in the palatal area (Figure 2A). All regions had plaque and calculus, and the patient claimed to have had the tartar cleaned off her teeth in the previous 3 months, illustrating that her oral hygiene was still poor.

Radiograph showed normal pulp chamber features at tooth 22, normal root canals, normal roots, dilated periodontal space, and interrupted lamina dura (Figure 2B). In addition, the periapical region showed diffuse, radiolucent lesions at the middle two-thirds of the root ±7 mm in diameter. Vertical alveolar bone resorption is shown in the mesial and distal regions. The patient presented with a major complaint of mobility of tooth 22 and no pain. Therefore, temporary splints were applied as fixation using fiber-reinforced composite material on tooth 22 that joined with 21 and 23. The materials used were Fiber Strands (Biodental TM Australia) and flowable composites (Kerr Dental, California USA).

After the splint was placed, root canal treatment started with an access cavity and was cleaned and shaped using ProTaper with sodium hypochlorite 2.5% and EDTA 17% as an irrigant (Figure 2C) . The canal was dressed temporarily with calcium hydroxide $(CaOH)_2$ and the access cavity sealed with temporary fillings. Scaling and root planing were performed after the root canal treatment. The patient returned again after 2 weeks with no pain or signs of inflammation, indicating that the final filling could be placed. Obturation was completed with gutta-percha and a root canal sealer (Figure 2D-F). Next, the tooth was restored with composite resin. The patient was stable at 1-month follow-up with no pain. At 6-month follow-up, the lesions were significantly improved, radiograph confirmed bone formation. Periodontal treatment was planned to obtain perfect marginal healing.

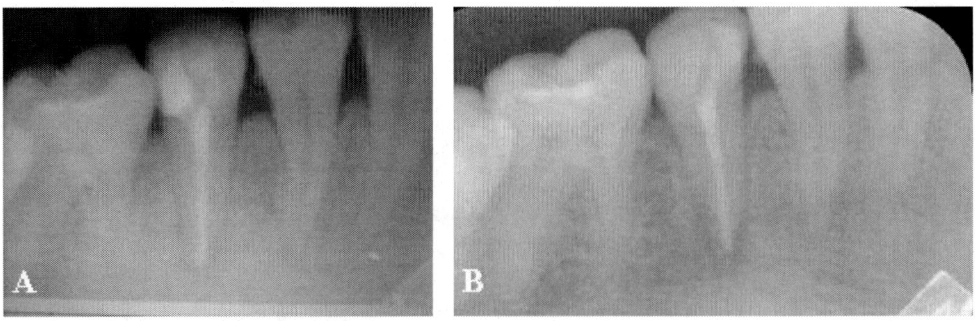

Figure 1. *Case 1*, Obturation showed the obturation material precisely at the apex (A); The tooth restored with composite onlay. The lesion was not completely healed at 1 month (B).

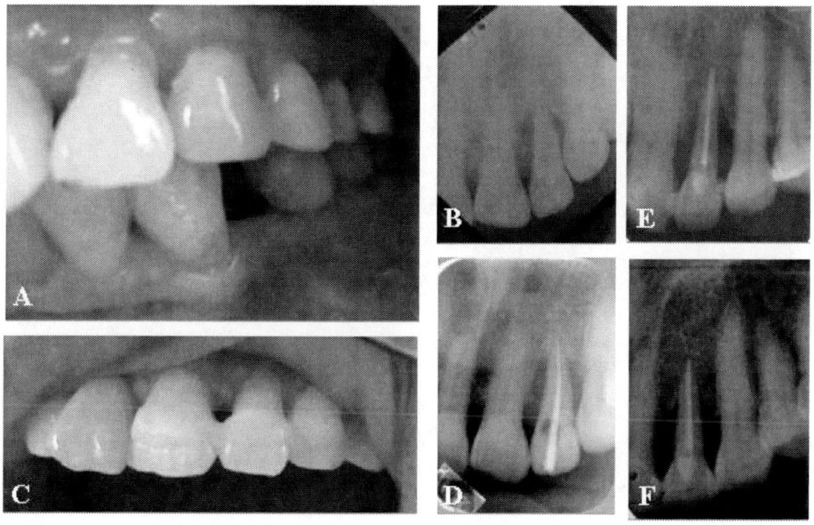

Figure 2. *Case 2*, Gingival recession (A); An overview of endo-perio lesions. On the mesial side, bone damage appears endo-perio lesions have met (pure combination). (B); Splint was placed to fixate the mobile tooth (C); Master cone adaptation during root canal treatment (D); Obturation was completed and the tooth restored with composite resin (E); Progressive healing process with bone formation (F).

3. DISCUSSION

Endo-perio lesions affect the pulp and periodontal tissue. Endo-perio lesions can occur because of the relationship or communication between the pulp and periodontal tissue [2]. Endo-perio lesions in these patients are classified as pure combination endo-perio lesions because the course of the disease is individual and finally the two lesions meet [1, 2, 3, 9, 10]. Periapical lesions due to pulp disease cause pressure on the periapical tissue and sinus tracts form in the periodontal tissue, resulting in epithelial attachment loss from apical to marginal. The disease condition is aggravated by the accumulation of plaque and calculus, which is exacerbated by the presence of palatogingival grooves on the tooth. The diagnosis in these patients is considered a pure combination endo-perio lesion, and endodontic treatment is planned, and the patient referred for periodontal treatment [1, 2, 4, 8].

A ProTaper file was chosen because of its large taper for facilitating irrigation for debridement. Considering the magnitude of periodontal tissue damage, preparation must be approached with care. The electronic apex locator was used to determine the working length to shorten time using initial file no. 20, and working length was confirmed radiographically after root canal preparation [1, 3].

2.5% NaOCl was used in the preparation to dissolve necrotic pulp tissue, and the root canal was prepared with a ProTaper hand file. The root canal was re-irrigated and given a $Ca(OH)_2$ medicament. The primary action of this material is achieved through dissociation of Ca^{2+} and OH ions, which can interact with vital tissue (in this case, the periodontal network) and can induce hard tissue deposition and antimicrobial effects [6]. On the second visit, the patient had no subjective complaints and was not sensitive to percussion or palpation testing. Next, it was decided to obtain obturation as soon as possible. The filler material used was size F4 gutta-percha with lateral condensation techniques. AH 26 sealer was used because of its density; thus, hermetic filling is expected to prevent bacterial invation [1, 5, 6, 7].

Conclusion

Endodontic treatment performed with proper cleaning and shaping, specific medication, followed by periodontal treatment could be successful in treating endo-perio lesions. Periodontal treatment needed to restore gingival attachment by scaling and root planing and reconstructing the attachment. Six-month follow-up showed new bone formation and no signs of mobility.

References

[1] Varma B, Nayak R. (2002). *Current concepts in periodontics.* New Delhi: Arya (Medi) Publishing House.

[2] Kerns D, Glickman G. (2010). Endodontic and periodontal interrelationships. In: Hargreaves K, Cohen S, editors. *Cohen's Pathways of the Pulp*. 10th ed. St Louis: Mosby Elsevier. pp. 655-670.

[3] Peeran SW, Thiruneervannan M, Abdalla KA, Mugrabi MH. (2013). Endo-perio lesions. *International Journal of Scientific and Technology Research*, 2(5):268-274.

[4] Singh P. (2011). Endo-Perio dilemma: a brief review. *Dental Research Journal*, 8(1):39-47.

[5] Barzilay I. (2000). Splinting teeth - a review of methodology and clinical case reports. *Journal of the Canadian Dental Association*, 66(8):440-443.

[6] Mohammadi Z, Dummer PMH. (2011). Properties and applications of calcium hydroxide in endodontics and dental traumatology. *International Endodontic Journal*, 44(8):697-730.

[7] Bruce R. (2002). Interrelationship of Pulpal and Periodontal Diseases. In: Kenneth M. Hargreaves (editor). *Seltzer & Benders Dental Pulpa.* Quintessence Publishing Co, Inc. pp. 411-422.

[8] Newman, Michael G et al. (2006). *Carranza's Clinical Periodontology*, 10th Ed. Philadelphia: W. B. Saunders Company. pp. 871-879.

[9] Nina Shenoy, Arvind Shenoy. (2010). Endo-perio lesions: Diagnosis and clinical considerations. *Indian J. Dent. Res.*, 21(4).

[10] Akreli KV. (2002). *Canal Preparation*. In: Johnson WT (Ed). *Color Atlas of Endodonthics*. Philadelphia: WB Saunders Co. pp. 70-80.

In: Clinical Reports in Dentistry
Editor: Lisa R. Amir

ISBN: 978-1-53617-328-4

Chapter 39

TREATMENT OF TRAUMA FROM OCCLUSION AND PERIODONTAL ABSCESS CAUSED BY IMPROPER SIZE OF PROSTHETIC CROWN: A CASE REPORT

Sandra O. Kuswandani*, Natalina and Yulianti Kemal
Department of Periodontics, Faculty of Dentistry,
Universitas Indonesia, Jakarta, Indonesia

ABSTRACT

Introduction: Application of fixed prosthetics can cause periodontal problems. Improper sizing and placement of fixed prosthetics can endanger the periodontal system in several ways, including causing gingival inflammation problems or trauma from occlusion that inhibits attachment and causes bony defects. We reported the treatment of occlusional trauma caused by improper prosthetic crown sizing.

Case report: A 75-year-old man presented with complaints of pain when chewing and eating. He underwent anamnesis, dental, periodontal examinations and radiography. Treatment planning was made from initial therapy through the rehabilitation phase. After 3 months he was re-evaluated. The patient's main complaint of pain disappeared after coronoplasty, but this treatment did not reduce the pocket depth. A flap operation that used a combination of DFDBA and pericardium membrane successfully reduced pocket depth, loss of attachment and intrabony defects after 3 months of follow-up.

Conclusion: Improper fixed prosthetic sizing can cause trauma from occlusion, pain, increased pocket depth and loss of attachment. In this case, coronoplasty successfully eliminated pain. Flap surgery is an effective means of reducing pocket depth and mitigating loss of attachment. Periodontal professionals should consider the prosthetic implant's size, placement and the occlusal loading of periodontal ligament as a result of prosthetic placement so as to prevent traumatic occlusion.

* Corresponding Author's Email: sandra.olivia01@ui.ac.id.

Keywords: coronoplasty, demineralized freeze-dried bone allograft, guided tissue regeneration

1. Introduction

One function of fixed prosthetics is the restoration of teeth after root canal treatments. When fabricating a fixed prosthesis, the practitioner must determine the periodontal status of the involved abutment teeth. This allows for the generation of a reliable and accurate prognosis for restoration. Periodontal disease is the major cause of tooth loss in adults, therefore it is important for dentists to be aware of basic periodontal concepts and available therapies to be able to develop an appropriate diagnosis and treatment plan [1].

Fixed prosthetics should address a number of periodontal considerations. First, from the patient's perspective, oral hygiene is an important factor. Second, the material and design of the fixed prosthesis should be carefully considered. Third, the preparation and placement of fixed prostheses require careful consideration, as do the maintenance and prognosis associated with fixed prostheses [2].

In the field of restorative dentistry, fixed prostheses are risk factors for periodontal disease. Many local factors can increase plaque deposition and retention, inhibit plaque control, and contribute to the development of gingivitis and periodontitis. These factors are termed *contributory* because they do not, by themselves, initiate gingival inflammation. Rather, they foster increased or long-standing plaque accumulation and make plaque removal more difficult [3]. The surface texture and contour of fixed prosthetics can increase the risk of gingival inflammation and periodontal disease. Improperly sized or placed fixed prosthetics can endanger the periodontium, causing gingival inflammation problems, and potentially traumatizing the tissue, loosening attachments and contributing to intrabony defects. Heavy occlusal forces can cause clinical tooth mobility and apparent bone loss on radiography. However, these changes involve periodontal ligaments and bone, and not the marginal gingival surface tissue. Trauma-induced pathologic lesions in the attachment apparatus can cause loss of the alveolar and crestal lamina dura and result in widening of the periodontal ligament space [4, 5].

Abscess formation can occur acutely. Coronoplasty and selective grinding are treatment options for trauma from occlusion. Flap surgery and bone grafting with demineralized freeze-dried bone allograft (DFDBA) and pericardium membrane are treatment options for intrabony defects. We reported coronoplasty for the treatment of trauma from occlusion caused by improper sizing of a prosthetic crown. Additionally, treatment of an intrabony defect using a combination of DFDBA and pericardium membrane was carried out.

2. Case Report

A 75-year-old male was referred to the Periodontology Department, Universitas Indonesia, complaining of pain in his mandibular right tooth when chewing (Figure 1). The initial examination revealed probing depths of the second molar mandible right tooth of 7mm on the mesial side and 5mm on the buccal side, with bleeding on probing (BOP) and no tooth mobility.

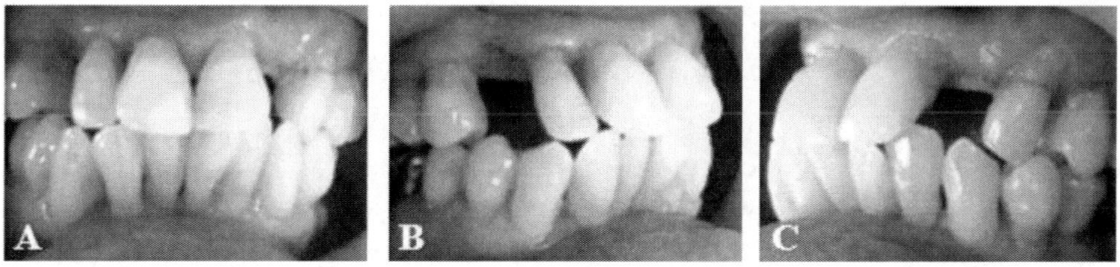

Figure 1. Initial clinical presentation

Suppuration was registered at the buccal side of the right mandibular second molar. In 2001, the patient underwent placement of a fixed prosthetic with a metal jacket crown, after root canal treatment of the first and second right mandibular molars. A tooth mobility between second and third degrees was noted on the anterior mandibular and maxillary teeth. Oral hygiene was already moderate and gingival inflammation was observed (full mouth score, plaque index: 1.2; and bleeding on probing index: 1.1). The patient was in good general health, had never smoked, and routinely took medication for high blood pressure (his hypertension was well-controlled). Almost all of his teeth exhibited gingival recession. Malpositioned teeth were apparent on the anterior side of both the maxillary and mandibular surfaces. He underwent periodontal surgery to the left mandibular side; however, the surgery was not successful, and he ultimately underwent tooth extraction. He had not received periodontal therapy since 2001 and denied any familial history of periodontitis.

After one appointment (including oral hygiene instructions, supragingival scaling, and polishing), we recorded the probing depth, clinical attachment level, furcation involvement, teeth mobility, plaque index, BOP, and the presence of suppuration. We obtained a panoramic radiograph and standard radiography of the right first and second mandibular molars (Figure 2A). Deep infrabony defects were seen in the mesial root of the second mandibular molar on the right, from the gingiva, to the furcation of the tooth. Based on the patient's main complaints, clinical diagnosis, periodontal examination and radiographic record, we confirmed the diagnosis of periodontal abscess and trauma from occlusion caused by root and crown imbalance and improper sizing of the fixed prosthetic. We addressed the patient's main complaint of pain.

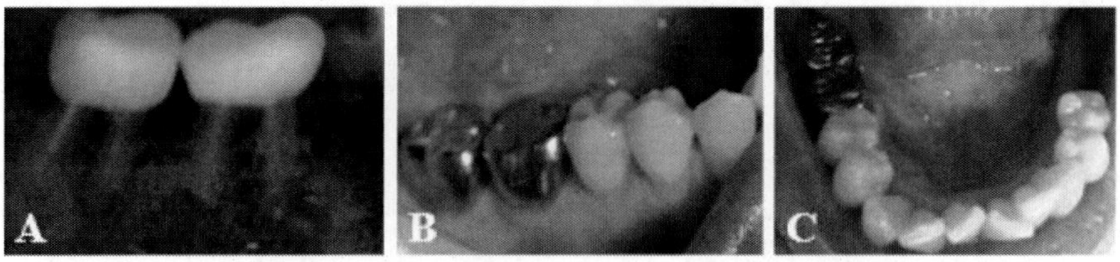

Figure 2. Dental radiograph before treatment (A); After coronoplasty (B); Maintenance therapy (C).

The abscess was drained using finger pressure to produce purulent drainage, through the otherwise intact surface of the mucosa. The treated sites were repeatedly irrigated with 3% hydrogen peroxide and we compressed the gingiva using cotton rolls. Treatment focused on eliminating the causes of trauma. Coronoplasty was completed and included selective grinding to reshape the occlusal surface of the teeth to improve the contact and balance ratio of the root and crown of the tooth (Figure 2B). We reshaped approximately 1 mm of the buccal and lingual surfaces of the metal jacket crown on the first and second right mandibular molar with a flame bur.

After addressing the patient's main complaint, we performed scaling and root planning (SRP) during a full mouth procedure. The patient was advised to rinse twice daily for 1 minute with 15ml of a 0.2% chlorhexidine solution (KIN) for 1 week. Starting with SRP, we prescribed systemic antibiotics (amoxicillin 500mg, metronidazole 250mg, both three times a day for 5 days), and an analgesic (mefenamic acid 500mg). The follow-up was performed one week after. By the patient's second visit (following coronoplasty), his main complaint of pain was resolved, and the abscess was healed, but there was no difference in pocket depth. Thus, planning for periodontal surgery commenced. Following 6 months of maintenance therapy, we observed no differences in probing depth (Figure 2C).

The vertical bone defect and the infrabony defect on the mesial root of the second right mandibular molar required a surgical intervention. We performed flap surgery using a combination of DFDBA and pericardium membrane to reduce the pocket depth, mitigate the loss of attachment, and treat the infrabony defects (Figure 3A). After anesthesia, sulcular incisions were placed using microsurgical blade #15, without a vertical incision. Using fine elevators, we elevated the mucoperiasteal flap. The infrabony defect and root surfaces were degranulated and cleaned with curretes, rinsed with saline, and dried with cotton swabs. After that, bone graft material was used to fill the defect, which was then covered with pericardium membrane. For wound closure, we used the sling-suturing technique. This suture was placed without tension before application of bone graft filling and pericardium membrane. After bone grafting and pericardium membrane, we tied the sutures.

After the patient's first visit, we were able to resolve his main complaint of pain resulting from trauma from occlusion. During his second visit, we addressed maintenance therapy. After periodontal surgery, we observed a negligible increase in gingival recession, and gingival edema and hyperemia (Figure 3B). He healed well, but gingival recession was still observed (Figure 3C).

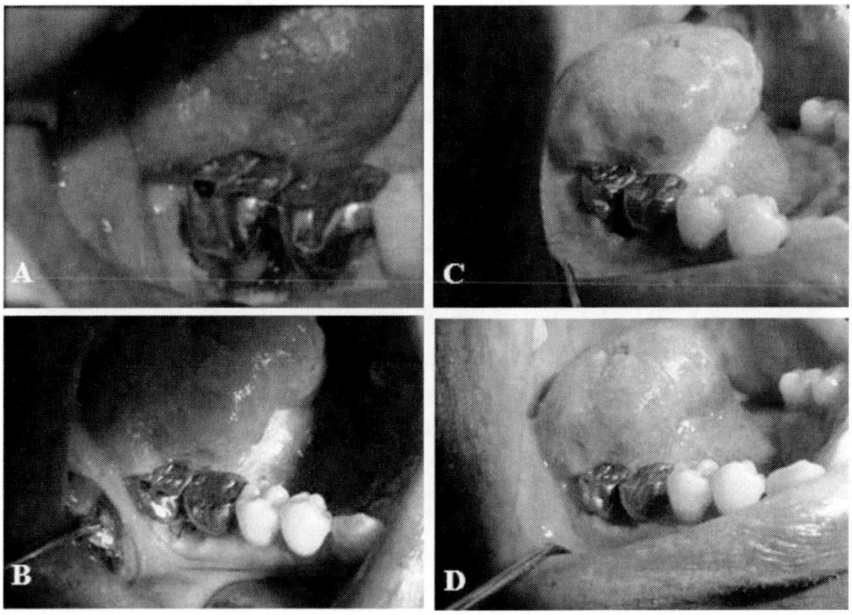

Figure 3. Flap operation (A); Control post flap operation, first control (B); second control (C); third control (D).

Three months after periodontal surgery, the patient underwent radiographic imaging to assess the results of bone grafting filling and pericardium membrane (Figure 3D). Suppuration was eliminated after the initial therapy and remained undetectable during the observation period.

3. DISCUSSION

A periodontal abscess, also called a lateral abscess, is the most common type of abscess involving the periodontium. This patient's main complaint was the pain when chewing and tenderness on percussion. These symptoms are in agreement with common complaints of patients reported in the literature, the most common of which are pain or discomfort, or the appearance of an area of swelling that is tender to touch, periodontal probing hewing, or tooth brushing. This area develops as a result of a bacterial infection that eventually leads to the formation of pus (suppuration) and is often associated with pre-existing periodontitis. In the case of this patient, there was involvement of the furcation, a common site for periodontal abscess formation, probably because of this area's anatomical limitations, which make oral hygiene and professional instrumentation difficult [6, 7].

An abscess may occur in anywhere throughout the periodontium by traumatic insertion of bacteria or a foreign body into the tissues, but most occur within the wall of a previously existing gingival or periodontal pocket. In this patient, there was an existing periodontal pocket, into which bacteria from dental calculus entered [7]. Microorganisms that colonize and are found in the exudates of periodontal abscesses are primarily Gram-negative anaerobic rods [8].

Treatment of periodontal abscesses is generally performed in two stages. The first stage involves management of the acute symptoms by drainage. If possible, drainage should occur through the lumen of the pocket. In this patient, this was done during the first visit. Next, the pocket is treated as soon as the acute symptoms have subsided and before the chronic stages are reached. Treatment may consist of nonsurgical therapy, or careful elevation of a mucoperiosteal flap. In this patient, treatment was performed after initial therapy, until the flap operation with DFDBA bone grafting and pericardium membrane [9].

Trauma from occlusion (TFO and sometimes referred to as occlusal trauma, or periodontal traumatism) is defined as injury to the attachment apparatus (bone, periodontal ligament, or cementum) as a consequence of normal or excessive occlusal forces applied to a tooth or teeth Occlusal forces are transmitted to the teeth and their supporting structures by tooth-to-tooth contact or through food or any other intervening material. When magnitude (size), direction, frequency, and/or duration of these forces exceed the reparative capacity of the attachment apparatus, the result is occlusal disease [4, 10]. There are two types of TFO, primary and secondary. Primary TFO results from excessive occlusal forces placed on a tooth with normal bone and attachment levels. Secondary TFO results from normal or excessive occlusal forces on a tooth with a reduced periodontium. Our case demonstrated secondary TFO. On radiography, secondary TFO is associated with reduced bone levels that are inadequate to support the tooth under normal loading without increasing mobility, migration, or fremitus [10].

In this case, trauma from occlusion resulted from magnitudinal (size) and durational forces that occurred secondary to the use of a metal jacket crown restorative material after root canal treatment. Here the occlusional forces exceeded the reparative capacity of the attachment apparatus. Radiographic imaging showed widening of the periodontal ligament that occurred as an adaptive response to excessive occlusal loading, potentially as a consequence of resorption of alveolar bone.

Placement of a fixed prosthetic, whether a crown or bridge, requires determination of the periodontal status of the involved the abutment teeth. The anatomy of gingival and periodontal tissue should be known before construction and placement of a fixed prosthetic [1]. Several points should be made relating to the planning of fixed prosthetics. First, in the planning and making of a fixed prosthetic, the patient's oral hygiene and condition of the individual teeth (periodontal disease and ratio of root and crown) are important considerations. The first priority should be to arrest the disease process and improve oral hygiene. Patients require oral hygiene education, including how oral hygiene affects periodontal disease progression. Any local periodontal problems should be assessed and treated. Root length (ratio of root and crown) should be measured to determine periodontal support, and the length of the root is important for retaining the installed crown [2].

Second, when designing crowns, care should be taken when considering material and periodontal tissue. In this case, the crown was constructed from metal. Dental casting metal is strong in thin sections and can be used to overlay and protect weakened cusps against occlusal forces. It is, however, ductile and can be distorted if it is too thin or if it is subjected to excessive forces. The shape of the crown margin (the cavosurface angle) should be designed so that the crown surface aligns with the tooth surface. Insufficient reduction at the margin can result in an overbuilt crown, which in turn produces a plaque retention area at the margin [2].

The pathogenesis of TFO is not the same as periodontal inflammation, because inflammatory cells like PMN, leukocytes are not released. TFO does not destroy the gingival margin tissue, but rather widens the periodontal ligament and hastens bone loss, often resulting in vertical bone loss. Once the trauma is removed, the tissue generally becomes healthier and will revert to its prior state. However, if trauma continues, the tissue will continue to degrade. The inter-relationship between trauma from occlusion and bone loss is still controversial. One theory asserts that there is no relationship between these factors. On the other hand, Glickman's theory of co-destruction postulates the existence of a relationship [5, 10].

Coronoplasty involves reshaping the buccal and lingual occlusal tables of teeth, in hopes of mitigating heavy forces. The balancing of root and crown can be achieved with this treatment. Coronoplasty relieves the patient's pain and discomfort while reducing tooth mobility, but not pocket depth. Flap surgery is recommended for reducing pocket depth and facilitate placement of regenerative material [5, 10, 11].

Flap surgery involves root surface debridement, exploration, plaque removal, removal of calculus and other plaque-retentive features, and placement of regenerative material [12, 13]. In this case, we used an intrasulcular incision with a full-thickness mucoperiosteal flap. The advantages of this flap include good access and visualization of root surfaces and alveolar bone. From a technical perspective, flap surgery is also less demanding, and associated with less post-operative recession [12].

In this case, after removal of all granulated tissue, subgingival calculus, and other debris, we were able to appreciate the morphology of the osseous defect. A wide three-wall defect had limited osseous regenerative potential, and bone replacement grafts were used to help regenerate tooth support structures. Bone grafting used DFDBA, tissue transplanted between persons of same species. Allografts function as osteoconduction templates that assist bone formation and deposition by undifferentiated cells in the wound.

Allografts create an additional surgical wound through which donor material is procured while still maintaining comparable osseous repair potential. pericardium membrane was used to further secure the bone graft material [14, 15].

CONCLUSION

In conclusion, improper sizing of fixed prosthetics can cause trauma from occlusion, pain, increased pocket depth, and loss of attachments. Coronoplasty can help eliminate the pain, while flap surgery is an effective means of reducing pocket depth and mitigating the loss of attachment.

REFERENCES

[1] Baima, R. F. (2001). Periodontal consideration. In S. Rosenstiel, M. F. Land, and J. Fujimoto, Editors (Eds.), *Contemporary fixed prosthodontics* (4th edition, pp. 145 - 173). St. Louis: Mosby Elsevier.

[2] Smith, B. G. N. (1998). *Planning and making crowns and bridges* (3rd edition). St. Louis: Mosby Elsevier; 41 - 45:87-90.

[3] Lang, N. and Lindhe, J. (2005). Dental calculus and local contributory factors. In J. Lindhe, Editor (Ed.), *Clinical periodontology and implant dentistry* (4th edition, pp. 102 - 156). UK: Blackwell Munksgaard.

[4] Jepsen, S, Caton, J. G. et al. (2018). Periodontal manifestations of systemic diseases and developmental and acquired conditions: Consensus report of workgroup 3 of the 2017 World Workshop on the Classification of Periodontal and Peri-Implant Diseases and Conditions. *J. Periodontol.,* 89 (Suppl. 1): S237 S248. https://doi.org/10.1002/JPER.17-0733.

[5] Hallmon, W. and Harrel, S. (2003). Occlusal trauma: effects and management. In G. Wilson Tomas, and K. Kornman, Editors (Eds.), *Fundamentals of periodontics* (2nd edition, pp. 531 - 538). Hong Kong: Quintessence Publishing Co, Inc.

[6] Herrera, D., Retamal-Valdes, B., Alonso, B., Feres, M. (2018). Acute periodontal lesions (periodontal abscesses and necrotizing periodontal diseases) and endo-periodontal lesions. *J. Clin. Periodontol.,* 45 (Suppl. 20):S78-S94. https://doi.org/10.1111/ jcpe.12941.

[7] Wilson, H. G. (2003). Acute lesions of the periodontium. In G. Wilson Tomas, and Kornman (Herrera, 2018 #24) Kenneth, Editors (Eds.), *Fundamentals of Periodontics* (2nd edition, pp. 491-495). Hong Kong: Quintessence Publishing Co, Inc.

[8] Singh, A. K., Saxena, A. (2015). The periodontal abscess: A review. *IOSR J. Dent. Med. Sci. (IOSR-JDMS),* (14);11: 81. e-ISSN: 2279 - 0853, p-ISSN: 2279-0861

[9] Gray, J. L. (2000). Periodontal emergencies. In Vernino, Gray, Hughes, Editors (Eds.), The Periodontic syllabus. Philadelphia: Lippincott William & Wilkins, 5th edition, pp. 242-243.

[10] Richetti, P. A. (1998). *Treatment of the periodontum affected by occlusal traumatism.* In M. M. Nevins, Editor (Ed.), Periodontal therapy clinical approaches and evidence of success. Japan: Quintessence Publishing Co, Inc,1: pp. 129-148.

[11] Harrel, W. and Hallmon, W. (2000). *Occlusion as a risk factor for periodontal disease.* In Vernino, Gray, Hughes, Editors (Eds.), The Periodontic syllabus. Philadelphia: Lippincott William & Wilkins, 5th edition, pp. 63-69.

[12] Saha, S. (2007). *Access flaps for surgical root surface debridement.* In G. Bateman, S. Shuva, and I. L. C. Chapple, Editors (Eds.), Contemporary periodontal surgery: an illustrated guide to the art behind the science. London: Quintessence Publishing Co, pp. 49-62.

[13] Yukna, R. A. (2000). *Management of soft tissue: flaps for pocket management.* In A. R. Vernino, J. L. Gray, and E. A. Hughes, Editors (Eds.), The Periodontic syllabus. Philadelphia: Lippincott William & Wilkins, 5th edition, pp. 169-176.

[14] Chapple, I. (2007). *Regenerative periodontal techniques.* In G. Bateman, S. Shuva, I. L. C. Chapple, Editors (Eds.), Contemporary periodontal surgery: an illustrated guide to the art behind the science. London: Quintessence Publishing Co. pp. 63-88.

[15] Yukna, R. A. (2000). *Management of osseous defects: bone replacement grafts.* In A. R. Vernino, J. L. Gray, and E. A. Hughes, Editors (Eds.), The Periodontic syllabus. Philadelphia: Lippincott William & Wilkins, 5th edition, pp. 195-200.

In: Clinical Reports in Dentistry
Editor: Lisa R. Amir

ISBN: 978-1-53617-328-4

Chapter 40

ESTHETIC CROWN LENGTHENING IN THE ANTERIOR AREA IN ALTERED PASSIVE ERUPTION PATIENT BEFORE ORTHODONTIC TREATMENT

***Sandra O. Kuswandani*[1,*] *and Luliek S. Handayani*[2]**
[1]Department of Periodontics, Faculty of Dentistry,
Universitas Indonesia, Jakarta, Indonesia
[2]Orthodontist, Private Practice, Jakarta, Indonesia

ABSTRACT

Introduction: It is believed that the smile represents personality and appearance. The common cause of excessive gingival display is altered passive eruption (APE), which was resulted from incomplete natural migration of the gingiva during tooth eruption.

Case report: A 30-year-old female was referred from Orthodontist in private practice. At the first visit, the patient chief complaint was her tooth arrangement, and asked any treatment to help her in order to minimize her gummy emergence when she was smiling. From the clinical examination, there was an excessive gum appearance of about 5 millimetres (mm) in her upper jaw. This case showed the unequal proportion of the teeth, including the square shape of central incisive, the proportion of lateral incisive and canine. The ratio of intra-tooth relationship for the central incisive was 8 mm:8 mm (height :width). In addition, the gingival zenith level was also not ideal. The management of this case was divided into the preparation phase, surgery phase and follow-up phase. In the preparation phase, we examined the biological width, anatomical consideration and esthetic consideration. In the surgery phase, we prepared for crown lengthening procedure with gingivectomy and bone reduction by 2 - 3 mm. From the result, the patient was very satisfied with her new tooth shape and smile.

* Corresponding Author's Email: Sandra.olivia01@ui.ac.id.

Conclusion: Crown lengthening procedure is one of the alternative treatments for altered passive eruption cases. Bone reduction estimation was calculated by the evaluation of biological width, anatomical and esthetic consideration.

Keywords: esthetic crown lengthening, altered passive eruption, gingivectomy, bone reduction, biological width

1. INTRODUCTION

The smile is believed to represent personality and appearance. For decades, the term "gummy smile" was used to explain excessive gingival display when the gingiva above the tooth margin appears while smiling [1]. Several conditions may cause excessive gingival display; these may be skeletal, alveolar, muscular, dental and periodontal in origin [2]. One cause of periodontal origin is altered passive eruption (APE), which is resulted from incomplete natural migration of the gingiva during tooth eruption. Although tooth emergence is complete, the gingival margin remains stable at the tooth coronal surface. Consequently, clinical crown height shortly in appearance and it will involve normal relationships of the bone to the cementoenamel junction (CEJ), usually 1.5 mm apical to the CEJ [1, 2]. Moreover, the biological width of these patients will be altered.

The prevalence of APE has been reported to be 7–14% compared to the normally defined gingival display space of 1–2mm between the gingival margin and upper lip. Another study showed that APE cases approximately 37.8% of the population and significantly more found in women than men. Another classification mentioned the excessive display of gingiva as ≥ 4mm from the upper lip [3, 4]. Many alternative treatments could be chosen for APE condition, that are crown lengthening procedure, orthodontic leveling of the gingival margin of maxillary teeth or in advance should add with lip reposition surgery. In advance case, the combination of all techniques could be improved for an optimum result [4].

The treatment plan of APE treatment should be based on analysis of biologic width, golden proportion, intra-tooth relationship, smile line, gingival zenith level, the thickness of attached and marginal gingiva [5]. The aim of crown lengthening is to provide the adequate biological width, optimizing the esthetic result, correcting gingival asymmetry or clinically short crowns. This can be performed with or without alveolar bone reduction, which is considering the adequacy of biological width of the clinical crown [6].

Lip repositioning, as the other alternative, is a conservative surgical technique used to treat excess gingival display. This limits lip elevation on smiling and increases lip fullness. However, orthodontic treatment for APE might perform as main treatment or combination with other techniques [7, 8]. Failure of APE treatment resulted as unsatisfying esthetic result, gingival inflammation or recurrent excessive gingival display. Treatment planning and preparation are the important keys of successful result. Moreover, this article reported the APE patient with a crown lengthening procedure.

2. Case Report

A 30-year-old female was referred by a private orthodontist. The patient was asked help to minimize her gummy appearance while smiling. She was in good physical health with good communication skills.

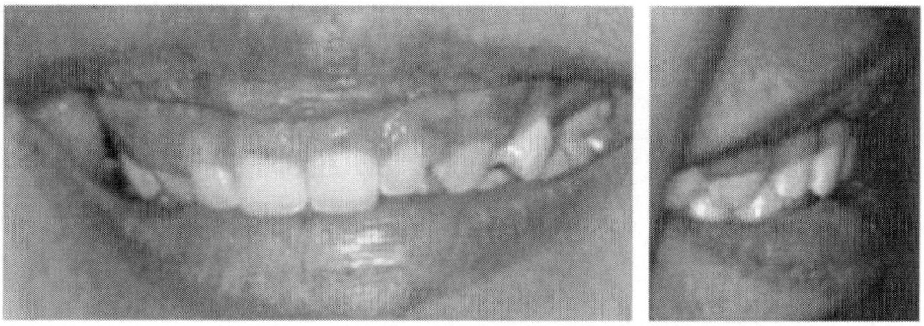

Figure 1. Clinical examination.

An extra-oral examination revealed no abnormality, but while smiling, she had approximately 5 mm of excessive gum appearance (Figure 1).

2.1. Preparation Phase

The analysis in the preparation phase were divided into two steps. First, extra-oral analyses, which included the smile line, lip line, and facial symmetrical analysis; and followed by intra-oral analyses.

From the extra-oral examination, we could analyze that her smile line was concave (based on the curve of the spee); her lip line was straight and above the gingival margin of maxillary teeth was about 5 millimeters.

The intra-oral analysis was including gingival tissue esthetic, interdental embrasures, the golden proportion of the teeth and gingival zenith level. The patient has an unequal proportion of the teeth, including the central incisive shape in a square, following by the proportion of lateral incisive was 65% from proportion of central incisive and then the proportion of canine was 85% from proportion of lateral incisive. The intra-tooth relationship for the central incisive in comparison with the height and width was about 8:8 mm.

The level of gingival zenith was far from ideal. One of the exemplified is the gingival level of the central incisive was below the gingival level of the lateral incisive. Biological width is one of the important biological considerations. Biological width defines as the amount of soft tissue that is attached to the tooth above the crest of the alveolar bone. Gargiulo stated that biological width should be at least 2.04 mm representing an epithelial attachment of 0.97 mm and a connective tissue attachment of 1.07 mm plus adding 1 mm for gingival sulcus depth. The gingival sulcus depth and bone level are measured to determine the surgery necessary to achieve adequate biological width.

From extra-oral, intra-oral analysis, and biological width calculation, the measurement for clinical crown, bone level depth, and anatomical/esthetic consideration is presented in Table 1.

Table 1. Measurement of crown lengthening procedure assessment (summary from intracoronal examination)

Tooth number	Clinical crown height (before)	Distance from gingival margin to sulcus depth	Distance from gingival margin to bone level	Clinical crown Height Needed (after)	Gingivectomy	Bone reduction
Unit	In milimetres (mm)					
14	9	2	3	10	2	-
13	7	1	2	10	2	3
12	5	1	1	8	3	3
11	8	2	3	11	3	3
21	8	2	3	11	3	3
22	6	1	1	8	2	2
23	8	1	2	10	2	2
24	9	2	3	10	1	-

2.2. Surgical Phase

After the preparation phase and treatment planning, the second step is performing the surgical treatment. Patient's oral hygiene should be in good condition. Infection control and asepsis should be done before the operation. Infiltration local anesthetic was injected over teeth 14 until 24. A pocket marker was used to mark the incision. Chu gauge was also useful for tooth proportion details (Figure 2A).

First step, gingivectomy was performed using the Orban-Kirkland knife with a 45-degree external bevel incision. Saline was irrigated to surrounding gingiva (Figure 2B). The second step, intra-sulcular incision was made and the gingival flap was reflected to visualize the bone (Figure 2C). Bone level reduction was performed with osteoplasty using bone bur, according to bone reduction assessment needs (Figure 2D). The flap was repositioned and the interrupted sutures were placed (Figure 2E, F).

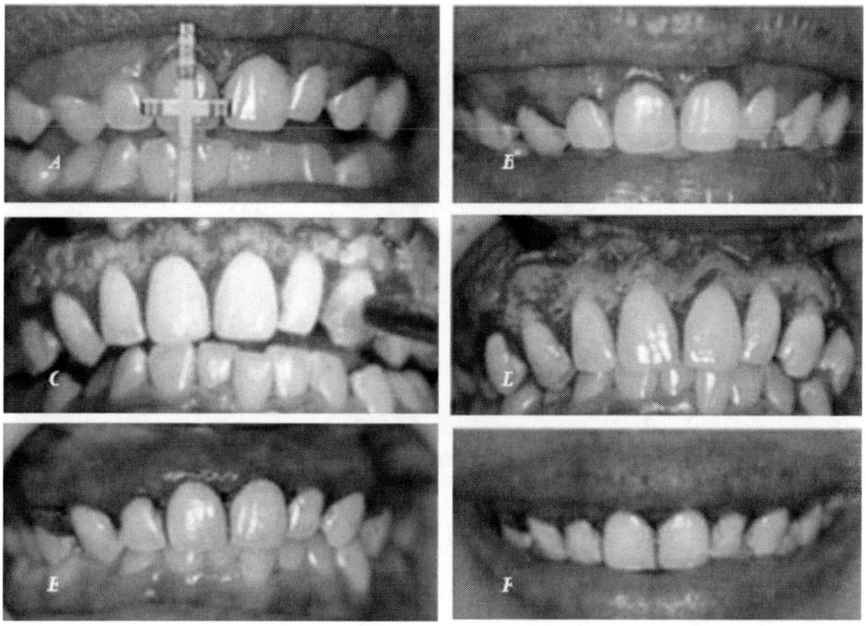

Figure 2. Crown lengthening with gingivectomy and bone height reduction operation procedures.

The patient was given the instruction for maintaining oral hygiene and instructed to do a follow-up visit one week after.

2.3. Follow-Up Phase

Based on the treatment result, the patient was very satisfied with her new teeth shape and smile. However, the smile line was above the gingival margin of the upper jaw by 1 millimeter (Figure 3). Orthodontic treatment with the aim to correct the malpositioned teeth and articulation after crown lengthening surgical treatment was carried out.

3. Discussion

The keys for successful and stable results from crown-lengthening procedures are accurate diagnosis and treatment planning. The management of this case is divided into preparation, surgery and follow-up phase. The preparation phase is the examination of biological width, anatomical consideration, and esthetic consideration. The treatment plan of crown lengthening procedure should be considered the biologic width as well as esthetic and anatomic factors. The role of biological width is preserving healthy gingival tissues and maintaining the gingival shape around restorations.

Esthetic consideration is including many factors, such as gingival zenith level, smile line, attached and marginal gingiva also intra-tooth analysis.

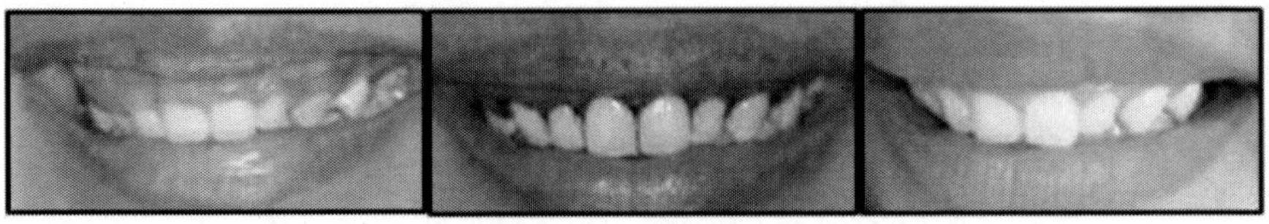

Figure 3. Comparison in clinical outcomes before treatment, after treatment and 6 months follow-up.

The anatomical consideration for altered passive eruption in adult patients may be assessed using Coslet classification. Firstly, based on gingival or anatomical crown relationship, there are; 1) type I, that is evaluated from gingival margin incisal to the CEJ, where there is a noticeably wider gingival dimension from the margin to the mucogingival junction; 2) type II, the dimension was assessed from the gingival margin to the mucogingival junction which appears to be within the normal mean width.

Secondly, based on the relationship of alveolar crest to CEJ and divided into 1) subtype A, the alveolar crest to CEJ distance is approximately 1.5 mm. This allows for normal attachment of the gingival fibers into cementum; 2) subtype B, where the alveolar crest is at the same level of the CEJ [9].

The details of preparation phase will impact treatment planning which leads to excellent result. The decision for esthetic crown lengthening may be established according to the esthetic crown lengthening classification developed by Lee [10].

Based on this case, the patient was classified as type III patient, which means bone sounding may reveal a scenario were repositioning the gingival margin will result in exposure of the osseous crest. This is an unacceptable complication that precludes the completion of any gingivectomy procedures prior to the surgical bone contouring.

A failure after crown lengthening procedure is requiring the combination with other treatment options, such as orthodontic treatment, veneer crown or lip reposition. A combination of treatments may enhance the best result of APE patient.

CONCLUSION

An altered passive eruption may be treated using the crown lengthening procedure. The decision for the bone reduction in crown lengthening procedure is depending on biological width, anatomical and esthetic consideration.

REFERENCES

[1] Omer, T. A., Mageet, A. O. (2016). Clinical Parameters of the Gummy Smile among Sudanese Female Sample. *Int. J. Dent. Oral Health,* 3(1).

[2] Silberberg, N., Goldstein, D., Smidt, A. (2010) Excessive gingival display – etiology, diagnosis and treatment modalities. *BDJ,* 208(10), 113.

[3] Bolívar, Londoño, Miguel Ángel and Botero Mariaca, Paola. (2012). The smile and its dimensions. *Revista Facultad de Odontología Universidad de Antioquia*, 23(2), 253-365.

[4] Ergezen, E. et al. (2017) Treatment of excessive gingival display with lip repositioning technique. *Inter. J. Oral Maxillofac. Surg.,* 46: 367.

[5] Pawar, B., Mishra, P., Banga, P., Marawar, P. P. (2011). Gingival zenith and its role in redefining esthetics: A clinical study. *J. Indian Soc. Periodontol.,* 15:135-138.

[6] Rossi, R., Benedetti, R., Santos-morales, Ri. (2008). *Treatment of Altered Passive Eruption: Periodontal Plastic Surgery of the Dentogingival Junction*, 3(3), 212-223.

[7] Nugala, B., Kumar, B. S., Sahitya, S. and Krishna, P. M. (2012). Biologic width and its importance in periodontal and restorative dentistry. *J. Conservat. Dent. JCD*, 15(1):12-17. doi:10.4103/0972-0707.92599.

[8] Landsberg, C. J. (2006). Management of excessive gingival display following adult orthodontic treatment: a case report. *Pract. Proced. Aesthet. Dent.,* 18(2), 89-96.

[9] Rossi, R., Brunelli, G., Piras, V. and Pilloni, A. (2014). Altered passive eruption and familial trait: a preliminary investigation. *Inter. J. Dent.*, 2014, 874092. doi:10.1155/2014/874092.

[10] Lee, A. E. (2004). Esthetic crown lengthening: consideration, biologic rationale, and treatment planning consideartions. *Pract. Proced. Aesthet. Dent.,* 16; (10):769-778.

SECTION 4: PEDIATRIC DENTISTRY AND ORTHODONTICS

In: Clinical Reports in Dentistry
Editor: Lisa R. Amir
ISBN: 978-1-53617-328-4

Chapter 41

SUCCESSFUL CONSERVATIVE MANAGEMENT OF INTRUSIVE LUXATION IN THE PRIMARY TEETH: A CASE REPORT

Andriani Octavia[1] and Eva Fauziah[2,*]
[1]Pediatric Dentistry Residency Program, Faculty of Dentistry,
Universitas Indonesia, Jakarta, Indonesia
[2]Department of Pediatric Dentistry, Faculty of Dentistry,
Universitas Indonesia, Jakarta, Indonesia

ABSTRACT

Introduction: An intrusive luxation is a severe type of dental trauma that may destruct the periodontal ligament, pulp, and alveolar bone. However, the position of the intruded primary teeth may be close to the developing permanent successors; thus, any traumatic injuries may result in multiple complications, and an appropriate treatment should be established, including waiting for spontaneous re-eruption, surgical repositioning, and extraction. This study aimed to present a successful conservative management of intrusive luxation in tooth 61 in a 23-month-old girl.

Case report: A 23-month-old girl and her parents were referred to the Pediatric Dentistry Clinic of Universitas Indonesia. The patient presented with a history of falling while playing, and she was then diagnosed with intrusive luxation in the left maxillary primary incisor. Spontaneous re-eruption was observed 4 weeks after injury. Periodic evaluation was conducted until 6 months after injury, and no complications were observed on the affected tooth.

Discussion: The successful treatment of intrusive luxation in the primary teeth was influenced by the child's age, severity and direction of intrusion, and/or involvement of permanent tooth bud. Conservative management, including waiting for spontaneous re-eruption, is a treatment option for intrusive luxation if the permanent tooth bud is not damaged.

* Corresponding Author's Email: eva.fauziah@ui.ac.id.

Conclusion: The intruded primary incisor was displaced away from the developing permanent tooth bud; therefore complete spontaneous re-eruption was observed 6 months after injury with no complications on the affected tooth clinically and radiographically.

Keywords: conservative management, intrusive luxation, primary teeth

1. Introduction

Dentoalveolar trauma is a common problem in children and young adults, which requires immediate treatment not only because of a possible severe injury but also due to emotional distress felt by the child and parents [1]. The prevalence rate of traumatic injuries in the primary teeth varies from 4% to 30%. Children aged 1 – 4 years are at high risk for injuries due to the fact that they are developing mobility skills, and during injuries, the maxillary incisors are the most frequently affected teeth [2]. Intrusive luxation is a dislocation of a tooth in an axial direction into the alveolar bone.

Based on the magnitude of the impact, intrusive luxation can be divided into three types: type I, >50% of crown exposure; type II, <50% of crown exposure; and type III, partial or total intrusion of the entire crown [3-5]. Intrusive luxation in the primary teeth accounts for 8% – 22% of all luxation injuries [1].

Individuals with such injury are more vulnerable due to large marrow space and incomplete grade of mineralization. Blunt force trauma against these teeth often causes them to move instead of break as they are not firmly supported [3, 4].

The primary teeth may present with several types of complications from dento-alveolar trauma, which include enamel discoloration, pulp obliteration, pulp necrosis, root resorption, inflammatory resorption, ankylosis, gingival recession, permanent displacement, and premature loss of primary tooth. Traumatic injuries in the primary teeth not only affect the primary tooth but also the development of the permanent tooth bud. The close anatomical relationship between the apices of the primary teeth and their developing permanent successors is a relevant factor as it promotes easy transmission of any impact from the primary teeth to the permanent tooth buds.

The extent of permanent tooth malformation caused by a traumatic impact significantly varies, which depends on the development of the permanent tooth, force impact, and direction of the traumatic collision on the primary teeth. Sequelae could manifest as pathological alterations, such as enamel discoloration and/or enamel defect, crown dilacerations, root dilacerations, odontoma-like malformation, partial or complete arrest of root formation, and disturbances in the eruption of the permanent teeth (ectopic or lack of re-eruption) [3, 4].

The routine use of a protocolized form has been to avoid missing out essential aspects of care, which include medical and dental history taking; a brief neurological examination; asking of mandatory questions of how, when, where, and why; and providing treatment, a protocol form should be used, which is considered extremely useful. The treatment of an intruded primary tooth depends on thorough clinical and radiographic examinations [5, 6].

When the primary teeth are damaged due to intrusive luxation, the treatment plan can be complex and it will depend on the magnitude of the trauma and on the displacement position. The recommendation of the American Academy of Pediatric Dentistry for managing intrusive luxation in the primary teeth include either extraction or waiting for a spontaneous re-eruption [7]. Herein, we present a successful conservative management of intrusive luxation in the primary incisor in a 23-month-old girl.

2. Case Report

A 23-month-old girl and her parents were referred to the Pediatric Dentistry Clinic of Universitas Indonesia. The parents stated that a front tooth had moved inside the jaw. The child was in good general health, and no neurologic problems were observed. No signs of head injury or trauma to the other body parts were observed. The child had a complete tetanus immunization. Furthermore, the girl sustained a dental injury due to falling while playing 2 days ago. After the injury, her parents took her to a clinic near their house. The dentist referred the patient to a pediatric dentist and prescribed analgesics and antibiotics.

Clinical and radiographic examinations were performed. Visual intra-oral inspection showed that the maxillary left central incisor was submerged into the alveolar bone away from the line of occlusion, and this is considered as type I intrusive luxation with approximately 2mm crown exposure (Figure 1A-C). The absence of tooth mobility and a palatal crown inclination indicated a buccal intrusion of the root away from the permanent successor. No signs of alveolar fracture were identified via gentle palpation of the mucosa in the traumatized area. Periapical radiograph of the maxillary anterior region showed the presence of an intruded incisor, which appeared foreshortened. No discontinuity in the follicle of tooth 21 was observed. This result indicated that the intruded tooth was displaced away from the developing permanent tooth bud.

Patient received conservative management, which involved the observation of spontaneous re-eruption without invasive treatment (Figure 2A,B).

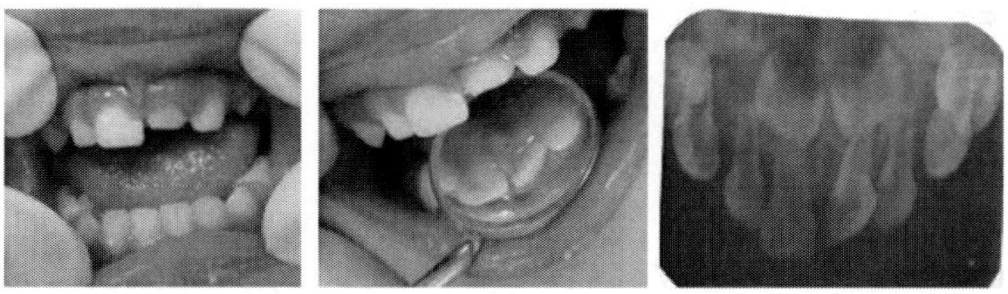

A B C

Figure 1. Clinical photograph during the 1st visit (A, B); Radiographic image (C)

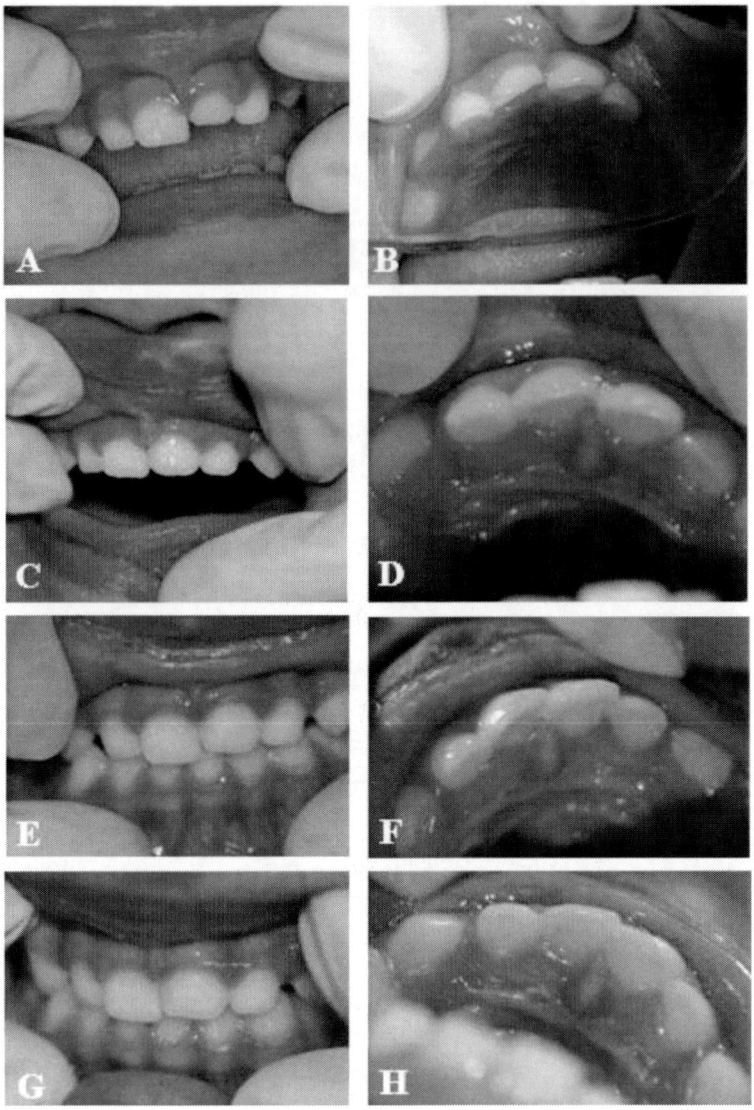

Figure 2. Clinical photograph during the 2nd visit (A, B); 5th visit, 4 months after injury (C, D);6th visit, 5 months after injury (E, F); 7th visit, 6 months after injury (G,H).

The parents were instructed about oral hygiene, non-use of a pacifier, and soft diet within the first week after injury. Moreover, they were advised to have the child undergo regular check-ups a week after injury and then monthly while waiting for a spontaneous re-eruption, which was observed 4 weeks after injury. The next dental appointments were 4 weeks after the injury and every month thereafter. After 5 months, tooth 61 presented with a better re-eruption than before (Figure 2C-D). Six months after the injury, no further re-eruption, tooth discoloration, or signs of inflammation on the affected tooth were observed (Figure 2E-F). Radiographic examination showed that the primary incisor did not present with any internal or external root resorption and that the permanent tooth bud had a normal development. The parents were instructed to have their child undergo clinical and radiographic examinations annually until the eruption of the permanent tooth.

3. Discussion

Intrusive luxation in the primary teeth is the most common dental trauma injury in early childhood that occurs between 12 and 24 months of age. The central upper incisors are the most commonly affected teeth. Accidental falls during walking or playing are considered the primary cause of these injuries. This is due to the fact that children begin to walk during this period, but they have not yet developed complete movement coordination [3, 4, 7]. Luxation is a more frequent cause of dental trauma than fracture. This could be explained by considering the flexibility, resilience, and medullary spaces of the growing bone. Indeed, an axial trauma intrudes the tooth into the alveolar bone, and such dislocation damages the periodontal ligament and vascular fibers [3].

A young child is often difficult to examine and treat due to the lack of cooperation and associated fear. Some of the important factors that influence the management of such injuries are the child's maturity and ability to cope with emergency situations, root resorption, severity and direction of intrusion, time period for the shedding of the involved tooth, and the relationship between the primary teeth and permanent tooth buds [1, 7]. The management of intrusive luxation in the primary teeth includes the observation of spontaneous re-eruption, surgical repositioning, and extraction [6]. The extraction or retention of the intruded primary tooth depends on the relative position of the root of the primary tooth and the permanent tooth bud. The root apex of the maxillary primary incisors has a labial curvature leading the root away from the permanent tooth germ in >80% of cases. Some clinical and radiographic findings support the diagnosis of labial alignment of the root, such as palatal inclination of the crown, which is characterized by a shortened and more opaque intruded primary teeth compared with an adjacent nondisplaced tooth and proper alignment of the permanent successor as observed on periapical radiograph. In cases when intrusive displacement occurs such that the primary tooth remains labial to the developing permanent tooth bud, the primary teeth are expected to re-erupt, and this normally occurs within a maximum of 6 months after injury. In agreement with the literature, the patient received conservative management, which includes the observation of spontaneous re-eruption, for intrusive luxation [1, 2, 6].

The follow-up schedules for individuals with traumatized primary teeth according to the guidelines of the International Association of Dental Traumatology are as follows: 1 week, clinical examination; 3 – 4 weeks, clinical and radiographic examinations; 6 – 8 weeks, clinical examination; 6 months, clinical and radiographic examinations; and annually, clinical and radiographic monitoring until eruption of the permanent successor. During each visit, a complete examination should be performed to check for any unusual symptoms, such as spontaneous pain, abscess, fever, fistula, and/or swelling of the soft tissues. Re-eruption begins within 2 – 3 weeks. However, it can be delayed for >6 months. If signs of re-eruption after 3 – 4 weeks from injury or physiological mobility are not observed, this may indicate ankylosis. Thus, the primary tooth should be extracted [1, 8]. In this case, the successful outcome was influenced by the child's age, severity and direction of intrusion, and/or involvement of the permanent tooth bud. During the re-eruption process of the intruded primary teeth, acute inflammation around the displaced tooth, which is characterized by spontaneous pain, tooth mobility, discoloration, or gingival swelling, is a risk [8]. Intrusive luxation accounts for a high number of pulp necrosis cases. The ratio of pulp vitality and pulp necrosis is approximately 50% in patients aged 0 – 3 years. When 90% of the intruded primary teeth have severe pulpal (necrosis and dystrophic calcification) and periodontal complications (inflammatory root resorption and ankylosis), extraction is preferred for the management of such case [3, 7]. In the present study, no tooth and/or periodontal complications were observed until the latest follow-up. This finding is in accordance with the literature showing that post-traumatic complications decrease with age. This can be explained by the high degree of vascularization, open radicular apex, and high resilience of the alveolar bone that allow a tooth to respond to possible infectious processes and maintain pulpal vitality of the intruded tooth during early stages [3]. Antibiotics and analgesics were prescribed to minimize the possibility of pulpal necrosis or pathological root resorption after intrusive luxation [8]. Histological response varies per patient, and in young children, a biological response is highly possible. Thus, the maturation stage of the traumatized root, health status of the damaged periodontal tissue, and degree of patient cooperation must always be evaluated [3].

CONCLUSION

The optimal treatment for intrusive luxation in the primary teeth involves the observation of spontaneous re-eruption and administration of antimicrobial medications, if injury in the developing permanent tooth bud is not suspected. In this case, the favorable relationship between the intruded incisor and the permanent tooth bud, the patient's age, and severity and direction of intrusion led to a successful outcome. Parents should be informed about the importance of periodic follow-ups so as not to overlook pulp infection of the affected tooth and disturbances in the development of the permanent teeth.

REFERENCES

[1] Gauba, K., Goyal, A., Bhatia, S. K. (2014). Intrusive dental injuries in children: Manifestations and management. *J. Postgrad. Med. Educ. Res.,* 48:53 - 62.

[2] Casamassimo, P. (2013). *Pediatric Dentistry: Infancy through Adolescence* (5th edition). St. Louis, Missouri: Elsevier.

[3] Caprioglio, A., Salone, G. S., Mangano, C., Caprioglio, C., Caprioglio, D. (2014). Intrusive luxation of primary upper incisors and sequelae on permanent successors: a clinical follow-up study. *Eur. J. Paediatr. Dent.,* 15(2):101 - 106.

[4] Carvalho, V., Ribeiro, D., Campos, V. (2010). Frequency of intrusive luxation in deciduous teeth and its effects. *Dent. Traumatol.,* 26:304 - 307.

[5] Mendoza-Mendoza, A., Gonzalez-mallea, E., Iglesias-Linares, A. (2015). Intrusive luxation in primary teeth: A case report. *J. Clin. Pediatr. Dent.,* 39:215 - 219.

[6] Gurunathan, D., Murugan, M., Somasundaram, S. (2016). Management and sequelae of intruded anterior primary teeth: A systematic review. *Int. J. Pediatr. Dent.,* 9(3):240 - 250.

[7] Charone, S., Kuchler, E., Costa, M., Maia, L. (2010). A successful outcome using a minimal invasive approach to manage a severe trauma to the primary maxillary incisor in a toddler. *Dent. Traumatol.,* 26:294 - 297.

[8] Gupta, M. (2011). Intrusive luxation in primary teeth–Review of literature and report of a case. *Saudi Dent. J.,* 23(4):167 - 176.

In: Clinical Reports in Dentistry
Editor: Lisa R. Amir

ISBN: 978-1-53617-328-4

Chapter 42

Direct Pulp Capping Using Mineral Trioxide Aggregate (MTA) - 6 Months Observation: A Case Report

Puspa D. Pratiwi[1] and Eva Fauziah[2,*]
[1]Pediatric Dentistry Residency Program, Faculty of Dentistry, Universitas Indonesia, Jakarta, Indonesia
[2]Department of Pediatric Dentistry, Faculty of Dentistry, Universitas Indonesia, Jakarta, Indonesia

Abstract

Introduction: Pulp capping in carious teeth has been considered unpredictable and therefore contraindicated. Mineral trioxide aggregate (MTA) known as new material can resist bacterial leakage and may provide protection for the pulp, allowing repair and continued pulp vitality in teeth when used in combination with a sealed restoration.

Case report: A 15-year-old boy patient reported to the Pedodontic Clinic at the Dental hospital Faculty of Dentistry Universitas Indonesia with an extensive destruction of coronal tooth on maxillary left second premolar.

Methods: Teeth were treated with MTA Angelus®. MTA material that has been manipulated according to the manufacturer's instructions was placed in the exposed area until closed. Upon completion, GIC material to cover the top surface of MTA was applied.

Results: MTA produced a white layer similar to hydroxyapatite in the upper layer and provide chemical bonds between the cavity wall and MTA layer. It was attached to the MTA surface and continues to grow. They also produce mineralized matrix on the MTA.

Conclusion: Case selection is necessary in determining the type of treatment that fits the caries conditions and the rest of the dental tissue. Exposure to the pulp due to caries involvement can be done with MTA material closure.

* Corresponding Author's Email: eva_dens@yahoo.com.

Keywords: caries, pulp capping, mineral trioxide aggregate

1. Introduction

Dental caries is a process of hard tissue damage that begins at the surface of the tooth. The condition of caries that does not get treatment will result in decalcification of the enamel layer followed by enzymatic organic structure lysis so that cavities (holes) are formed and involve the pulp chamber [1]. In pulp conditions exposed due to caries or mechanics, the dental pulp has the basic ability to form a physical barrier by decreasing dentine permeability, forming tertiary dentine and inflammatory and immune reactions. The permeability degradation process of dentine occurs with an increased of intratubular dentine deposition and mineral crystal deposition in the dentine tubules, as characterized by the formation of dentin sclerosis [2].

The formation of tertiary dentine occurs longer than dentin sclerosis and depends on the characteristics of the stimulus. A mild stimulus will activate the odontoblasts around the stimulus and form the physiological dentine. In advanced stimulation, the process will lead to the formation of a reparative dentine containing atubular, regular/irregular, and cuboidal cell-associated fibrodentine cells [2]. This can be observed in cases with direct pulp capping or pulpotomy treatments. During the reparative procedure, exposed odontoblasts will be damaged and replaced by odontoblast-like cells. Caries that already involve the pulp area are a dilemma in the determination of treatment. Direct pulp capping is one of the procedures by which the exposed pulp is coated with a biocompatible material. This treatment aims to form tissue formation from dentinal bridges to close off stimulation and maintain healthy pulp tissue [1].

Some studies suggest that conditions that have a good success rate in direct pulp capping are the result of mechanical trauma when compared with caries. Penetration of caries to the pulp will cause bacterial invasion resulting in pulp inflammation. Adequate laying of materials and restoration of pulp capping is the key to successful treatment [1, 2]. Pulp bleeding control is another important factor in the treatment of direct pulp capping. Bleeding is an indicator of increased degree of inflammation in the pulp. In addition, moist conditions and contamination of surrounding tissues with blood cause the difficulty of doing the restoration properly. Bleeding can generally be controlled by placing a moisturized cotton pellet on the exposed area. Some of the solutions that can be used are saline, sodium hypochlorite (concentration of 0.12-5.25%), hydrogen peroxide, ferric sulfate, and chlorhexidine [3].

There are various materials for pulp protection such calcium hydroxide, GIC, Zinc Oxide Eugenol, amalgam and IRM. Calcium hydroxide has some disadvantages such as mild antibacterial, short term seal ability, and marginal leakage [2, 4]. Mineral Trioxide Aggregate (MTA), a new material currently being used in pulp therapy, has been demonstrated to provide an enhanced seal the vital pulp and is non-resorbable. MTA is a bioactive material currently recommended as a communication cover between the root canal area and the periodontium tissue [5]. Therefore, this material is used as a root canal filler, the healing agent under perforated furcation and apical conditions, apical plugs. MTA is also recommended as a direct pulp capping and pulpotomy agent [6]. Various studies have shown that MTA induces the formation of hard tissue, and previous studies have shown the effect of MTA on sementoblasts and odontoblasts. Boezman, the use of MTA produces a white layer similar to hydroxyapatite in the upper layer and provide chemical bonds between the cavity wall and MTA layer [6]. The odontoblasts are attached to the MTA surface and continues to grow and producing mineralized matrices on the MTA. Some studies also suggest that MTA has an anti-inflammatory effect on the pulp area [7]. In MTA placement in the pulp area will result in the proliferation, migration, and differentiation of odontoblast-like cells that produce collagen matrix [8-10]. The process of matrix formation, mineralization and will result in osteo-dentin initials followed by dentinal bridge tertiary formation after several months of pulp capping procedure.

2. Case Report

A 15-year-old boy patient reported to the Pedodontic Clinic at the Dental hospital Faculty of Dentistry Universitas Indonesia with an extensive destruction of coronal tooth on maxillary left second premolar. The tooth was decayed and had been restored less than 6 months ago but the restoration was broken (Figure 1). Patient has good general health and obtained approval from parents. During the first visit, bleeding control with cotton pellet application was done to increase visibility in the determination of exposed areas. MTA Angelus® for direct pulp capping contains of MTA powder and 1 drop of distilled water. The mixture should be homogeneous and with a consistency similar to wet sand and applied on the selected site with a sterilized instrument in the exposed area [6]. GIC material (Figure 2).

During the second visit, post-direct pulp capping controls, no subjective complaints were reported. Clinical examination showed normal gingival areas and negative percussion tests. The tooth restoration was replaced by composite resin. During recall appointment 6 months after restoration, radiographical image showed the improvement of the dental tissue.

There were no subjective complaints. Clinical examination showed normal gingival areas and negative percussion tests. Resin composite restoration also adapt well (Figure 2A-C).

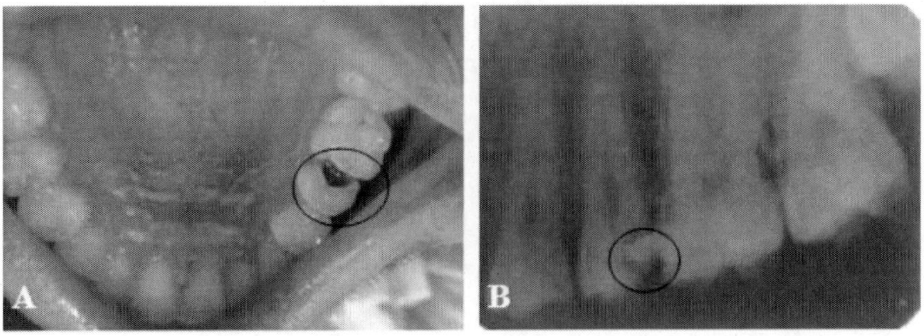

Figure 1. Intraoral and periapical rontgen of teeth 25 (A); Radiolucency was observed in the middle third of the distal crown that has not reached the pulp horn (B).

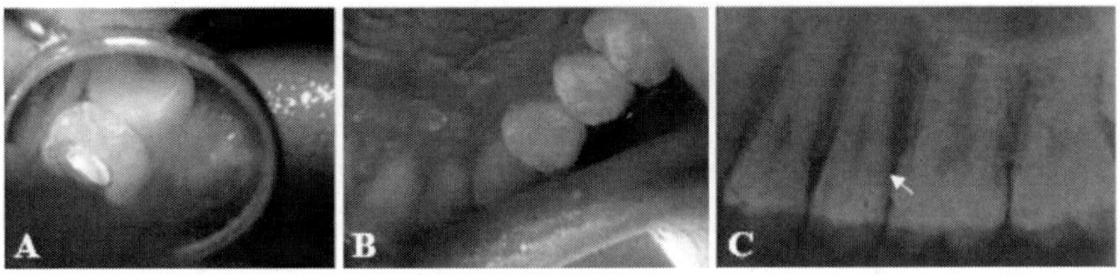

Figure 2. Placement of MTA materials in exposed areas in #25 tooth (A) followed by GIC restoration; Periapical radiograph showed good adaptation of MTA. Note that thin layer was observed (white arrow).

3. Discussion

In this case the tooth of exposure to the pulp due to the caries tissue cleaning procedure is carried out by the pulp capping process using a MTA that will be restored with a composite resin. In accordance with the literature, pulp capping treatment is an action that aims to maintain the vitality and function of the dental pulp from the outside environment of the tooth. The selection of pulp capping also aims to allow the pulp to demonstrate the basic ability to form a physical barrier by decreasing dentin permeability, forming tertiary dentine and inflammatory and immune reactions.

The use of MTA as a pulpcapping material can stimulate the pulp cells both cytologically and functionally in the formation of fibrodentine and reparative dentin. MTAs contain calcium oxide, which is formed when calcium hydroxide is mixed with water. The reaction that occurs in calcium hydroxide and carbon dioxide from pulp tissue will form calcite crystals. The role of calcite and fibronectin calcium will initiate the formation of hard tissue barriers [8].

The use of MTA has since been introduced by Ford et al. (1996) as pulp capping material. The study was conducted on animal teeth comparing calcium hydroxide and MTA, where treated teeth showed inflammation-free condition and dentin bridge formation was established after 5 months.

Aeneichi et al. (2003) performed a direct pulpcapping with MTA and calcium hydroxide in third molar with an open pulp due to caries and mechanics. Histologically, the dentine bridge formation was accompanied by mild chronic inflammation after 2 months of MTA placement. Teeth treated with calcium hydroxide were observed to form thin and thin bridges irregularly after 3 months but accompanied by hyperemia conditions. Aenechi et al. concluded that MTA is better for the treatment of exposed pulp [9].

Bogen et al. (2008) reported that a success rate of 97.96% in treated teeth of pulpcapping was directed against caries-related MTA. Evaluation of the success of the treatment should take up to 1 year to determine changes in the pulp area [10].

Conclusion

Case selection is necessary in determining the type of treatment that fits the caries conditions and the rest of the dental tissue. Exposure to the pulp due to caries involvement can be done with MTA material closure. After direct pulp capping treatment has been completed, a radiographic view of the absence of lesion formation in the area as well as on percussion and palpation examination is negative. Based on subjective examination also no complaints. In this case, direct pulpcapping treatment with MTA followed by composite resin restorations successfully defended the dental tissue well.

References

[1] Glossary of Endodontic Terms. (2003). American Association of Endodontists. Chicago, IL, USA.

[2] Baume, L. J., Holz, J. (1981). Long-term clinical assessment of direct pulp capping. Inter. Dent. J., 31(4):251 - 260.

[3] De Sousa Costa, C., Edwards, C., Hanks, C. (2001). Cytotoxic effects of cleansing solutions recommended for chemical lavage of pulp exposures. Amer. J. Dent., 14:25 - 30.

[4] Rowe, A. H. (1967). Reaction of the rat molar pulp to various materials. Br. Dent. J. 122: 291 - 300.

[5] Cirstescu Ioana, Liliana, R. M. (2001). Mineral Trioxide Aggregate (MTA): An Update Review. Oral Health Dent. Pract. Retrieved from: https://www.oralhealth group.com/features/product-profile-mineral-trioxide-aggregate-mta-an-updated-review/.

[6] Butt, N., Talwar, S., Chaudhry, S., Nawal, R. R., Yadav, S. et al. (2014). Comparison of physical and mechanical properties of mineral trioxide aggregate

and Biodentine. Department of Conservative Dentistry and Endodontics, Maulana Azad Institute of Dent. Sci., 25(6):692-697.

[7] Sarkar, N. K., Caicedo, R., Ritwik, P., Moiseyeva, R., Kawashima, I. (2005). Physicochemical Basis of the Biologic Properties of Mineral Trioxide Aggregate. J. Endod., 31(2):97-100. 8

[8] Kuratate, M., Yoshiba, K., Shigetani, Y., Yoshiba, N., Ohshima, H., Okiji, T. (2008). Immunohistochemical Analysis of Nestin, Osteopontin, and Proliferating Cells in the Reparative Process of Exposed Dental Pulp Capped with Mineral Trioxide Aggregate. J. Endod., 34 (8):970-974.

[9] Aeinehchi M, Eslami B, Ghanbariha M, Saffar AS. Mineral trioxide aggregate (MTA) and calcium hydroxide as pulp-capping agents in human teeth: a preliminary report. Int Endod J. 2003 Mar;36(3):225-231.

[10] Bogen G, Kim JS, Bakland LK. Direct pulp capping with mineral trioxide aggregate: an observational study. J Am Dent Assoc. 2008 Mar;139(3):305-315.

In: Clinical Reports in Dentistry
Editor: Lisa R. Amir
ISBN: 978-1-53617-328-4

Chapter 43

INITIAL TREATMENT OF CLASS II DIVISION I MALOCCLUSION WITH TWIN BLOCK FUNCTIONAL APPLIANCE IN 10 YEAR OLD GIRL: A CASE REPORT

***Aprillia P. Rachmadani*[1], *Sarworini B. Budiardjo*[2,*] *and Mochamad F. Rizal*[2]**

[1]Pediatric Dentistry Residency Program, Faculty of Dentistry, Universitas Indonesia, Jakarta, Indonesia
[2]Department of Pediatric Dentistry, Faculty of Dentistry, Universitas Indonesia, Jakarta, Indonesia

ABSTRACT

Introduction: Class II division 1 malocclusion is the most frequent problem in the orthodontic practice. It is characterized with a retrognathic mandible, and repositioning the mandible forward is needed to enhance its growth and improve dentoskeletal relationships. Functional twin block appliance is a widely used functional appliance for the management of Class II malocclusion.

Case report: a 10-year-11-month old girl patient attended Dental Hospital of Faculty of Dentistry, Universitas Indonesia with a chief complaint of her upper anterior teeth were more protrude than lower anterior teeth. On clinical examination, her facial profile is convex, symmetry. She had proclined maxillary anterior teeth with a 10mm overjet and a 5mm overbite. The lateral cephalometric radiography indicated a skeletal class II pattern with hyper-divergent growth which was due to mandibular retroposition and maxillary protrusion. The initial treatment objective was reduce overjet by skeletal improvement, thus promoting mandibular growth by correction class II relationship, attain normal overjet and overbite by using functional twin block appliance and then consider fixed orthodontic treatment after functional appliance treatment. The use of twin block functional appliances have skeletal effects such as increase mandibular growth

* Corresponding Author's Email: sarworinibagio@yahoo.com.

(increase height of mandibular ramus and length of mandible), the SNB value was improved to 2°. The ANB value was reduce 2°, decrease overjet 4.5mm and overbite 1mm.

Conclusion: This case has demonstrated the successful management of the first phase of treatment of a patient with Angle Class II Division 1 malocclusion using the Twin Block appliances in 6 months. The Second phase of treatment will be continued with fixed appliances.

Keywords: Class II division 1 malocclusion, twin block, functional appliances

1. INTRODUCTION

Malocclusion is frequently associated with discrepancies in arch relationship due to underlying skeletal and soft tissue factors, resulting in unfavourable cuspal guidance and poor occlusal function. The proprioceptive sensory feedback mechanism controls muscular activity and provides a functional stimulus or deterrent to the full expression of mandibular bone growth. The unfavourable cuspal contacts of distal occlusion represent an obstruction to normal forward mandibular translation in function, and as such does not encourage the mandible to achieve its optimum genetic growth potential [1]. Angle defined Class II division 1 malocclusion as characterized by a distal relation of the lower teeth to the upper to the extent of more than one-half the width of one cusp and the maxillary incisors being protrusive [2, 3]. Class II division 1 malocclusion, most of the times is caused by a retrognathic mandible.Retrognathic mandible, maxillary prognathism and reduced vertical skeletal jaw relationship are the most common characteristics of Class II division 1 malocclusion [4]. Functional appliances have been widely used to correct a Class II division malocclusion [5]. Various types of functional appliances (e.g., Activator, Bionator, Frankel and Herbst appliance) are used for the correction of class II skeletal and occlusal disharmonies. During the last ten years twin block appliance has gained increasing popularity [6]. Functional twin block appliance, originally developed by Clark, is a widely used functional appliance for the management of Class II malocclusion [7].

The appliance consists of maxillary and mandibular acrylic plates with bite blocks that posture the mandible forward on closure [6]. Functional appliances were developed to correct muscle deviation and jaw relationship to attain facial balance through functional repair of muscle and bone. Functional twin block appliance treatment aims to improve functional relationship of dento-facial structure by eliminating undesirable development and muscle function which affects occlusion by changing tooth position and support tissues [8]. This article demonstrated the skeletal correction using a twin block appliance for a girl who was 10 years 11 months of age with a severe skeletal class II (overjet 10mm) caused by a retrognathic mandible.

2. Case Report

A 10-year-11-month old girl patient attended Dental Hospital of Faculty Dentistry, Universitas Indonesia with a chief complaint of her upper anterior teeth were more protrude than lower anterior teeth. Her facial profile was convex and symmetry. She had incompetent lips with lower lips behind the maxillary central incisors when in rest position. Intra-orally, she had proclined maxillary anterior teeth with a 10mm overjet and a 5mm overbite. She showed end-on Class II molar on the left side. She had mild crowding in both arches, and the maxillary dental midline to the mandibular dental midline was deviated 2mm to the right (Figure 1).

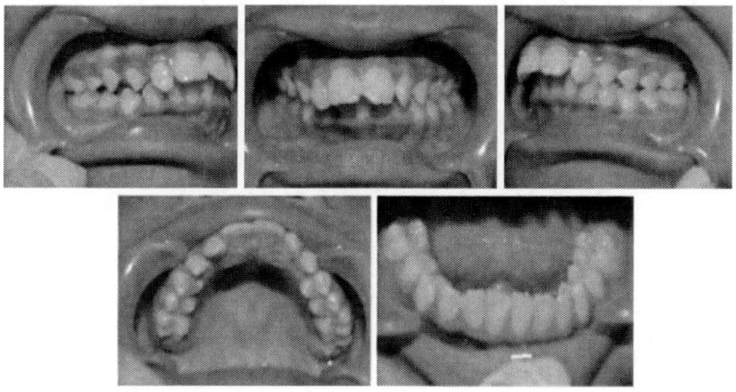

Figure 1. Pre-treatment intra oral photographs.

The lateral cephalometric analysis indicated a skeletal class II pattern. Maxillary and mandibular relationship (ANB) is 5° with hyperdivergent growth which was due to mandibular retroposition and maxillary protrusion. The height of mandibular ramus ArGo is 38mm and the length of mandible GoMe is 60mm. Both of height mandibular ramus (<38mm) and length of mandible (<60mm), less than normal (Figure 2). Since the patient was still growing, the initial treatment objective was reduce overjet by skeletal improvement, thus promoting mandibular growth by correction class II relationship, attain normal overjet and overbite by using functional twin block appliance and then consider fixed orthodontic treatment after functional appliance treatment.

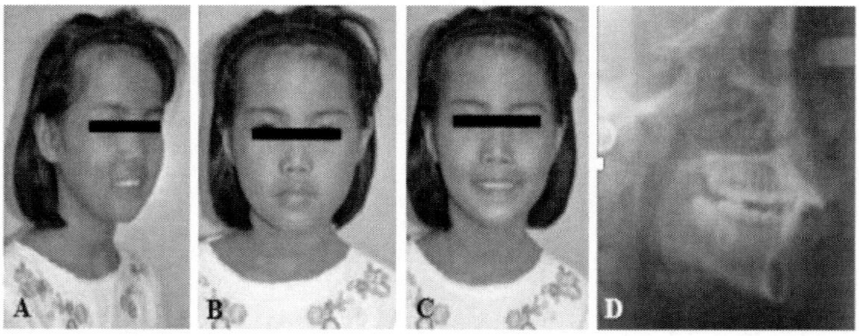

Figure 2. Pre-treatment clinical photographs (A,B,C); Pre-treatment Cephalometric Radiograph (D).

The treatment began with twin block appliances. The design of maxillary component, twin block component with acrylic baseplate covered palatal area and occlusal surfaces of second premolar and first molar. There was inclined plane in the mesial ends of acrylic bite block. Mandibular component consists of an acrylic baseplate which covers lingual surface (Figure 3).

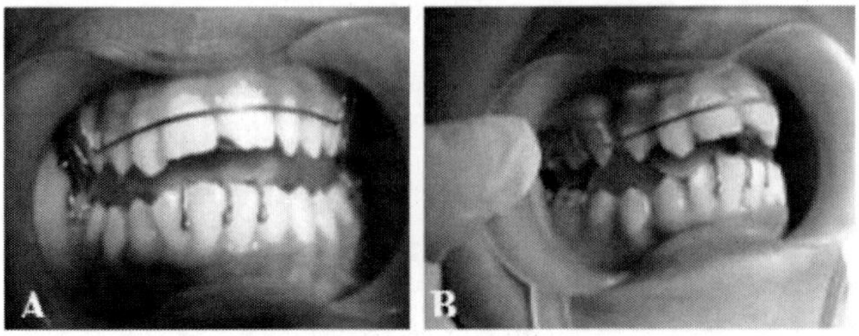

Figure 3. Twin block appliances design (A, B).

Table 1. Cephalometric Measurement

Measurement	Bjork	Before	After 6 Months of Therapy
< N-S-Ar	123° ± 5°	128°	128°
< S-Ar-Go	143° ± 6°	127°	130°
< Ar- Go-Me	130° ± 7°	136°	137°
Sum	396°	391°	395°
SN	71 ±3mm	63mm	68mm
SAr	32 ±3mm	40mm	40mm
< ArGoN	52°-55°	65°	70°
ArGo	44 ±5mm	38mm	45mm
GoMe	71 ±5mm	60mm	67mm
GoMe/SN	1	0.95	1
< SNA	83°	83°	83°
< SNB	78°	78°	80°
< ANB	5°	5°	3°
< GoGnSN		32°	33°
Y axis		68°	69°

Both block had Adam clasps on first molar. Twin block are designed to be worn 24 hour per day including meal time and activate the expansion screw in once per two week and control in every months. During adjustment, acrylic was removed by slicing from the undersurface of the posterior bite blocks to allow for the eruption of the mandibular premolar and molar.

During treatment, the SNA value was no change and the SNB value was improved to 2°. The ANB angle value was reduce 2°, and increase the height of mandibular ramus from 38 mm to 45 mm and length of mandible from 60mm to 67mm, ratio of length mandible to basis cranii (GOMe/SN) is being normal from 0.95 to 1 (Table 1).

Maxillary incisors inclination was reduced although the proclination was still exist. The vertical proportion was improved during treatment (Figures 4, 5).

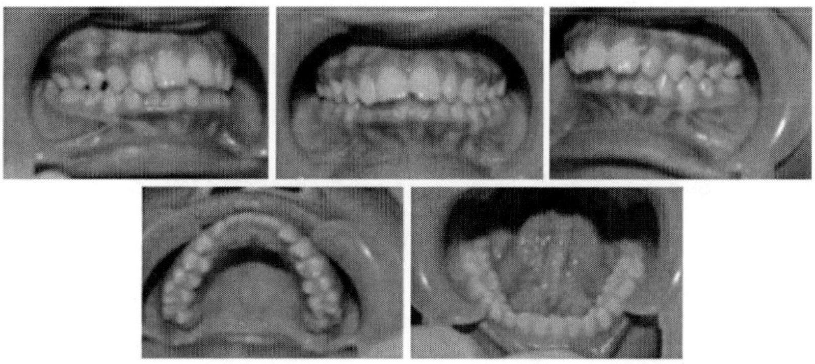

Figure 4. Intra-oral photograph, 6 months after continous use of twin block appliances.

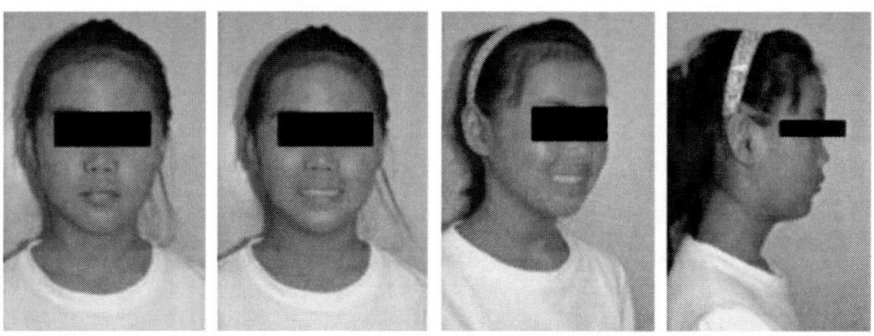

Figure 5. Post treatment clinical photograph.

3. Discussion

Growth and development are continuous processes that occur from intra uterine and continue until adulthood. Growth and development are relatively fast in infants and will slow down during childhood and then increase again during puberty and eventually the rate of growth becomes slower until maturity.

The growth velocity occurs due to secretion of Growth Hormone Releasing Hypothalamus (GHRH) produced by the hypothalamus which stimulates the secretion of Growth Hormone (GH) from the adenohypophysis [9].

A 10-year-11 months girl was diagnosed class II division 1 malocclusion and treat with functional twin block appliance. Patient was in the onset of pubertal peak. Girls experienced experience accelerated growth earlier than boys. The chronological age of pubertal peak in growth velocity varies between individuals [9, 10]. In this case, the twin block appliance treatment used during early permanent dentition. Lee at al conclude that to achieve the best outcomes, the correction of a Class II malocclusion should be started using the Twin block during adolescence rather than during the mixed dentition [5]. Bacetti et al. also mentioned that the optimum treatment timing for twin-block therapy of a class II disharmony appears to be during or slightly after the onset of pubertal peak in growth velocity. In their study, they reported that when compared with treatment before the peak, late twin block treatment produces more favorable effects that include the greater increments in total mandibular length and height of the ramus, and skeletal changes for the correction of molar relationship [5, 11, 12].

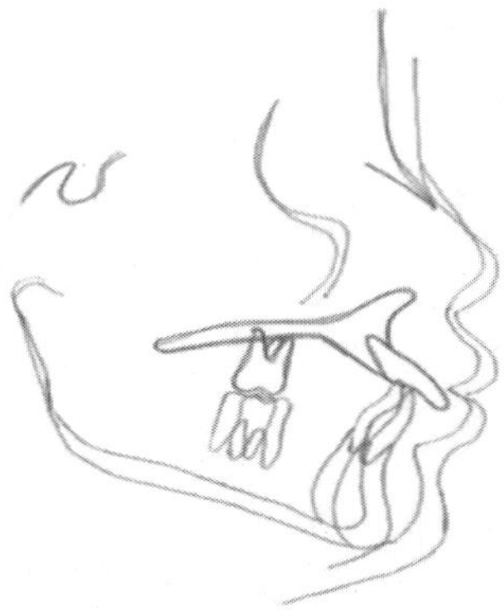

Figure 6. Superimposed after 6 months of continuous use of twin block (Green Line: before treatment; Red Line: Post 6 months of treatment).

In the present case the use of removable functional orthopedic appliances in growing individuals with class II division 1 malocclusion doing by 2 phase treatment using functional twin block appliance and then continuous using fixed orthodontic treatment after functional appliance treatment. Illing et al. and Jena et al. also mentioned the use of removable functional orthopedic appliances in growing individuals with skeletal class II has demonstrated to have some advantages promoted by treatment of class II malocclusion in two stages (functional orthopedics and fixed appliance). Reduction in overjet at early ages, better relationship between the jaws, reduction in facial convexity and shorter treatment time with fixed appliances are factors that encourage treatment of Class II malocclusion in two stages [7].

The occlusal inclined plane is the fundamental functional mechanism of the natural dentition. Cuspal inclined plane play an important part in determining the relationship of the teeth as the erupt into occlusion. If the mandible occludes in a distal relationship to the maxilla, the occlusal forces acting on the mandibular teeth normal function have a distal component of force that is unfavorable to normal forward mandibular development. The inclined planes formed by the cusps of the upper and lower teeth represent a servo-mechanism that locks the mandible in a distally occluding functional position [1].

In the present case twin block have been worn for more than 20 hours per day during 6 months to obtain functional forces which distributed to teeth, include mastication force. Interlock bite block of maxilla and mandibula is in 70° when worn in close position to edge to edge position with maxilla, which gives comfort for patient. This appliance consist maxillary and mandibular bite block that function not only for retracted maxilla with expansion screw. Twin block appliance are simple bite blocks that are designed for full-time wear. They achieve rapid functional correction of malocclusion by the transmission of favorable occlusal forces to occlusal inclined planes that cover the posterior teeth. The forces of occlusion are used as the functional mechanism to correct the malocclusion [8].

In the first control, a reduction of maxillary bite block to stimulate the eruption process of mandibular molars and also reduced overjet. In the next visits the maxillary bite block is gradually reduced to free the occlusion of mandibular molar teeth. According the literature, maxillary block was reduced in occluso-distal and remained a 2-3mm space in mandibular molars relieved from occlusion with mandibular molars allowing the eruption until all acrylic removed from occlusal surface of maxillary molars followed by removal of mandibular part to allow total eruption when occlusion [8]. Like the study of Bacetti et al, in our patient after 6 months of twin block therapy, the greater increase in length mandibular body (Go-Me, 7mm) and height of mandibular ramus (Ar-Go, 7mm). According the literature, the use of twin block functional appliances have skeletal effects such as increase mandibular growth, SNB value, restriction maxilla growth, changes in vertical direction, and stimulus condylar growth [1].

Most of the functional appliances are designed to enhance the forward growth of the mandible by encouraging a functional displacement of the mandibular condyles downward and forward in glenoid fossa. This is balanced by an upward and backward pull in the muscles supporting the mandible. Adaptive remodeling may occur on both articular surface of the temporomandibular joint to improve the position of the mandible relative to the maxilla [12].

Several advantage of the twin block appliance is its relatively small size that is easy wear by patient, thus that distraction while taking is minimal, easily repaired, and suitable for use in mixed and permanent dentition periods. Functional appliance section depends on few factors which is categorized as follow: age and patient's compliance, and also habitual factor [13].

Conclusion

This case has demonstrated the successful management of the first phase of treatment of a patient with Angle Class II Division 1 malocclusion using the Twin Block appliances in 6 months. The effect of Twin Block functional appliances is mostly dento-alveolar with small skeletal component. It is important that functional appliances are used in a growing patient to achieve the maximum benefit and very important prepared to the goal treatment planned.

References

[1] Clark, W. (2004). *Twin Block Functional Therapy: Applications in Dentofacial Orthopaedics*. 2nd ed. Mosby Elsevier, United Kingdom.

[2] McNamara, J. A. Jr. (1981). Components of Class II malocclusion in children 8-10 years of age. *Angle Orthod.,* 1(51):177-202.

[3] Patel, P., Shanthraj, R., Garg, N., Vallakari, A. (2017). Skeletal Class II division 1 malocclusion treated with twin- block appliance. *Int. J. Orthod. Rehabil.*, 8:31-37. doi:10.4103/2349-5243.200217.

[4] Sharma, B. P., Xin, C. (2014). Comparative Cephalometric Analysis of Angle Class II Division 1 Malocclusion Between Nepalese and Chinese Subjects. *Orthod. J. Nepal,* 4(1):17-21.

[5] Lee, K. Y., Park, J. H., Tai, K., Chae, J. M. (2016). Treatment with Twin-block appliance followed by fixed appliance therapy in a growing Class II patient. *Am. J. Orthod. Dentofac. Orthop.,* 150(5): 847-863. doi:10.1016/j.ajodo.2015.10.033.

[6] Sidlauskas, A. (2005). The effects of the Twin-block appliance treatment on the skeletal and dentolaveolar changes in Class II Division 1 malocclusion. *Medicina,* (Kaunas), 41(5):392-400.

[7] Saikoski, L. Z., Cançado, R. H., Valarelli, F. P., Freitas, K. M. S. de. (2014). Dentoskeletal effects of Class II malocclusion treatment with the Twin Block appliance in a Brazilian sample: A prospective study. *Dental Press. J. Orthod.,* 19(1):36-45. doi:10.1590/2176-9451.19.1.036-045.oar.

[8] Achmad, H. (2017). An Overjet Reduction of Class II, Division 1 Malocclusion in Twin Block Dentofacial Orthopedic and Fixed Orthodontic Treatment: Case Report. *J. Int. Dent. Med. Res.,* 10(3): 1010-1017.

[9] Proffit, W. (2013). *Contemporary Orthodontics*. 3rd ed. St. Louis: Mosby.

[10] Vinaya, S. (2014). Two Phase Orthodontic Treatment: A Case Report. *IJSS Case Reports Rev.,* 1:26-30.

[11] Ehsani, S., Nebbe, B., Normando, D., Lagravere, M. O., Flores-Mir, C. (2014). Short-term treatment effects produced by the Twin-block appliance: A systematic review and meta-analysis. *Eur. J. Orthod.,* 37(2):170-176. doi:10.1093/ejo/cju030.
[12] Chavan, S. J., Bhad, W. A., Doshi, U. H. (2014). Comparison of temporomandibular joint changes in Twin Block and Bionator appliance therapy: a magnetic resonance imaging study. *Prog. Orthod.,* 15(1):1-7. doi:10.1186/s40510-014-0057-6.
[13] Jazaldi, F., Handayani, E. D., Damayanti, U. et al. (2016). A Potential Bioindicator of Class II Malocclusion. *Journal of International Dental and Medical Research,* 9:351-355.

In: Clinical Reports in Dentistry
Editor: Lisa R. Amir

ISBN: 978-1-53617-328-4

Chapter 44

MANAGEMENT OF INTRUSIVE LUXATION INJURIES OF THE PRIMARY INCISOR: A CASE REPORT

***Eva Fauziah*[1,*] *and Cahyanti W. Susilo*[2]**

[1]Department of Pediatric Dentistry, Faculty of Dentistry, Universitas Indonesia, Jakarta, Indonesia
[2]Pediatric Dentistry Residency Program, Faculty of Dentistry, Universitas Indonesia, Jakarta, Indonesia

ABSTRACT

Introduction: Intrusive luxation is commonly seen in primary dentition as young children have wide medullar spaces in their alveolar bone. The management of intruded primary incisors recommended by the American Academy of Pediatric Dentistry is to wait for spontaneous re-eruption or extract the tooth, depending on the degree and the direction of intrusion as well as the presence of alveolar bone fracture. Comprehensive examination is essential for determining the most appropriate approach. Here we report our experience with a case of intrusive luxation in the left maxillary lateral incisor of a 6-year-old patient.

Case Report: Intrusive luxation of left maxillary lateral primary incisor (tooth #62) was diagnosed, the tooth was in contact with the underlying permanent tooth and the treatment of extraction of the intruded tooth was performed. Recall examination was regularly conducted to monitor the eruption of the permanent successor. Direct trauma caused by simulation of deciduous teeth can impact the permanent successor. By extracting tooth #62, direct trauma to permanent successor tooth #22 was minimized so the development can be continued normally. Recall examination post extraction on week 1 and 4 revealed no unusual symptoms such as abscess, fever, fistula or soft tissue swelling.

Conclusion: Intrusive injuries need a careful examination owing to their close anatomical association with the developing permanent successors. In the case of intrusive

* Corresponding Author's Email: eva_dens@yahoo.com.

luxation of tooth #62, due to the root impacting the underlying permanent tooth, extraction was selected as the ideal treatment approach.

Keywords: dental trauma, intrusive luxation, primary teeth, extraction

1. Introduction

Children and adolescents form the largest group that experiences dental injuries. Approximately 50% of children under the age of 15 years experience orofacial injuries, especially dental trauma. Various studies have reported that 30%-40% of children had experienced at least one dental trauma at the preschool age. Such high prevalence may be due to the incomplete development of physical and emotional aspects. The lack of experience exacerbates the consequences of the activity and the possibility of injury [1-3].

Dental injuries at the preschool age may interfere the development of primary and permanent teeth. Moreover, injuries can impact the structure of hard tissue supporting the teeth and directly or indirectly affect the child's speech and appearance [3]. Mendoza et al., have identified that the most common injuries in primary dentition were subluxation (47.29% of the injuries affected the periodontal ligaments), intrusion (23.15%) and avulsion (13.63%)[2]. The predominant injury is subluxation and not dental fracture since the alveolar process in primary dentition is characterized by large bone marrow spaces and is relatively flexible. Intrusive luxation is a type of subluxation that is often seen in primary dentition and can cause complications of both the primary and permanent teeth buds. Traumatic intrusion pushes deeper into alveolar socket, resulting in damage to the pulp and periodontal tissues. Intrusion contributes to 8%-22% of all traumatic injuries in the primary teeth anterior whereby the upper jaw incisor teeth are most often affected by this condition accounting for 93.47% of all dental intrusions [4, 5]. The management of intrusion of the primary teeth depends on several factors, including its direction and severity as well as the presence of alveolar bone fracture [4]. Therefore subjective, objective and complete investigations are imperative to arrive at the diagnosis and determine the most appropriate case management approach. This case report presented the management of 62 tooth intrusion in a 6-year-old girl who fell down from the second floor of her house.

2. Case Report

A 6-year-old girl and her mother visited the pediatric dental clinic of Universitas Indonesia, with a chief complaint of a front tooth displaced into the jaw. The mother reported that the child had suffered from trauma in her oral region approximately 2 weeks ago. The child was immediately taken to the nearest hospital, emergency care was provided and tetanus vaccine was injected. As per the information provided by her parents, the ankle bone had shifted and cracked and the girl was wheelchair-bound for 2 weeks.

The child's general health was good and she had no neurological defects. Upon extra-oral examination, there was a facial asymmetry due to a bluish swelling (hematoma), with clear boundaries on the forehead that was painful during palpation. In intra-oral examination, the lower lip appeared reddish. Lacerations in the upper frenulum regions of maxillary central primary incisors along with the other surrounding anatomical structures were observed.

Visual intra-oral inspection revealed that the left maxillary lateral incisor was submerged in the alveolar bone away from the occlusion line, with <50% of the crown being visible (Figure 1A). The tooth was not mobile and was not tender to percussion. No signs of alveolar fracture were detected upon gentle palpation of the mucosa of the traumatized area.

Following clinical examination, radiographs and photographs were obtained to assess the degree of intrusion and to decide the best treatment strategy. From the periapical radiograph, it appeared that the left maxillary lateral primary incisor (tooth #62) was present above the occlusion line, with resorption in 1/3 root apical and the growth of left maxillary lateral permanent incisor bud (tooth #22) had reached 1/3 middle of the root (Figure 1B). The anterior occlusal radiograph revealed that tooth #62 appeared elongated compared with the contralateral tooth (tooth #52) and the panoramic radiograph indicated that it was situated below the occlusion line and was overlapping with the tooth bud #22.

Clinically, the intruded tooth #62 was noticed to be submerged in the alveolar bone and located above the occlusion line, with no mobility upon palpation. The tooth produced a dull sound in response to percussion and <50% of the crown was visible. A radiographic examination was performed, in which the tooth appeared elongated and was present above the occlusion line, overlapping with bud #22. The treatment plan was to extract the tooth.

On the next visit, the procedure was performed under local anesthesia. The tooth, with the root pointing in the labial direction, was extracted using pediatric forceps by applying minimal pressure (Figures 2). Post-extraction instructions were given to the patient's family. Recall examination was performed after 1 week, 1 month and 6 months. On 1-week and 1-month post extraction examination, there were no unusual symptoms such as abscess, fever, fistula and soft tissue swelling. Clinical and radiographic monitoring was performed until the eruption of the permanent successor.

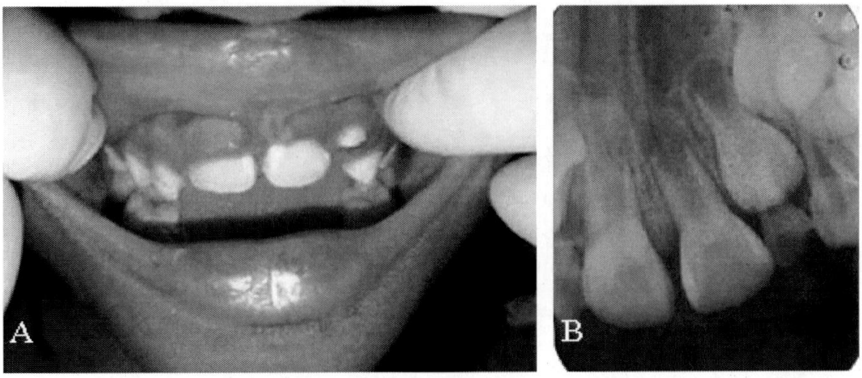

Figure 1. Intra-oral photograph (A); Periapical radiograph of the intruded tooth #62 (B).

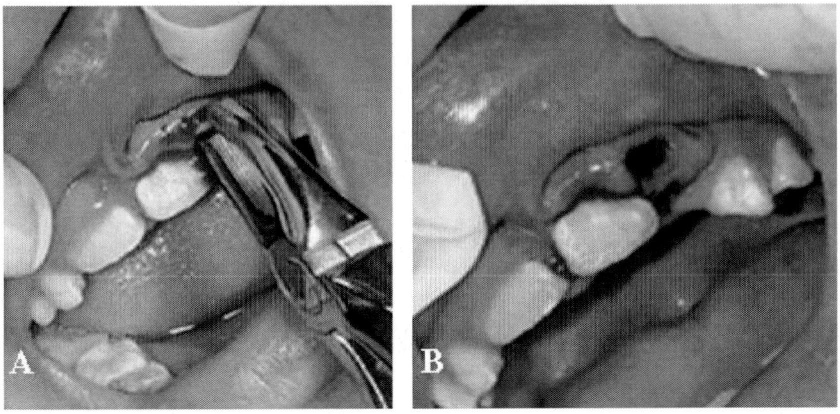

Figure 2. Extraction procedure for tooth #62.

3. Discussion

Traumatic dental injuries to the primary incisors are extremely common. The highest incidence occurs in children in the first 3 years of life and in preschool children because of poor motor coordination, lack of experience, physical and emotional underdevelopment, failure to understand the consequences of different activities and inability to evaluate risks [1, 3]. Falls while playing in home or school, riding a bicycle, or indulging in extreme sports activities have been reported as the primary causes of dental injury in young children and teenagers worldwide [4]. In primary dentition, luxation or avulsion occurs more often than fractures as the alveolar bone in young children has wider medullar spaces and tends to be more flexible [6, 7]. Large bone marrow spaces result in an increased elasticity of the alveolar bone surrounding the primary teeth and the primary teeth become more susceptible to displacement than to fracture accordingly. It was previously reported that the most frequently intruded primary teeth are the maxillary incisors (93.47%) [5].

After a comprehensive clinical and radiographic assessment, intrusive luxation of tooth #62, with the root pointing in the palatal direction, was diagnosed. Clinically, the intruded tooth was found to be submerged in the alveolar bone and located above the occlusion line, without mobility during palpation and producing a dull sound in response to percussion. Radiographic examination indicated palatal displacement, suggesting that the follicle germ of the permanent tooth was at risk. Radiographic examination in this case was extremely essential because it allowed the medical team to identify the degree of injury, the direction of displacement, the presence of alveolar bone fractures, the degree of root formation, and the association between the injured tooth and its permanent successor [8].

In cases involving the intrusion of the primary teeth, it is important to determine the direction of the displaced tooth to devise a treatment plan to prevent the occurrence of sequelae in the permanent dentition. Owing to the close association of the primary tooth apex with the underlying permanent tooth germ and its mechanical impact, such injuries may cause disturbances in the permanent successor [9]. In this case, intrusion of #62 resulted in contact with the underlying permanent tooth; therefore, extraction was performed. Developmental disturbances in permanent teeth caused by trauma in their predecessors are prevalent in 12%-74% cases [6]. Impacts on the permanent teeth that are attributed to trauma in their predecessors include white, yellow, or brown enamel discoloration; enamel hypoplasia; crown malformation; root dilacerations; partial or complete arrest of root formation; and eruption disturbances [6, 10]. Therefore, it is important to inform the parents regarding the possible effects of trauma on the developing teeth.

Considering the degree of intrusion, tooth extraction was decided. Whenever the intrusion is moderate or severe (grade II or III), the tooth rarely re-erupts and may become necrotic, indicating the need for extraction [5]. In our case, the degree was grade II, which is a moderate partial intrusion, with <50% of the crown being visible. The preferred management was to carefully remove the intruded tooth and relieve the pressure on the developing follicle of tooth #22. Treatment commenced with the application of topical anesthetics and administration of local anesthesia. The tooth was grasped with narrow forceps without elevators and removed with the root pointing in a labial direction (Figure 3). Subsequently, the palatal and facial bone plates were repositioned with slight digital pressure. An adequate oral hygiene instruction was given, and a soft diet was prescribed. A minimal pressure was applied, and a careful removal was executed to decrease the risk of damaging the developing follicle. The use of elevators is contraindicated as they may enter the follicular space and harm the tooth germ [5].

Post-extraction visits were scheduled for complete examination according to the guidelines of the International Association of Dental Traumatology to check for unusual symptoms, such as abscess, fever, fistula, and soft tissue swelling, and to assess the growth of the permanent tooth bud. The schedule of the follow-up visits was as follows:

after 1 week for clinical examination, after 3-4 weeks for clinical and radiographic examinations, after 6-8 weeks for clinical examination, after 6 months for clinical and radiographic examinations, and after 1 year for clinical and radiographic examinations [11]. In this case, recall examination after 1 week and 4 weeks post extraction showed a good soft tissue healing and didn't show any pathological findings. In each subsequent year post extraction, the patient was scheduled for evaluation clinically or radiographically until the eruption of the permanent successor [5]. Hence, even after the primary tooth is extracted or avulsed, the growth of the tooth bud and its eruption should be followed-up to detect any possible damages to the permanent successor [9].

Conclusion

Intrusive luxation of the primary central incisor in a 6-year-old girl is reported. Children of preschool age are at the highest risk of traumatic dental injuries because they are physically and emotionally underdeveloped and lack awareness regarding the consequences of their risky activities. Intrusive luxation of a primary tooth is extremely likely to cause damage to the permanent tooth germ owing to its close anatomic association with the apex of the primary incisor. Comprehensive clinical and radiograph examinations are required to determine the management approach to intrusive luxation. In this case, with the root impacting the underlying permanent tooth, extraction was the preferred treatment choice. A periodic follow-up visits and proper maintenance of oral hygiene were advised.

References

[1] Emerich K, Wyszkowski J. (2010). Clinical practice: Dental trauma. *Eur. J. Pediatrics*, 169:1045-1050.

[2] Mendoza-mendoza A. (2015). Prevalence and complications of trauma to the primary dentition in a subpopulation of Spanish children in southern Europe. *Dental Traumatology: Official Publication Inter. Assoc. Dent. Traumatol.* 31:144-195.

[3] Choi SC, Park JH. (2010). Retrospective study on traumatic dental injuries in preschool children at Kyung Hee Dental Hospital, Seoul, South Korea. *Dental Traumatology: Official Publication Inter. Assoc. Dent. Traumatol.,* 26:70-75.

[4] Gupta M. (2011). Intrusive luxation in primary teeth - Review of literature and report of a case. *Saudi Dent. J.,* 23:167-176.

[5] Carvalho V, Ribeiro D, Campos V. (2010). Frequency of intrusive luxation in deciduous teeth and its effects. *Dental Traumatology: Official Publication Inter. Assoc. Dent. Traumatol.,* 26:304-307.

[6] Altun C, Cehreli ZC, Güven G, Acikel C. (2009). Traumatic intrusion of primary teeth and its effects on the permanent successors : A clinical follow-up study. *Oral Surg., Oral Med., Oral Pathol., Oral Radiol., Endodont.,* 107:493-498.

[7] Diaz JA, Bustos L, Brandt AC. (2010). Dental injuries among children and adolescents aged 1-15 years attending to public hospital in Temuco, Chile. Dental Traumatology: *Official Publication Inter. Assoc. Dent. Traumatol.,* 26:254-261.

[8] Mendoza-mendoza A, Gonzales-Mallea E, Iglesias-Linares A. (2015). Intrusive luxation in primary teeth: A case report. *J. Clin. Pediatr. Dent.,* 39:215-219.

[9] Miranda C, Killian B, Luiz M, Miranda C. (2012). Consequences of dental trauma to the primary teeth on the permanent dentition. *Revista Sul-Brasileira de Odontologia*, 9:457-463.

[10] Bardellini E, Amadori F, Pasini S, Majorana A. (2017). Dental anomalies in permanent teeth after trauma in primary dentition. *J. Clin. Pediatr. Dent*., 41:5-10.

[11] Malmgren B, Jens O, Flores MT et al. (2012). International Association of Dental Traumatology. International Association of Dental Traumatology guidelines for the management of traumatic dental injuries : 3. Injuries in the primary dentition. *Dental Traumatology: Official Publication Inter. Assoc. Dent. Traumatol*., 28:174-182.

In: Clinical Reports in Dentistry
Editor: Lisa R. Amir
ISBN: 978-1-53617-328-4

Chapter 45

MANAGEMENT OF CLASS I MALOCCLUSION WITH BILATERAL CONSTRICTION OF THE UPPER AND LOWER ARCH: A CASE REPORT

Sharah Syam[1] and Miesje K. Purwanegara[2,*]
[1]Orthodontics Residency Program, Faculty of Dentistry, Universitas Indonesia, Jakarta, Indonesia
[2]Department of Orthodontics, Faculty of Dentistry, Universitas Indonesia, Jakarta, Indonesia

ABSTRACT

Introduction: The goals of orthodontic treatment are correcting the malocclusion especially bilateral constriction of upper and lower arch, achieving good occlusion and also improve the esthetic. *Case report*: This case report described the treatment of class I malocclusion with bilateral arch constriction. The 33-year-old female patient presented with class I malocclusion, mesofacial, retrognathic chin, convex profile, and bilateral constriction of both arch. She was treated by pre-adjusted appliances and no teeth was extracted. The upper arch had 2 phases treatment, segmental method and continuous method to correct the constriction. After 18 months of treatment, the malocclusion was corrected with successful aesthetic improvement, class I canine and molar relationship in the left and right side, and also ideal overjet and overbite. *Conclusion*: Treatment for bilateral arch constriction could be corrected by pre-adjusted appliances. An accurate examination will result in a proper diagnosis and an effective and efficient treatment plan. However, expansion for bilateral arch constriction should consider the limits of expansion because excessive expansion leads to instability.

Keywords: constriction, pre-adjusted, orthodontic treatment, expansion

* Corresponding Author's Email: miesjekar@gmail.com.

1. INTRODUCTION

Malocclusion can be defined as a deviation from an ideal which is considered aesthetically and functionally [1]. In the 1980s, Angle classified malocclusion into 3 classes, namely class I, class II, and class III. According to Angle the maxillary first molars were key to occlusion. The maxillary and mandibular molars had to be related so that the cusp mesiobuccal maxillary molars occluded with the buccal groove of the mandibular molars. Angle described 3 classes of malocclusion based on occlusal relationships in the first molar where class I malocclusion is described as a normal molar relationship but not ideal occlusion line due to malocclusion, rotation, or other causes [2].

Malocclusions occur not only in the anteroposterior and vertical directions but in the transverse direction. One of malocclusions that can occur in the transverse direction is the constriction of the dental arch. Constriction of dental arches may occur in the maxillary, mandible or both with clinical signs of narrowed dental arch, crowding teeth, impaction, and incisive proclination [2]. Increasing the size of the dental arch by expansion, reducing the size of the tooth with interproximal reduction and tooth extraction is the preferred treatment in overcoming the constriction of the dental arch [2]. Tooth extraction is an efficient way to deal with crowding, but has a detrimental effect on facial aesthetics if done carelessly. In addition, extraction of the teeth does not guarantee better stability compared to anteroposterior and transversal arch expansion [3]. Increased dental arch dimensions, both in the anteroposterior and transverse planes can create space. However, the problem that can arise is if the tooth moves excessively in either buccal or labial direction, the tooth will move out of the equilibrium zone and can affect the stability of the tooth because there is a force imbalance that makes the teeth tend to return to the previous position [2].

Constriction of the dental arch in the maxilla and mandible require expansion to increase the dimensions of the dental arch in the transverse direction. Orthodontic treatment with non-extraction in narrow dental arches and crowded teeth requires increased arch perimeter for leveling aligning stages [4]. This can be achieved by distalizing the posterior teeth, transverse expansion and proclination of the incisors [5]. The appliances that can be used include maxillary expansion appliances such as quad-helix, mandibular expansion appliances, conventional bracket, and self-ligating bracket such as Damon bracket [5]. Ricketts et al. reported that 1 mm of proclination increasing arch length of 2 mm, 1 mm of canine expansion increasing arch length of 1 mm and 1 mm of molar expansion increasing arch length of 0.25 mm [4].

Proper diagnosis in determining constriction of dental arches will result in an appropriate treatment plan. There are several analyzes and calculations that can be used in diagnosis and treatment planning for dental arch constriction. As for some analysis that can be used is the analysis of Howes and Pont. Both of these analyzes will assist the operator in determining whether the treatment plan should be expansion or extraction [6].

Ashley Howes stated that crowding teeth occurs due to deficiency of arch width rather than arch length. Howes analysis is useful for make the treatment plan and helping determine whether the treatment plan needs expansion or extraction. Howes stated that there was a relationship between the total mesio-distal width of the teeth in the M2 area and the width of the dental arch in the P1 area. Howes stated that the maxillary width in the premolar area is at least 43% of the tooth material [6]. Another analysis that can be used is Pont analysis. In 1909, Pont suggested that measuring 4 maxillary incisors could determine the width of the dental arch in the premolar and molar areas. The Pont index describes the estimated width or narrowness of the dental arch and the amount of lateral expansion required to accommodate the teeth in a perfect arrangement [6].

There are two mechanics in orthodontic treatment, that is continuous mechanics and segmental mechanics. The use of continuous mechanics in moderate and severe crowding will cause the incisor proclination during the leveling aligning stage. This condition is undesirable because it will make facial aesthetics worse, increase overjet and require longer time to retract the teeth. One solution is the use of segmental mechanics by placing the bracket only in the posterior and canine segments. This mechanic will overcome crowded teeth without incisive tooth proclination during leveling and aligning [7]. Orthodontic treatment with segmental mechanics is usually used to align the initial anterior and posterior segments, creating better anchor, leveling using intrusion and extrusion methods, space closure with differential movements in the anterior and posterior segments, and for additional torque. The advantage of using segmental mechanics is more able to control the movement of teeth and can perform tooth movements that cannot be carried out by continuous methods. The disadvantage of using segmental mechanics is that the application is more complex and in some cases the amount of visit time is longer [2]. This case report discussed the case of class I malocclusion patients with bilateral dental arch constriction treated with non-extraction using segmental methods. The patient has given permission to use photographs of her case for publication.

2. Case Report

The 33-year-old female patient came to the orthodontic clinic of Universitas Indonesia Dental Hospital complained about her crowding teeth. Her profession was a model that required her to have good aesthetics of the teeth. Her body weight was 49 kg and height was 165 cm. An extra-oral clinical examination showed the patient's face is mesofasial, asymmetrical, unbalanced and convex soft tissue profile (Figure 1). An intra-oral examination showed poor oral hygiene and gingival without tooth mobility, high palate and medium tongue size (Figure 2). Maxilla and mandible showed bilateral dental arch constriction. Moderate crowding was observed in the maxillary teeth whereas mandibular teeth showed severe crowding and filling at tooth #11 and #21. The first molar relationship was class I while canine relationship was class II. The patient's overjet is 3 mm from distal 21 to 41 with 3 mm overbite. She had normal curve of spee, the upper midline is normal whereas lower midline is shifted 2 mm to the right. The shape of upper arch was oval and lower arch was triangle (Table 1).

The intercanine and intermolar widths of the maxilla were 30 mm and 48 mm, respectively. The intercanine and intermolar widths of the mandible were 23 mm and 40 mm, respectively. There was a scissor bite between 24, 34 and 15, 45 (Figure 2). Functional examination showed no abnormalities in the temporomandibular joint. The results of the cephalometric analysis concluded that the patient had an orthognathic jaw to the cranial base, class I skeletal pattern and straight profile. Position of the chin to profile was retrognatic. The upper incisive position to profile was protrusive. The lower incisive position to the mandible is protrusive. The position of the chin to the alveolar process is retrusive. The upper and lower lips are behind the E-line (Table 1). The OPG showed normal bone height, root alignment was not parallel, radiopaque appearance on mesial teeth 11 and 21 (Figure 3).

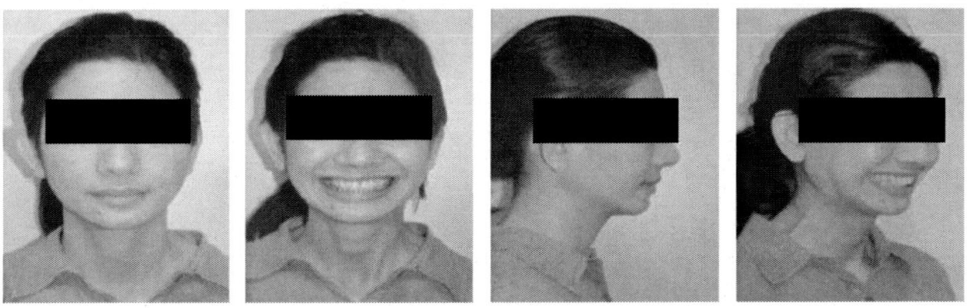

Figure 1. Extra-oral photographs of pre-treatment.

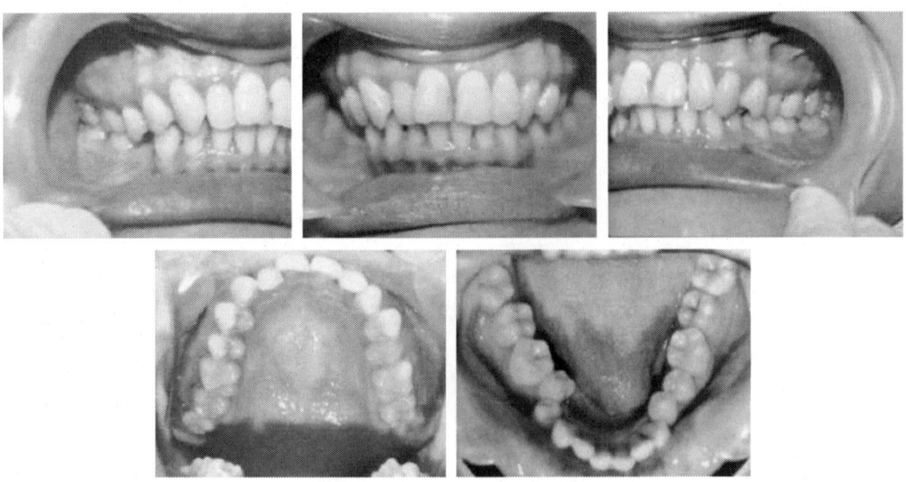

Figure 2. Intra-oral photographs of pre-treatment.

Table 1. Cephalometric values for pre-treatment

	Mean	*Patient's value*	*Description*
Skeletal Parameter (horizontal)			
SNA	82° ± 2	84°	Relationship of maxilla to cranial base is normal
SNB	80° ± 2	80°	Relationship of mandible to cranial base is normal
ANB	2° ± 2	4°	Skeletal relationship is orthognathy
The Wits	F: (-2)-(-4) M: (-1,5)-(-4,5)	0.5 mm	Skeletal pattern is class I (AO in front of BO)
Facial Angle	87° ± 3	82°	Position of the chin to profile is retrognathy
Angle of Convexity	0° ± 10	4°	Profile of the skeletal is straight
Skeletal Parameter (vertikal)			
Y-axis	60° ± 6	65°	Direction of the mandibular growth is normal
Go angle	123° ± 7	123°	Direction of one third of lower face is normodivergent
SN-MP	32° ± 3	32°	Vertikal growth of middle and lower face is normodivergent
MMPA	27° ± 4°	27°	Vertikal growth o flower face is normodivergent
Dental Parameter			
Interincisal Angle	130°	120°	Inclination of the upper incisive to lower incisive is normal
UI-SN	104° ± 6	109°	Inclination of the upper incisive to cranial base is normal
UI-PP	109° ± 6	104°	Inclination of the upper incisive to palatal plane is normal
UI-NA	4 mm	4 mm	Position of the upper incisive to maxilla is normal
UI-Apg	4 mm	8 mm	Position of the upper incisive to profile is protrusive
LI-Apg	2 mm	4 mm	Position of the lower incisive to profile is normal
LI-MP	90° ± 4	100°	Inclination of the lower incisive to mandibular plane is protrusive
LI-NB	4 mm	8 mm	Position of the lower incisive to mandible is protrusive
Pg-NB	4 mm	1 mm	Position of the chin to processus alveolaris is retrusive
Soft Tissue Parameter			
Upper lip-E line	1 mm	-6 mm	Upper lip is behind the E-line
Lower lip-E line	0 mm	-5 mm	Lower lip is behind the E-line

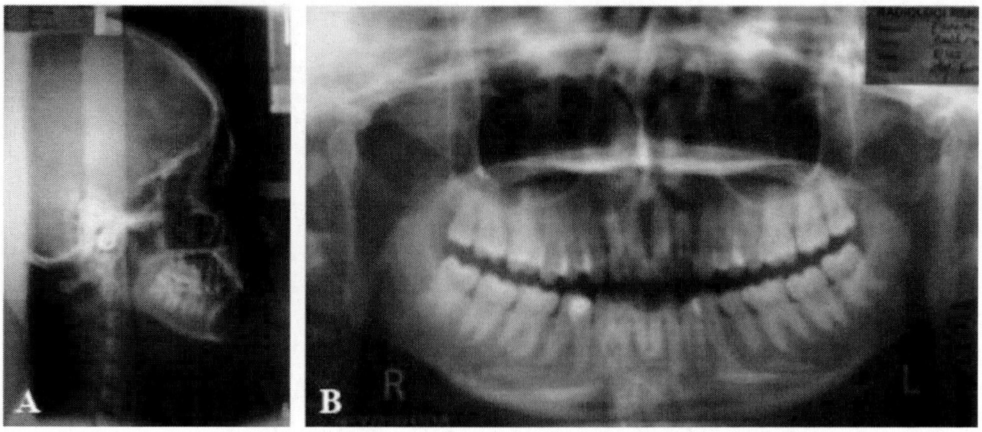

Figure 3. Lateral cephalometry (A); pre-treatment orthopantomograph (B).

Lundstrum analysis showed space deficiency 5 mm and 4 mm in the maxilla and mandible, respectively. The Bolton analysis showed that there was an excess of tooth size in the anterior mandible that was 2.8 mm (anterior ratio) while the overall ratio showed a normal range that was 93.55% (normal range 87.5-94.8). Pont analysis showed that the Calculated Premolar Value/CPV and Calculated Molar Value/CMV is less than Measured Premolar Value/MPV and Measured Molar Value/MMV at both maxilla and mandible. Howes analysis shows the value of Premolar Basal Arch Width greater than the Premolar Diameter of the maxilla and mandible. Kesling analysis was calculated by performing a 1 mm protraction and expansion in the lower dental arch and shifting the mandibular midline 2 mm to the left while in the maxilla are planned for uprighting the inclination of posterior teeth toward the buccal. Therefore, the space requirement was -3 mm in the region of 1, -1.5 mm in the region of 2, 0 mm in region 3, and -2 in region 4.

2.1. Etiology

Skeletal factors that play a role in this case is skeletal relationship class I tendency class II with maxillary has a tendency to be prognatic relative to cranial base. Lateral constriction of the mandible due to linguo-version of tooth 45 causes the dental arch become smaller and narrower and the shape of the arch becomes a triangle. Linguo-version of tooth 45 was probably caused by premature tooth loss 85 causes the tooth 45 to grow more lingually and result in scissor bite teeth between 15 and 45 and midline shifting of the to mandible to the right. Lateral constriction and triangular shape of the lower arch cause adaptation of the maxillary teeth resulting in lateral constriction of the upper arch.

2.2. Diagnosis

The 33-year-old female patient came to the orthodontic clinic of Universitas Indonesia Dental Hospital with a chief complaint of her crowding teeth. She has a model that required her teeth to be good. Extra-oral examination showed the facial type of the patient is mesofacial, not symmetrical and unbalanced. Intra-oral examination showed poor dental hygiene and gingival. Skeletal relationship was class I tendency class II with prognatic maxillary related to the cranial base. Skeletal pattern is class 1 with straight profile. Position of chin to profile was retrognathic. The upper incisive position to profile was protrusive. The incisive inclination of the mandible was protrusive. The lower incisive position to mandible was protrusive. The position of the chin to alveolar process was retrusive. The upper and lower lips are behind the E-line. Molar relationships was class I whereas canine relationship was class II. Overjet 3 mm and overbite 3 mm. Scissor bite between 24, 34 and 15, 25. Midline of the mandible was shifted 2 mm to the right. The shape of the upper arch was oval while the lower arch was triangle.

2.3. Treatment Planning

Orthodontic treatment was performed using a 0.022 "MBT slot bracket with non-extraction. Space deficiency will be obtained from lateral expansion and slicing. Constriction in the upper arch will be corrected by uprighting posterior tooth to buccal with segmental method. After that a bracket will be placed on the maxillary anterior teeth and will be re-aligned and re-leveled. The canine relationships will be class I and the class I molar relationship will remain class I. Midline of the lower teeth was corrected together with the use of open coil spring to create space for the tooth 45. Finishing was done until obtained good inter-digitation between the teeth. Retention was planned using Essix retainer in the maxilla and mandible.

2.4. Treatment Result

After 18 months of treatment, a debonding bracket was performed. Overjet and overbite become 2.5, relationship of canine and molar was class I, maxillary and mandibular teeth had level and align, upper and lower midline teeth in line with the midline face (Figure 4-6). Good inter-digitation at left and right posterior. After debonding bracket, patient use Essix Retainer to maintain the stability. Pont analysis in post-treatment shows that the Calculated Premolar Value/CPV and Calculated Molar Value/CMV values are smaller than the Measured Premolar Value/MPV and Measured Molar Value/MMV in the upper and lower jaws. Howes Analysis shows the value of the

Premolar Basal Arch Width is bigger than the Premolar Diameter in the upper and lower jaws (Table 2).

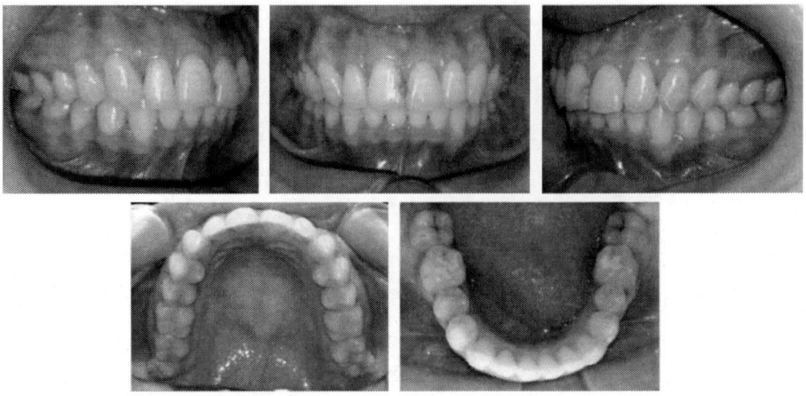

Figure 4. Intra-oral photos after debonding.

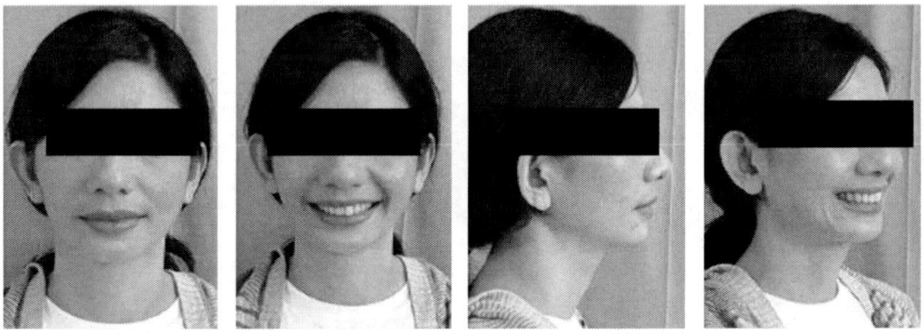

Figure 5. Extra-oral photographs of post-treatment.

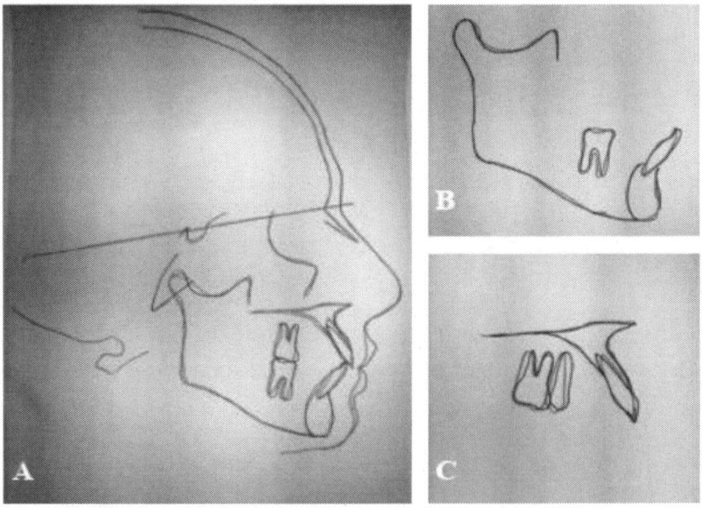

Figure 6. Superimposition of lateral cephalometry. SN plane (left); mandible (middle); palate (right). Note: Black colour shows cephalometry before treatment and blue colour shows cephalometry after treatment.

Table 2. Comparison of cephalometric value before and 18 months after treatment

	Mean	*Pre-treatment*	*After treatment*
Skeletal Parameter(horizontal)			
SNA	82° ± 2°	84°	84°
SNB	80° ± 2°	80°	80°
ANB	2° ± 2°	4°	4°
The Wits	F: (-2)-(-4) M: (-1,5)-(-4,5)	0.5 mm	- 0.5 mm
Facial Angle	87° ± 3°	82°	84^0
Angle of Convexity	0° ± 10°	4°	4°
Skeletal Parameter (vertikal)			
Y-axis	60° ± 6°	65°	64°
Go angle	123° ± 7°	123°	123°
SN-MP	32° ± 3°	32°	32°
MMPA	27° ± 4°	27°	27°
Dental Parameter			
Interincisal Angle	135° ± 10°	120°	113°
UI-SN	104° ± 6°	109°	109°
UI-PP	109° ± 6°	104°	105°
UI-NA	4 mm ± 2 mm	4 mm	4 mm
UI-Apg	4 mm ± 2 mm	8 mm	9 mm
LI-Apg	1 mm ± 2 mm	4 mm	6 mm
LI-MP	93° ± 6°	100°	102°
LI-NB	4 mm ± 2 mm	8 mm	8 mm
Pg-NB	4 mm ± 2 mm	1 mm	0 mm
Soft Tissue Parameter			
Upper lip-E line	1 mm ± 2 mm	-6 mm	-2 mm
Lower lip-E line	0 mm ± 2 mm	-5 mm	-1 mm

3. Discussion

In this case, bilateral dental arch constriction occurs in the upper and lower arch. The upper arch of the patient is oval but it appears that the crown of the posterior teeth is tipping to the palatal. In contrast to the upper jaw, the lower arch is triangular. It showed that the constriction of the lower arch is greater than the upper arch. Bilateral dental constriction of the lower arch was caused by linguoversion of tooth 45 which causes the dental arch to become smaller and narrower and the arch becomes a triangle. The main etiologies of upper dental arch constriction are mouth breathing, bad habits such as fingers sucking, and abnormal speech and swallowing patterns [8]. However, the etiology factor of lower arch constriction is due to position of the teeth, agenesis teeth, and impacted teeth [8]. In this patient, the possibility of upper arch constriction occurs because the adaptation of lower arch constriction and also because of crowding teeth in the maxilla.

It is important to determine whether the constriction that occurs in the upper and lower arches can be corrected by expansion or not. Accurate examination and diagnosis will result in an appropriate treatment plan. One of the analyses to determine whether the treatments can be expansioned or not is the analysis of Pont and Howes. The results of the Pont and Howes analysis showed that expansion on the upper and lower arches can be performed. Therefore, in the new Kesling dental analysis was made with anterior protraction and lateral expansion of the lower teeth while in the upper teeth molar uprighting was performed. Consideration of the absence of extraction in this patient because the patient has a sharp nose but has a convex profile due to the chin position to the profile is retrognathic and the position of the chin position to the alveolar process is retrusive. In addition, on the soft tissue parameters, the upper lip and lower lip of the patient are far behind the E-line. Then, when viewed on cephalometric examination, the position and inclination of the maxillary teeth tend to be normal.

The first treatment plan of upper arch is by molar uprighting with segmental mechanics followed by aligning and leveling of the anterior teeth with continuous mechanics. Segmental mechanics of the maxilla are selected to avoid proclination or flaring of the anterior teeth in the aligning leveling stage as is common in continuous mechanics [7]. However, the lower jaw is used continuous mechanics because the flaring or proclination effect of the mandibular anterior teeth is expected and lateral expansion is obtained following the available wire form. Results of cephalometric analysis after 18 months of treatment showed a change in skeletal parameters i.e., facial angle. Position of the chin to profile became normal probably caused by mandible rotation to the front due to class II elastic wear. Another major change is in dental parameters. It appears that the incisive inclination of the maxilla to the palatal plane turns to be more protrusive but still within the limits of normal inclination ($109^{o}\pm6^{o}$). Inclination changes also occur in the mandible incisive to the mandibular plane. Incisive inclination of the mandible increases 2° to become more protrusive. Increased inclination of the maxilla and mandible may be due to the effects of crowding teeth correction during the leveling and aligning stages. In addition, the inclination changes in the maxilla and mandible make the interincisal angle decrease. However, these incisive inclination changes make the patient's soft tissue profile better. It can be proofed by the value of soft tissue parameters on cephalometric examination after bracket debonding. The upper lip and lower lip previously far behind the E-line became close to the E-line.

The inter-canine width of upper arch increased from 30 mm to 33 mm while the intermolar width increased from 48 mm to 51 mm. The inter-canine width of lower arch increased from 23 mm to 27 mm and the inter-molar width increased from 40 mm to 42 mm. Increased inter-kaninus and inter-molar width is caused by lateral expansion and molar uprighting to the buccal segment of the maxilla and mandible. The lateral expansion and molar uprigting to the buccal segment of the maxilla is done by segmental method first. This is done to prevent the flaring or proclination of the maxillary anterior teeth. Post-treatment analysis of Pont and Howe showed that expansion does not exceed the maximum expansion limit or in other words does not cross the basal curve. The lateral expansion and molar uprighting to the buccal segment of the maxilla was performed for 5 months until the NiTi wire installation was 0.017 "x 0.025." The lateral expansion of the mandible is performed by a continuous method because of the flaring or proclination effects of the mandibular anterior teeth are expected. Flaring or proclination of the mandibular anterior teeth also aims to reduce the overjet. The reduction of overjet is also done by the use of class II elastics from the maxillary canines to the mandibular first molars hook. Ackerman and Proffit suggest that the mandibular expansion limit is 0 mm at the intercanine and 2-3mm in the intermolar [9]. The intercanine width of the lower arch increases 4mm while the intermolar width increases 2mm. Although some studies suggest that it is difficult to maintain the stability of the expansion in the lower arch, many studies say otherwise [4, 9-13].

At the end of the treatment, it was seen that the crowding teeth had been corrected, the overjet and the overbite were reduced to 2.5mm, interdigitation was good with class I canine and molar relationship. The soft tissue profile of the patient also improved. The preferred retainer for final stabilization is Essix retainer. Several studies suggest that fixed retainer from canine to canine is sufficient for post-expansion treatment stabilization [4, 12]. However, this patient used Essix retainer to maintain post-treatment stability until second molars. Relapse in this patient may be due to an increased of incisive proclination of the lower teeth with a large relapse tendency [10]. However, an increase of inclination in mandibular incisive is necessary to compensate patient's skeletal relationship (SNA 84º, ANB 80º). Relapse prevention can be done with the retainer check-up every 3 months.

CONCLUSION

Class I malocclusion patients with bilateral dental constriction may be corrected with MBT slot 0.022" bracket. This case report concluded that bilateral dental constriction of upper and lower arches can be corrected by conventional bracket. An accurate examination will result in a proper diagnosis and an effective and efficient treatment plan. The choice of treatment for bilateral constriction of the dental arch depends on the severity of the constriction, whether it includes dental arches, jaws, or both. Flaring or proclination of incisive teeth because of leveling aligning stages can be prevented by the use of segmental methods during the early stages of treatment. The expansion in patients with bilateral dental constriction should consider the limits of expansion because excessive expansion leads to instability. One of the retainers that can be used to maintain the stability of the treatment is Fixed and Essix retainer.

REFERENCES

[1] Cobourne MT, Dibiase AT. (2010). Handbook of Orthodontics. *Mosby Elsevier*, London.

[2] Proffit W, Fields H, Sarver D. (2013). Contemporary Orthodontics. 5th ed. *St Louis: Mosby.*

[3] Sabri R. (2010). Treatment of a severe arch-length deficiency with anterposterior and transverse expansion: Long-term stability. *Am J Orthod Dentofac Orthop,* 137(3):401-411. doi:10.1016/j.ajodo.2007. 08.040.

[4] Neto JV, Evangelista K, Pithon M et al. (2016). A 22-year Follow-up of the Nonsurgical Expansion of Maxillary and Mandibular Arches in a Young Adult: Are the Outcomes Stable, Relapsed, or Unstable with Aging?. *Am J Orthod Dentofac Orthop,* 159:521-532. doi:10.1016/j. ajodo.2015.10.030.

[5] Atik E, Ciğer S. (2014). An assessment of conventional and self-ligating brackets in Class i maxillary constriction patients. *Angle Orthod,* 84(4):615-622. doi:10.2319/093013-712.1.

[6] Stifter J. (1958). A study of pont's, Howes' Rees,' Neff's and Bolton's Analyses on class 1 adult Dentitions. *Angle Orthod,* 28:215-225.

[7] Road PH. (2010). The segmental mechanics - An efficient method to reduce treatment duration in severely crowded cases. *Virtual J Orthod,* 8(4):10-18.

[8] Helena R, Belluzzo L, Junior KF et al. (2012). Maxillary constriction : Are there differences between anterior and posterior regions?. *Dental Press J Orthod,* 17(4):1-6.

[9] Ackerman JL, Proffit WR. (1997). Soft tissue limitations in orthodontics. Treatment planning guidelines. *Angle Orthod,* 67(5):327-336.

[10] Burke SP, Silviera AM, Goldsmith LJ et al. (1997). A Meta-Analysis of Mandibular Intercanine Width in Treatment and Postretention. *Angle Orthod*, 68(1):53-60.

[11] Motoyoshi M, Hirabayashi M, Shimazaki T. (2002). An experimental study on mandibular expansion : increases in arch width and perimeter. *Eur J Orthod*, 24(2002):125-130.

[12] Housley JA, Nanda RS, Currier GF, McCune DE. (2003). Stability of transverse expansion in the mandibular arch. *Am J Orthod Dentofac Orthop*, 124:288-293. doi:10.1016/S0889-5406(03)00450-5.

[13] Sharda J, Sharma G, Shetty P, Sharda A. (2011). Mandibular Arch Expansion- A New Treatment Approach by Transverse Transforce: A Case Report. *Int J Dent Clin,* 3(1):98-99.

SECTION 5: FORENSIC DENTISTRY

In: Clinical Reports in Dentistry
Editor: Lisa R. Amir
ISBN: 978-1-53617-328-4

Chapter 46

THE ROLE OF TOOTH DEVELOPMENT AND ATTRITION ANALYSES IN BURNT VICTIM AGE ESTIMATION: A CASE REPORT

Jessica Jessica[1], Vanessa Vanessa[1], Denys P. Alim[2], Fitri A. Sari[2] and Nurtami Soedarsono[3,*]

[1]Dentistry Master Program, Faculty of Dentistry,
Universitas Indonesia, Jakarta, Indonesia
[2]Department of Forensic and Medicolegal, Faculty of Medicine,
Universitas Indonesia, Jakarta, Indonesia
[3]Department of Oral Biology, Division of Forensic Odontology,
Faculty of Dentistry, Universitas Indonesia, Jakarta, Indonesia

ABSTRACT

Introduction: A case of age estimation on burnt victim using tooth development and attrition analyses was reported. *Case Report*: A burnt body was brought to Forensic Department of National Cipto Mangunkusumo Hospital (RSCM), Jakarta, for identification. The authorities instructed minimal invasive identification procedure to avoid more damage to the body. Teeth were the only evidence available in the victim that could be used for age estimation. Victim's age was estimated from the third molar eruption status and attrition severity.

Discussion: All teeth had reached the occlusal plane except the left lower third molar, which had not fully erupted. Attrition was found on almost all teeth especially on all first molars, but not on any third molar. By comparing these findings to American Dental Association (ADA) eruption diagram and the findings of Firdaus (2014) and Tuteja (2012) studies and by analyzing the severity of the attrition, it could be concluded that the estimated age range of victim was 20 to 30 years with a clenching or bruxism habit.

* Corresponding Author's Email: drtamy@gmail.com.

Conclusion: This case illustrated the importance of tooth development and attrition analyses in burnt victim age estimation.

Keywords: age estimation, attrition, burnt victim, dental analysis, third molar eruption

1. Introduction

Age can be estimated through skeletal analysis and dental analysis. Skeletal analysis such as diaphyseal long bone length analysis can be used to determine juvenile's age, while analyses of pubic symphysis can be used to determine adults 'age [1, 2]. Teeth have a very important role in human identification, especially in conditions where the victim is found in a very deceased state and no body parts or other evidence can be used for identification. Visually, a dental examination can provide information of estimated human age. Age estimation can be observed and analyzed through the stages of dental development and degenerative changes that occur in the teeth and supporting tissue [3-5]. This paper reported a case of age estimation on burnt victim with locked jaw using dental analysis based on third molar eruption status and attrition severity. This highlighted the role of dental analysis in burnt victim age estimation.

2. Case Report

A body was found inside a burnt building on July 26th, 2018 and brought to the Forensic Department of National Cipto Mangunkusumo Hospital (RSCM), Jakarta for identification. The case investigators requested age and sex determination under minimal invasive procedure to avoid more damage to the body. Body examination revealed a fourth-degree burn, according to the University of Rochester classification [6]. All extremities and the whole posterior part of the skull were destroyed, while chin, neck and the face was found with a hole on left cheek next to the lip corner. The body to the genitalia area remained intact. Male sexual characteristic was found on genitalia area, indicating that the victim was a male.

On examination of the facial area, a hole in the left cheek was found next to the left lip. The lower jaw was locked with the upper jaw and the teeth were maximally occluded with the tongue bitten, causing the difficulties to open the mouth and analyzed all teeth. Non-invasive experiments to open the victim's mouth were unsuccessful, so the *M. Masseter* incisions were made with a V-shaped modification technique that started from the hole in the left cheek until the upper and lower left third molars were seen. In the right region, the V-shaped incision was started from about 1 cm to the right of the lip until the right upper and lower third molars were visible. After the V-shaped incision, the lower jaw could be slightly pushed down and the tongue pushed in, so the view to examine the teeth became clear and an extra-oral photograph could be taken. Based on the examination, it was found that the left lower third molar had not fully erupted while all other third molars had reached the occlusal plane. Attrition was found on all teeth, especially on all first molars (score 2 or 3 on Kim's scoring) [3, 7] but no attrition was found on any of the third molars. Comparing the third molar eruption status to American Dental Association (ADA) eruption diagram (Figure 1) with the previous reports [9,10], and by analyzing the severity of the attrition, the range of age was estimated to be 20 to 30 years old [8-10].

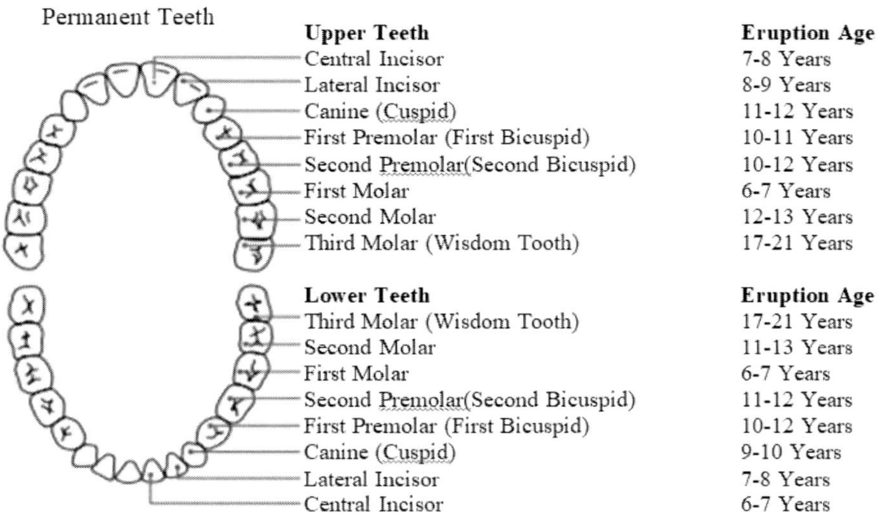

Figure 1. American Dental Association (ADA) eruption diagram (8).

Later on, our conclusion was confirmed after the case investigators received information from someone claiming as the relative of the victim stating that the victim was a 26 years old male.

3. DISCUSSION

Age determination can give a valuable clue in personal identification [11,12]. Skeletal or dental analysis is commonly used as a method for age estimation. In juvenile, age estimation through skeletal analysis can be performed by examining diaphyseal long bone length, while in adults, pubic symphysis can be employed (Suchey-Brooks method) [1,2]. Dental analysis such as analysis of the stages of tooth eruption or degenerative changes that occur in the teeth and the surrounding tissue can visually be observed for dental age estimation [3,4,7,8]. In this case, the victim suffered severe burn throughout the body resulting in the destruction of the long bones (categorized as a fourth-degree burn according to the University of Rochester classification) and only minimal invasive procedure was allowed, so that age estimation could not be made through skeletal analysis and could only be done through dental analysis. Teeth often stand as the only evidence available for a disaster victims identification, because they have the strongest mineral structures and their position is protected by surrounding tissues [13,14].

In this case, the victim's lower jaw was found very stiff and locked into the maxilla with a maximum occlusion of the teeth, and a bitten tongue. A *M. masseter* incision with V-shaped technique was needed as the non-invasive attempt to open the victim's mouth was unsuccessful. We modified the V-shaped incision by not performing the incision until the auricular region as introduced by Luntz and Luntz, but only up to third molars [15]. This minimal incision was aimed to open the mouth slightly, enough to analyze the teeth and stages of tooth eruption, and also to avoid any major facial damage. Tooth development/eruption stage analysis is a simple and non-invasive age estimation procedure, but it is limited for individual having at least one developing tooth such as children and juvenile [9,16]. In this case, all teeth of the victim had reached the occlusal plane, except the left lower third molar, which had not fully erupted, so age could be estimated by comparing this eruption status to the references. Based on the American Dental Association (ADA) diagram (Figure 1), the lower third molar in general has a complete eruption at the age of 17-21 years [8]. But on their study on Indian population, Tuteja et al. (2012) found that male's upper and lower third molar reach the occlusal plane by the age of 16.58-26.25 years [10]. Studies on Indonesian population also found that Indonesian third molars reach the occlusal plane by the age of 21.5 years ±12 months (Putri) and could have their complete eruption at the age of 25 years (Firdaus) [9,17]. This eruption age difference shows that the third molar eruption age might differ between different populations, and indicates that third molar might erupt after someone reaches 21 years old. In a limited view, tooth attrition was observed visually by buccal cusp/incisal edge screening and occlusal surface/lingual cusp probing. Tooth attrition was found in almost all teeth especially in all first molars (surface or band-like wear facet more than 1 mm, score 2 or 3 on Kim's scoring on each first molar), but not in any of the third molars. Attrition is teeth regression change, which progressively increases with advancing age [4]. Attrition in almost all teeth might be due to the advanced age of the victim, but estimating the age only by attrition analysis might lead to inaccurate age estimation, because attrition also depends on dietary habit and bad habit, such as bruxism [4]. In our case, no attrition was found in any third molar. This finding might be because the right third molars and the upper left third molar had just fully erupted not long before, giving no time for attrition to occur. From these data, the examiners estimated that the victim's age ranged from 20-30 years and with a clenching or bruxism habit. Later on, this estimated age was confirmed after the case investigator received information from someone claiming as the relative of the victim stating that the victim was a 26 years old male. Previous report of burnt victim dental analysis performed removal of the maxilla and the mandible [18]. In the present case, as the case investigator requested minimal invasive procedure, it was not possible to perform removal of the maxilla and the mandible. Despite the limitation, the examiners could conclude an accurate age estimation range. This report showed that accurate age estimation in burnt victim could be achieved without such invasive procedure, which would be more acceptable for victim's relatives.

CONCLUSION

By comparing the findings on dental analysis and references, we concluded that the estimated age was 20-30 years old with a clenching or bruxism habit. This case illustrates the importance of tooth development and attrition analyses in burnt victim age estimation especially if minimal invasive procedure is requested.

REFERENCES

[1] Danforth ME, Wrobel GD, Armstrong CW, Swanson D. (2009). Juvenile age estimation using diaphyseal long bone lengths among ancient Maya populations. *Lat. Am. Antiq.*, 20(1):3-13. http://www.jstor.org/stable/40650073.

[2] Savall F, Rérolle C, Hérin F, Dédouit F, Rougé D, Telmon N, et al. (2016). Reliability of the Suchey-Brooks method for a French contemporary population. *Forensic Sci. Int.*, 266:586.e1-586.e5.

[3] Faillace KE, Bethard JD, Marks MK. (2017). The applicability of dental wear in age estimation for a modern American population. *Am. J. Phys. Anthropol.*, 1-12.

[4] Lu CK, Yee MCS, Ravi SB, Pandurangappa R. (2017). Forensic age estimation of Chinese Malaysian adults by evaluating occlusal tooth wear using modified Kim's index. *Int. J. Dent.*, 41-50.

[5] Rózyło-Kalinowska I, Kalinowski P, Kozek M, Gali I, Ró I, Cameriere R. (2018). Validity of the third molar maturity index I 3M for indicating the adult age in the Polish population. *Forensic Sci. Int.*, 290:352.e1-352.e6.

[6] Health Encyclopedia: Classification of burns [Internet]. (2018). University of Rochester Medical Center. http://www.urmc.rochester. edu/encyclopedia. Accessed 2018 Aug 6.

[7] Suchita S, Kulkarni PG, Keerthi M, D SPR, T MR. (2014). Occlusal wear - An age determinant. *Ind. J. Dent. Adv.*, 6(2):1523-1528. http://rep.nacd.in/ijda/06/02/06.02. 11523.pdf.

[8] ADA. (2016). Tooth eruption: the permanent teeth. *J. Am. Dent. Assoc.*, 137:127.

[9] Firdaus. (2014). Estimated age of 8-25 years based on the third molar calcification stage (application of Demirjian method) in a population in Indonesia. Thesis. University of Indonesia.

[10] Tuteja M, Bahirwani S, Balaji P. (2012). An evaluation of third molar eruption for assessment of chronologic age: a panoramic study. *J. Forensic Dent. Sci.*, 4(1):13-18.

[11] Krishan K, Kanchan T, Garg AK. (2015). Dental evidence in forensic identification - An overview, methodology and present status. *Open Dent. J.*, 9:250-256.

[12] Mittal S, Nagendrareddy S, Sharma M, Agnihotri P, Chaudhary S, Dhillon M. (2016). Age estimation based on Kvaal's technique using digital panoramic radiographs. *J. Forensic Dent. Sci.*, 8(2):115.

[13] Vandrangi S, Radhika M, Paremala K, Reshma V, Sudhakara M, Hosthor S. Adjunctive role of dental restorations in personal identification of burnt victims. (2016). *J. Oral Maxillofac. Pathol.*, 20(1):154-161. http://www.jomfp.in/text.asp?2016/20/1/154/180981.

[14] Shahin KA, Chatra L, Shenai P. (2013). Dental and craniofacial imaging in forensics. *J. Forens. Radiol. Imaging*, 1(2):56-62. http:// dx.doi.org/10.1016/j.jofri.2012.12.001.

[15] Heit O, Silva R, Franco A. (2014). Improving traditional dental autopsies in postmortem examinations of intraoral gunshot wounds. *J. Forensic Leg. Med.*, 23:87-90.

[16] Boaz K, Nagesh K, Srikant N, Gupta N, Nandita K, Manaktala N, et al. (2015). Demirjian's method in the estimation of age: A study on human third molars. *J. Forensic Dent. Sci.*, 7(2):153-157.

[17] Putri AS. (2014). Age forecast based on radiographic root resorption, calcification, and tooth eruption in Indonesia's population aged 5-23 years. Thesis. University of Indonesia.

[18] Stavrianos C, Kafas P, Stavrianou I. (2008). Forensic dentistry: Post-mortem jaw resection for dental evaluation. *Res. J. Med. Sci.*, 2(4):197-199.

In: Clinical Reports in Dentistry
Editor: Lisa R. Amir
ISBN: 978-1-53617-328-4

Chapter 47

THE ROLE OF FORENSIC ODONTOLOGY IN A CHILD FIRE VICTIM IDENTIFICATION: A CASE REPORT

Vanessa[1], Jessica[1], Aria Yudhistira[2] and Nurtami Soedarsono[3,*]
[1]Dentistry Master Program, Faculty of Dentistry,
Universitas Indonesia, Jakarta, Indonesia
[2]Department of Forensic Medicine and Medicolegal, Faculty of Medicine,
Universitas Indonesia, Jakarta, Indonesia
[3]Department of Oral Biology, Division of Forensic Odontology,
Faculty of Dentistry, Universitas Indonesia, Jakarta, Indonesia

ABSTRACT

Introduction: Forensic odontology is primarily concerned with dental findings or evidence analysis which can help investigators determine victim identification including gender, race, and age in a justice context. According to studies, the accuracy is high enough (up to 43-89%) because of the dental resilience from the decomposition process and its ability to survive an extreme conditions such as high temperature in burn cases.

Case report: The postmortem procedure in this child fire victim case was done as requested by the police department by only examining the overall external body as well as the extra-oral and intra-oral conditions, taking routine photographs, and estimating victim's age by using the dental eruption chart. As there was no radiograph caused by the limited postmortem procedure, clinical examination with dental chart method was used and the estimation result was then matched to the victim's document.

Conclusion: Forensic odontology could give better information with more detailed antemortem data and postmortem procedure.

Keywords: dental evidence, burns, age estimation

*Corresponding Author's Email: drtamy@gmail.com.

1. INTRODUCTION

Burn case ranked the 4th utmost common trauma case in the world, following traffic accidents, falls and interpersonal violence [1]. Fire and Rescue Service (DPKP) at Jakarta city, Indonesia alone reported 2.055 fire cases with about 1.017 families as fire victims in 2017 which was mostly caused by electricity shortages [1]. Visual facial recognition and fingerprint identification in fire victims are often impossible to do due to the degree of destruction of the bodies, whereas Indonesian Health Act No. 36/2009 has mandated the identification of unknown bodies to fulfill the victims' rights to be returned to their families and to be properly buried according to their religion and beliefs [3, 4].

Forensic odontology is a field combined with forensic medicine science, dentistry, and legal studies which primarily aims in human identification by analyzing the case from dental findings or evidence [5]. This identification method is useful when the victim body is fragmentized and/or visual recognition can not be done such as in burn cases since the dental structure are considered to be the hardest structure and could resist decomposition and high temperatures [6].

Dental analysis usually requires a postmortem and antemortem dental records comparison to confirm one's identity. Radiograph in dental identification procedure is often useful to depict the tooth development stages, external and internal anatomical features such as root curvatures, bony anatomical landmarks, dental history of restorations, root canal treatments, surgical plates, dental prosthesis or dental implants. A postmortem dental findings could provide information of the deceased such as ancestry background or race, sex or gender, and age estimation [7,8].

2. CASE REPORT

Eastern Jakarta Police Department along with the family delivered a female child fire victim body to the Forensic Department of Cipto Mangunkusumo National Hospital (RSCM) Jakarta on 26th July 2018. Police investigation reported a house fire incident caused by electricity shortage which took place at the victim's home located in the Tambora area, Jakarta city that occurred on 26th July 2018 at 04.25 am. The victim's family described that the incident happened while the other members of the family were outside the house, leaving only the victim and her father trapped inside. Police requested forensic medicine along with forensic odontology department of the hospital to confirm the victim's death and determine the age estimation of the child victim for the issue of legal death certificate.

Postmortem examinations of the child fire victim were performed in Cipto Mangunkusumo National Hospital (RSCM) by a forensic medicine resident (Department of Forensic Medicine of Universitas Indonesia) and two forensic odontology residents (Department of Forensic Odontology of Universitas Indonesia). In this case report, only external inspections were carried out due to the victim's family financial constraints, so there was neither full postmortem procedure nor any radiograph taken from the anatomical and dental structures.

The full postmortem examination rejection statement form was signed by the family. Therefore, only standard postmortem forensic procedure was performed consisting of general external examination of victim body and routine photograph which were done by the forensic medicine resident and dental examination such as an extra-oral and intra-oral visual inspection and dental photograph which were performed by forensic odontology residents (Figure 1).

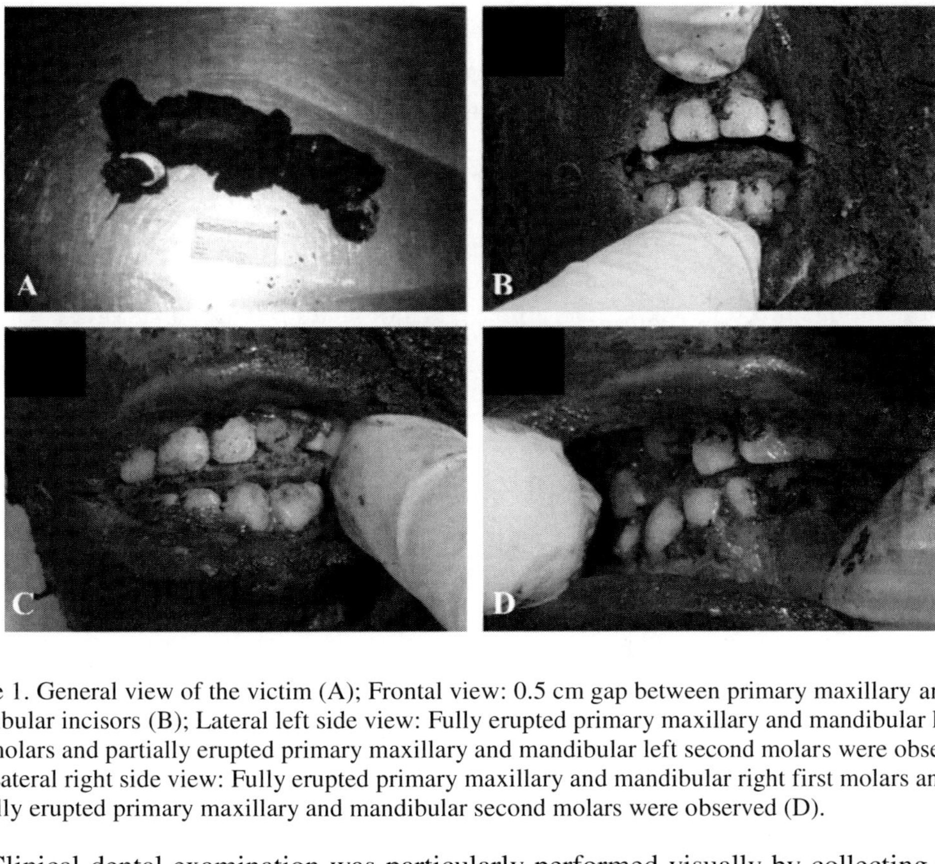

Figure 1. General view of the victim (A); Frontal view: 0.5 cm gap between primary maxillary and mandibular incisors (B); Lateral left side view: Fully erupted primary maxillary and mandibular left first molars and partially erupted primary maxillary and mandibular left second molars were observed (C); Lateral right side view: Fully erupted primary maxillary and mandibular right first molars and partially erupted primary maxillary and mandibular second molars were observed (D).

Clinical dental examination was particularly performed visually by collecting dental findings or evidence such as the teeth presence, specific characteristics, the degree of attrition, the occlusion, the color of the teeth, the supporting structures, the dental hygiene status, and any pathologic conditions that would possibly influence the assessment. The dental eruption chart based on the American Dental Association (ADA) Development Tooth Chart revised by Schour and Massler on 1982 was used to estimate the child fire victim's age [9]. External body examination showed fourth-degree burns on the victim's entire body surface without any fabric or clothes on.

The cranial bone was damaged and all parts of the victim's extremities comprising legs and arms were capitated and about 5cm long left. An extra-oral examination showed open lips about 2cm wide with clearly visualized and intact anterior teeth. Furthermore, while doing the intra-oral examination, we found it difficult to open the victim's mouth due to the suspected muscle stiffness.

There was no antemortem dental data as the family stated that the child has never gone to the dentist before. Intra-oral examination was done by clinical or visual inspection by retracting the right and left m. masseter. We observed 16 fully erupted teeth (primary maxillary right first molar, canine, lateral incisor, central incisor; primary maxillary left central incisor, lateral incisor, canine, first molar; primary mandibular left first molar, canine, lateral incisor, central incisor; primary mandibular right central incisor, lateral incisor, canine, first molar). Four partially erupted primary second molars (primary maxillary right second molar, primary maxillary left second molar, primary mandibular left second molar, primary mandibular right second molar). All teeth were seen in a good condition, no attrition, yellowish-white in color, and no sign of burnt or charred teeth, no calculus, no staining, good periodontal condition, good dental hygiene, no caries, and no pathology condition. According to the American Dental Association (ADA) Development Tooth Chart, the primary mandibular second molars erupt at 25-33 months old for the maxilla and 23-31 months for the mandible.

3. Discussion

The most commonly used methods in age estimation in forensic medicine are by using skeletal age and dental age. Skeletal age estimation includes cranial sutures, femur, elbow and joint, hand-wrist, and pubic symphysis [6].

Dental age is considered as an accurate tool in estimating age. It is because of the uniqueness and high reliability based on dental calcification, growth, and development stage [8].

In this case report, fingerprints identification could not be done because of the severely burnt deceased and the capitated body. It became more complicated to estimate the victim's age by using damaged skeletal and without any radiograph taken. Moreover, DNA profiling was thought to be expensive and time-consuming procedure [10]. While in this burn case, all teeth were still in a very good shape and they could provide better information compared to the burnt long bones. Bone maturity itself was commonly affected by nutrition and endocrine status during one's life, in contrast to the teeth, they are not significantly affected by these systemic factors [6].

Dental maturity is grouped into three classifications; prenatal-neonatal-postnatal child, children-adolescents, and adults. Histological examination can be used to determine the stage of tooth development in prenatal-neonatal-postnatal child by using the incremental line as the indicator. The radiological age estimation method is used to determine tooth eruption and tooth calcification in children-adolescent and adulthood [11]. The most simple way to determine adult dentition is by examining the shape and size of the teeth in the oral cavity [5]. According to Dostalova, the age estimation method is more accurate by examining the apical resorption, transparency of roots, and the size of the pulp chamber using radiograph, compared to the use of a dental eruption chart alone. This makes radiograph a more accurate method in age estimation compared to clinical examinations without any radiographs [6].

Based on this highlighted dental evidence which were 4 partially erupted primary second molars, according to the London Atlas by AlQahtani (2009) the age estimation was 1.5- 2.5 years old, ADA chart by Schour and Massler (1982) was 23-33 months old, and Age Estimation Guide by Uberlaker (1989) was 1.4-34 years old [12-14]. AlQahtani et. al., studies the accuracy of three dental chart from London Atlas, ADA chart, Age Estimation Guide, they showed that the London Atlas performed to be the most accurate. It can be seen from the mean difference of ADA, Age Estimation Guide, and London Atlas In the midpoint of 1.5 year old children was 0.36; 0.36; and 0.37 respectively. While in the midpoint of 2.5 year old children the mean difference was 0.61; 0.61; and 0.43 respectively [9].

CONCLUSION

This case report confirmed that forensic odontology could play an important role as an aid in victim identification in extreme cases such as the child fire victim case and even in a limited post-mortem procedure (no radiograph) we could still provide the child fire victim's age estimation as requested by police department, i.e., 2-2.5 years old. This estimation was matched and confirmed by the victim's family member. Forensic odontology could have possibly provided more detail and accurate information whenever the antemortem, radiograph, and other examinations were present in the case.

ACKNOWLEDGMENTS

The authors would like to thank Dr. Denys Putra Alim and Dr. Septia Eva Lusia resident of Forensic Medicine and Medicolegal of Universitas Indonesia and the authors of various scientific articles published as reference journals.

REFERENCES

[1] Peranantham, S., Manigandan, G., Shanmugam, K. (2014). Forensic approach to a case of death due to burn injury : a case report. *Int. J. Res. Med. Sci.,* 2(3):1214-1216. doi:10.5455/2320-6012.ijrms20140866.

[2] BPB area. *Jakarta Fire Report*. [Internet] (2017) http://data.jakarta.go.id/dataset/data-kejadian-kebakaran-di-provinsi-dki-jakarta-tahun-2017 Assesed on 2018 August 10.

[3] Martin-de, A. V. S., Marques, H. T., Bohoyo, N. E. J. M. (2000). The application of dental methods of identification to human burn victims in a mass disaster. *Int. J. Leg. Med.,* 113:236-239.

[4] *Undang-Undang Republik Indonesia No.36 Tahun 2009 tentang Kesehatan* [Internet]. (2009) as [*Law of the Republic of Indonesia No.36 of 2009 concerning Health*. [Internet]. (2009).] http://binfar.depkes.go.id/dat/lama/1303887905_UU%2036-2009%20Kesehatan.pdf Accessed 2018 June 20.

[5] Krishan, K., Kanchan, T., Garg, A. K. (2015). Dental evidence in forensic identification – an overview, methodology and present status, *Open Dent. J.,* 31(9):250-6.

[6] Dostálová, T., Eliášová, H., Seydlová, M. et al. (2008). Forensic dentistry – identification from the dentist's point of view. *Prague Medical Report,* 109(1):14-18.

[7] Cunha, E., Baccino, E., Martrille, L. et al. (2009). The problem of aging human remains and living individuals: a review. *Forensic Science International,* 193:1-13. doi:10.1016/j.forsciint.2009.09.008.

[8] Vijay, G., Augustine, J., Urs, A. B. (2015). Journal of forensic and legal medicine forensic considerations when dealing with incinerated human dental remains. *J. Forensic Leg. Med.,* 29:13-17. doi:10.1016/j.jflm.2014.10.006.

[9] Hector, M., Alqahtani, S. J., Hector, M. P., Liversidge, H. M. (2014). Accuracy of age estimation using three dental development schemas accuracy of dental age estimation charts: schour and massler, ubelaker, and the london atlas. *Am. J. Phys. Anthropol.,* 154(1):70-8. doi:10.1002/ajpa.22473.

[10] Martin-de, A. V. S., Marques, H. T., Bohoyo, N. E. J. M. (2000). The application of dental methods of identification to human burn victims in a mass disaster. *Int. J. Legal Med.,* 113(4):236-9.

[11] Shamim, T., Student, P. (2006). Age estimation: A dental approach. *Journal of Punjab Academy of Forensic Medicine and Toxicology,* 6(1):14-16.

[12] Alqahtani, S. J., Hector, M. P., Liversidge, H. M. (2010). Brief communication: the london atlas of human tooth development and eruption. *Am. J. Phys. Anthropol.,* 142:481-490. doi:10.1002/ajpa.21258.

[13] Goltz, R. A. (2016). A comparison of four methods of dental age estimation and age estimation from the risser sign of the iliac crest. Thesis. Eastern Michigan University. *https://commons.emich.edu/honors/493* Accesed 2018 August 11.

[14] Blenkin, M., Taylor, J. (2012). Age estimation charts for a modern Australian population. *Forensic Sci. Int.,* 221:106-112.

Editor's Contact Information

Lisa R. Amir, DDS, PhD
Faculty of Dentistry Universitas Indonesia
DKI Jakarta, Indonesia
Email: lisa.amir@gmail.com

INDEX

#

A

B

C

D

E

F

G

H

I

N

O

P

Q

R

S

T

U

V

W

X

Y

Z